"If you have any tendency to worry about the physical conditions in your baby or child—and who doesn't?—this is the encyclopedia to have on your shelf."
—DR. BENJAMIN SPOCK

"By decoding the ominous-sounding polysyllabic terms that doctors use so often to label many innocent findings in newborn babies, the authors have performed a much-needed service for bewildered parents—their new offspring are demystified."
—WILLIAM A. SILVERMAN, M.D.
Former head of the Premature Nursery
Babies Hospital
Columbia-Presbyterian Medical Center

"[This] is a book that every pediatrician will want the families in his practice to possess. Instead of his having to give the same explanations day after day to such common entities as birthmarks, turned-in feet, sore throats, colds and fevers, *The Parent's Pediatric Companion* provides scientifically sound explanations in an eminently readable fashion."
—ABRAHAM B. BERGMAN, M.D.
Director of Pediatrics, Harborview Medical Center
Professor of Pediatrics, University of Washington

"Well written! Should be an excellent guide for mothers and fathers alike."
—HUGO A. KEIM, M.D.
Professor of Orthopedics
Columbia University

The Parent's Pediatric Companion

GILBERT SIMON, M.D., F.A.A.P.,
and MARCIA COHEN

WILLIAM MORROW AND COMPANY, INC.

New York

Library of Congress Cataloging in Publication Data

Simon, Gilbert.
  The parent's pediatric companion.

  Bibliography: p.
  Includes index.
  1. Pediatrics—Popular works.   I. Cohen, Marcia.
II. Title.   [DNLM: 1. Pediatrics—popular works.
WS 200 S5945p]
RJ61.S6328   1985   618.92   84-27302
ISBN 0-688-03791-7

Printed in the United States of America

First Edition

1 2 3 4 5 6 7 8 9 10

BOOK DESIGN BY ELLEN LO GIUDICE

To parents who want to know more
and pediatricians who wish they had time
to tell them

· ACKNOWLEDGMENTS ·

Our thanks are due to hundreds of people whose names cannot be mentioned here. They are the parents of Dr. Simon's patients, his former colleagues on the faculty of the Columbia University College of Physicians and Surgeons, and many individual doctors throughout the country—men and women who were once called "community doctors" and who are now known as "providers." The first group—concerned parents—gave impetus to the book by insisting on answers, often even refusing to leave the office until they had received a complete explanation of what was (and was not) wrong with their children. The second group—dedicated teachers—provided concepts and the standards that are, hopefully, adhered to throughout the book. And we are in debt to the practicing physicians for many illustrations of common conditions and much of what we hope is a commonsense approach to medical problems.

We are also grateful to the distinguished pediatricians who so unselfishly donated their time and expertise to reading and commenting on the manuscript. These generous physicians include the incomparable Dr. Benjamin M. Spock, author of *Baby and Child Care,* and Dr. Abraham B. Bergman, professor of pediatrics at the University of Washington and director of pediatrics, Harborview Medical Center, Seattle, Washington.

Many other eminent pediatric authorities reviewed those sections of the book that dealt directly with their own specialties and offered interesting and helpful suggestions. Our deep thanks, therefore, to:

Dr. Mary Jane Jesse, former professor of pediatric cardiology at the University of Miami; former director of the Division of Heart and Vascular Disease at the National Heart, Lung and Blood Institute, National Institutes of Health; and past president of the American Heart Association, who reviewed our writing on children's hearts and blood pressure.

Dr. Neils Low, clinical director, Blythedale Children's Hospital, Valhalla, New York, and professor of clinical neurology and pediatrics, Columbia University College of Physicians and Surgeons; and Dr. Sidney Carter, former chief of Division of Pediatric Neurology and professor emeritus of Neurology and Pediatrics, Columbia University College of Physicians and Surgeons, who reviewed our references to neurology.

Dr. William A. Silverman, former director of the Prenatal Division at Children's Hospital, San Francisco, and former director of the Premature Nursery at Columbia–Presbyterian Medical Center, who read and commented on the chapters on the newborn.

Dr. Myron Wynick, director of the Institute of Human Nutrition, editor of *Current Concepts in Nutrition,* and professor of pediatrics, Columbia University College of Physicians and Surgeons, who reviewed the pages on nutrition.

Dr. William Heird, associate professor of pediatrics, Columbia University College of Physicians and Surgeons; director of the Division of Pediatric Gastroenterology; and member of the editorial board of the *Journal of Pediatrics,* who examined the portions pertaining to gastroenterology.

Dr. John Kingsley Lattimer, former director of the Squire Urologic Clinic, former chairman of the Urology Department of Columbia University College of Physicians and Surgeons, former chairman of the American Academy of Pediatrics' Committee on Pediatric Urology, and past president of the Society of Pediatric Urology, who reviewed all references to children's urinary tracts and genitalia.

Dr. Robison Dooling Harley, editor of *Pediatric Ophthalmology* and former chairman and professor of ophthalmology at Temple University School of Medicine, who read the passages on the eyes.

Dr. Charles D. Bluestone, professor of otolaryngology at the University of Pittsburgh School of Medicine and co-author of *Pediatric Otolaryngology,* who read and commented on the sections dealing with children's ears, noses, and throats.

Dr. Judson Graves Randolph, professor of surgery and child health at George Washington University Medical School and surgeon-in-chief at Children's Hospital, Washington, D.C., who reviewed the entries on pediatric surgery.

Dr. Lynn T. Staheli, professor of orthopedics at the University of Washington and director of orthopedics at Children's Orthopedic

Hospital in Seattle, Washington, who reviewed the sections on children's bones and joints.

Dr. Ellin Leiberman, associate professor of pediatrics at the University of Southern California School of Medicine and head of the Division of Nephrology at Children's Hospital in Los Angeles, who reviewed the sections dealing with the kidneys.

Dr. Melvin Malcolm Grumbach, director of pediatric services and chairman of the Pediatric Department at the University of California in San Francisco and former head of the Pediatric Endocrinology Division at the Columbia–Presbyterian Medical Center, who reviewed all references to endocrinology.

Dr. James Alexander Wolff, director of the Valerie Center for Cancer and Blood Disorders in Summit, New Jersey, and former chairman of pediatric hematology at Columbia–Presbyterian Medical Center, who read and commented on the references to hematology.

Dr. Hugo A. Keim, director of spine services and professor of orthopedics at Columbia–Presbyterian Medical Center, who reviewed the section on scoliosis.

Special thanks as well to the many reference librarians coast to coast who helped gather documentation for the material in the book. In particular: Barbara Walcott of the Columbia–Presbyterian Medical Center Library; Arlene Buda and K. Lindner of the Engelwood Hospital Medical Library in New Jersey; and Ms. K. D. Proffit of the Sacramento–Eldorado Medical Society Library in Sacramento, California. Ms. Proffit's role was especially appreciated in the preparation of the index.

We are also grateful to Mary Ann Stackpole, who not only typed the manuscript but gave so much to the project in the way of organization and encouraging commentary. Our thanks to our editor, Maria Guarnaschelli; to Ellen Levine, editor of *Woman's Day;* to Dick Kaplan, editor of *Us* magazine; to Dr. John Bloom, associate clinical professor of pediatrics at the University of Cincinnati; and to our agent, Kathy Robbins, for their inspiration and support.

And on a more personal note, we would like to express our appreciation to our long-suffering families.

From Dr. Gilbert Simon, a grateful husband: Thanks to my incredibly tolerant and very beautiful wife, Maggy, for allowing me the freedom to devote as much time as was needed to complete this labor of love. While I ate and then ran back to the office to the excitement of working at my desk, she stayed home to the much less exciting chores of washing the dishes and putting our babies to bed. This book could not have been written without her support.

And from Marcia Cohen, a working wife: Thanks to my husband, Larry, for smoothing things over with friends and relations when I was too busy writing to attend to them, for running both the vacuum cleaner and myriad errands, for thoroughly earning his nickname, "Mr. Darling." To my children, Betsy Marrion and Jesse Cohen, my gratitude for oceans of sensitive, loving encouragement.

· NOTE ON AUTHORSHIP ·

Although *The Parent's Pediatric Companion* employs the first-person pronoun *I*, reflecting my viewpoint, the book represents a collaborative effort by Marcia Cohen and myself.

We chose to use the first-person pronoun because we wanted to give our readers the feeling that they were actually hearing the voice of a doctor.

GILBERT SIMON, M.D.

Contents

PART ONE   THE NEWBORN—

From Birth to Six Months

Physical Conditions

Functional Conditions

PART THREE   **THE OLDER CHILD—**
From 6 to 16 Years

Physical Conditions

Introduction

When I was a young smart aleck, I used to delight in telling the younger kids on the block that their epidermis was showing. It never failed to drive them crazy. They would look themselves over, scurry around, and worry about how they could cure this awful condition. Some would ask for a "second opinion." Still others wouldn't relax until they learned that *epi* meant on top of, and *dermis* meant skin. Most would be thoroughly upset until they learned that their epidermis was nothing more than the outer layer of their skin and that *everybody's* epidermis shows.

By now, some of those younger kids on the block have children, with epidermises of their own. The odds are that as parents they, like you, will witness many other childhood conditions that are just as innocent and just as universal as having a visible epidermis. And when your pediatrician gives one of them a name—especially a nice long Latin one—you may worry and wonder just like my old friends on the block.

In my 20 years as a pediatrician, I've seen parents fret themselves sick over every condition discussed in this book. Yet their children were normal, happy, and thriving, and the parents had nothing to worry about. Usually, all this needless anxiety started this way:

I would examine the baby in the hospital—or the toddler in the office. I would mention that the child had one or another of these conditions, tell the parent that the condition was perfectly normal, give a short explanation, and wave good-bye till the next time. Or so I thought.

Soon the phone calls would begin.

"Are you sure it's normal?" an anxious voice would ask. "What does it mean?" "When will it go away?" "How many children have it?" And so on. It seemed, at times, that I'd raised more questions than I'd answered.

As the years went on, I began to realize that the very active minds of these very active parents needed more information than I was able to provide during the office visit. (As you'll read in the section on innocent heart murmurs, one of these anxious parents was my own wife!) Often the worry was perfectly understandable, but the sad truth was that anxiety over these normal, harmless conditions was blocking the way to what should have been the parents' pure enjoyment of their wonderful, exuberantly healthy children.

The birth and development of a healthy child is one of the greatest joys in the world, and no needless worry should be allowed to interfere with it. Today's well-educated, serious parents, it seemed to me as I tried to answer their questions, needed more knowledge than they could get from an office visit to help them understand not the illness, but the true health of their children. As a result, about five years ago, I decided to write a book that would accompany and support a parent's relationship with her pediatrician. *The Parent's Pediatric Companion* is the outcome. It is not a substitute for regular examinations by your pediatrician, but an adjunct to them, and on page 33 you'll find out how to use it to your greatest advantage. For now, however, you should know that a careful reading of the book will help you avoid needless worry when your pediatrician isn't available at the exact moment that a question pops into your head. *The Parent's Pediatric Companion* is designed to help you retain your peace of mind—even as you go off to work in the morning—and to gain all the pleasure you should from each stage in your child's normal growth and development. After you read it, you'll understand why doctors say that a normal, healthy child isn't "spotless" or "perfect," and that the conditions mentioned here are just part of growing and changing. Almost every normal child will have a number of them.

I often describe the conditions you'll find in *The Parent's Pediatric Companion* as growing pains, although many physicians use the specific medical term *nondiseases*. Doctors call these conditions nondiseases because, though they may appear to be diseases, i.e., mimic diseases, they are not. They're harmless, benign, and require little or no treatment. They're also so common that the odds are overwhelming that your child will have many of them.

Some of these conditions have surprising and unexpected characteristics. For example, your baby's skin may get a purplish, mottled look when he's cool (p. 54) or, during a physical exam, your doctor's stethoscope may pick up the sound of an innocent murmur in your infant's heart (p. 82). Like the rest of the conditions in *The Parent's Pediatric Companion,* these are absolutely harmless.

No one wants to be be frightened and worried about his child, and the worry is an awful waste if the child is perfectly normal. One "Wow, what a relief!" is one reason—and for you, perhaps, reason enough—to learn about these conditions.

Sometimes, however, parents who are still worried after their visit to the pediatrician take their children elsewhere and I, like most other pediatricians, have seen much unnecessary surgery and overtreatment as a result of this misunderstanding.

I've seen children with insignificant tongue-tie (p. 75), adherent labia (p. 193), lumps that are the normal result of DPT injections (p. 149), lymph nodes that are swollen from a cold (p. 171), tonsils that are appropriately enlarged for the child's age (p. 165), normal one-sided breast buds (p. 178), ordinary harmless breast cysts (p. 256), and too many others to mention undergo needless surgery to correct these perfectly normal conditions.

I've seen children faithfully marched to medical-center tumor clinics week after week to have what were *assumed* to be slowly growing tumors carefully monitored. What the children had was nothing more than the normal thickness at the root of a baby's nose (p. 69), or the bulge in a teenager's midsection caused by a vigorous regimen of sit-ups (p. 258). It wasn't hard to imagine how both children and parents felt about those trips!

Children with normally speckled eyes (p. 65) or single creases in their palms (p. 104) have undergone chromosome analyses because both of these conditions appear in children with Down's syndrome, and so these perfectly normal children were suspected of having Down's.

The parents or grandparents of babies with harmless Mongolian spots, which do indeed resemble bruises (p. 39), have accused doctors of dropping the babies in the delivery room. Worse yet, well-meaning persons have accused the parents of child abuse!

Children with commonplace white milk curds (p. 74) in their mouths have been treated with antifungal medication in the mistaken notion that the milk curds were thrush.

Children have received antibiotics for the injury that comes from sucking on Popsicles (p. 157), for normally healing circumcisions (p. 92), and for normal vaginal discharges (p. 204). Children who tend to hold their breath (p. 213) or have fainting spells (p. 307) have been treated with anticonvulsants. I've seen children with trivial and self-correcting intoeing wearing bars on their feet (p. 101), and children whose normally tight foreskins have been forcefully peeled back (p. 92) or whose perfectly functioning urinary openings were made wider because they appeared too small (p. 262).

Nursing babies with typical soft stools (p. 127) have been suspected of having diarrhea. Or, when the stools were infrequent, babies have been given sugar or had objects inserted in their rectums.

All this worrisome attention to perfectly healthy children!

Aside from all the unnecessary treatment, there is, or surely ought to be, the pocketbook to consider—either the parents' or the health insurance company's. Not satisfied by the pediatrician's diagnosis that the condition is normal, some anxious parents seek outside opinions: the ophthalmologist's when the child looks a bit cross-eyed (p. 67), the gynecologist's when she has irregular early menstrual cycles (p. 263), the endocrinologist's for ordinary familial short stature (p. 324), the urologist's for a testicle that appears not yet descended (p. 190), the hematologist's for pale skin (p. 146), the otolaryngologist's for a hoarseness that comes from shouting (p. 292), the cardiologist's for an innocent heart murmur (pp. 82, 181). Of course in all these cases everybody goes home happily reassured, but someone has to pay the bill. How much of our national health bill is spent on these needless consultations is anybody's guess.

Expensive or risky tests and hospitalizations can be another pitfall when parents worry that their child's normal condition is a disease. CAT scans have been performed or time spent in the hospital to investigate what was simply the child's normal, hereditarily large head (p. 155), for the altogether commonplace urinary retention (p. 223) that's merely the toddler's way of resisting toilet training, for the yellow skin that comes from eating lots of vegetables with carotene in them (p. 145), for "failure to thrive"—which is simply the child's changing growth rate (p. 231)—for a little boy's supposedly too-small penis that just seemed that way because his prepubic fat was hiding his perfectly normal organ (p. 193), for high blood pressure that came from some cold medicine the child took (p. 111), and so on.

Sometimes worried parents restrict a child's activity—in the case of an innocent heart murmur for instance. The poor—though perfectly healthy—child then perceives herself as less than healthy, as somehow stigmatized, and her restricted activities may delay her developing normal agility and strength.

And then there's the emotional cost to the child who believes that something isn't quite right because a single reading of his blood pressure was higher than expected (p. 283), or that he's freakish because his breasts are enlarging (p. 254) or he's much slower to mature than his friends (p. 329).

I certainly don't mean to suggest by all this that a parent should never seek a specialist's opinion. Pediatric cardiologists, neurologists, and so on are among the great healing experts in modern medicine, and all pediatricians are grateful for their advice, particularly their invaluable help in the diagnosis of real illness. Sometimes, even in treating some of the nondiseases described in *The Parent's Pediatric Companion*, a specialist's opinion will be very helpful, but your pediatrician will know when that's the case. Too often parents spend considerable sums on second opinions and laboratory tests that weren't requested by their pediatrician. If you read about your child's condition in this book, you'll find out whether or not a specialist's view would be valuable and you can help your pediatrician make that decision.

How common are these nondiseases?

"Non-disease is more common than disease. Common conditions and variations of those common conditions are more likely than rare diseases," states R. S. Illingworth in *Common Symptoms of Disease in Children.*

With a few exceptions, *every* baby will have swollen breasts (p. 81), and every breast-fed baby will have loose stools (p. 127). Most fair-skinned babies will have salmon-colored patches at the bases of their skulls (p. 40), and most dark-skinned babies, blue-gray splotches on their lower backs (p. 39). Half of all normal, full-term babies will have yellow skin during the first week of life (p. 46); two fifths of all black infants will have protruding navels (p. 88); one fifth of all healthy infants will cry a lot more than expected (p. 129).

Almost every toddler will have swollen neck glands (p. 171), and sometime during his childhood, his doctor will pick up the sounds of an innocent heart murmur (p. 181).

Most teenage girls will have stretch marks (p. 235), and the breasts of most teenage boys will swell (p. 254). One tenth of all teenage boys will develop a soft swelling in the left side of the scrotum (p. 260); one tenth of all teenage girls will have really painful menstrual periods (p. 266) and a routine urinalysis will show protein in a tenth of normal teenagers (p. 321). One entirely healthy girl in 40 will be late in having her first period (p. 329).

Are all these conditions really benign? After all, one person's view of what is benign may be different from another's. You may be excused if you see nothing particularly benign about the sleepless nights you've been spending with your colicky baby.

The conditions in *The Parent's Pediatric Companion* are all benign for one important reason: They have no effect on the health of your child. The child who has one of them was healthy to begin with, and the latest growing pain he shows up with won't make him any less so.

Most of the conditions described in *The Parent's Pediatric Companion* are just ordinary eventualities in the everyday life of a child. Some of them are included simply because they're hard for parents to interpret. An adolescent's dieting, for example, can be tough to assess. Is it anorexia or just successful weight loss? (You'll find the answer on p. 304.) When is a child too short (p. 324)? Or too tall (p. 327)?

Others, so visually obvious that you can't miss them, are equally innocent. A red strawberry mark (p. 41), for example, is benign, despite its rapid growth during the baby's first year, because 90 percent of all strawberry marks eventually disappear.

Some of these growing pains do well with a bit of supportive treatment. Vomiting due to reflux (p. 125), for example, improves with thickened feedings and gentle handling. Persistent hoarseness due to voice abuse (p. 292) improves with voice training.

Some conditions are innocent for the time being and come with a limited warranty. Crossed eyes are perfectly OK up till the time the baby reaches 6 months of age (p. 67), tears and mucus that drain from the eyes are tolerable until 12 months (p. 66), and the little water-filled sac that sometimes appears in a baby's scrotum (p. 95) should, to be perfectly safe, disappear by 12 months.

A few of these conditions look so much like "something else," i.e., some real disease, that they can send parents into an awful tizzy. Examples of such out and out imposters are: the brick-dust stain that often appears on a baby's diapers (p. 140) and looks a lot like—but absolutely is not—blood, a movable lump in a child's belly (it feels like a growth but it's only fecal matter, as explained on p. 257), or bright red bowel movements that come from red food coloring (p. 212).

Other conditions are at the limits of normal, or else are normal for a particular family. Examples of the first are babies with small heads (p. 156), and of the second, babies with large heads (p. 155).

Still others just aren't as bad as they seem to be. A baby who's colicky and cries a lot (p. 120), for example, or a normal infant who occasionally has convulsions (p. 136), or one who, after a head injury, can't see for a short time (p. 314) are among these.

Reading about these conditions in *The Parent's Pediatric Companion* will not only put your mind to rest about all these growing pains, but might also help you keep your visits to your pediatrician down to a sensible number and your relationship with him productive. It will help you understand how and why all of these conditions are harmless. When you fully realize that your child's innocent heart murmur or strawberry mark is just a part of normal growing, your worries will vanish. At that point, you can, as you should, get on with the fun of raising and enjoying your wonderful, healthy child.

And don't let anyone tell you that your child's epidermis is showing!

How and When to Use This Book

Your relationship with your pediatrician is an important one for both you and your child. *The Parent's Pediatric Companion* is designed to aid and support this relationship and the information in it should be used both prior to and after your office visits or phone calls. After reading about some of these conditions—heat rash (p. 45), for example, which is the result of overproduction of sweat, or carotenemia (p. 145), which is easily traceable to the child's diet—you may decide to forgo phoning the doctor at all. In most situations, however, you'll want to read about your child's condition *after* your pediatrician has made the diagnosis (and before calling him back for a further explanation).

Why do you need to know more than the doctor told you during that examination?

Because, even assuming that your pediatrician had all the ramifications of your child's nondisease on the tip of her tongue, she would need the combined skills of a dozen research scientists and an auctioneer to convey them to you thoroughly. (You may notice here that I've alternated the gender of the personal pronouns. You'll find this to be true throughout *The Parent's Pediatric Companion.* After all, children come in both the male and the female gender and so do physicians.)

During every pediatric examination, particularly those of the newborn, your doctor will spend a considerable amount of time running through a list of observations about your child, then giving you a timetable for their predicted disappearance. If you ask how the condition arose, why it will go away, or what may be done meanwhile, the time allotted for the exam will permit the doctor only two choices: one, to give you a simplified description; the other, to refer you to a jargon-laden, probably morbid medical text.

Furthermore, the pediatric examining room is hardly the place to learn the whole story. Kids are screaming, squirming, bubbling, burping, and otherwise doing what comes naturally. Bedlam is the order of the day—a far cry from the hushed halls of academia.

But you *still* want to know. Perhaps you want to know more than the busy doctor had time to convey, or perhaps you simply want a chance to absorb the same information in the quiet of your home.

This is where *The Parent's Pediatric Companion* comes in. It's a manual for parents who want the whole story, the one they can't always get from their busy physician. ("Did the doctor say that Johnny has an innocent heart murmur? Doesn't that mean something's wrong with his heart?" If this is one of your questions, *please* see pp. 82, 181.)

The book is divided into three parts reflecting the three developmental stages of the child: "The Newborn" (from birth to 6 months), "The Preschooler" (from 6 months to 6 years), and "The Older Child" (from 6 to 16 years). Within each of these parts are two subsections, one on the physical conditions of the child and one on the functional conditions.

Physical conditions are just that—what you might see or feel on the child's body. Consequently, you'll find in the "physical" section separate chapters on various parts of the body, such as the head, ears, neck, mouth, and so on. Within each of these chapters appear the nondisease conditions that occur on that part of the body. Sucking blisters, for example, are discussed in the chapter entitled "Mouth," in the part called "The Newborn."

The term *functional conditions* refers primarily to the workings of the child's body. Included here, therefore, are chapters on the respiratory system, digestive system, nervous system, and so on. The harmless condition known as sleepwalking, for example, is listed in the chapter entitled "Nervous System," in the "Older Child" part.

If you read the book straight through from beginning to end, you'll certainly be prepared for any nondisease that may show up on the horizon. That long journey really isn't necessary, though, because *The Parent's Pediatric Companion* is designed as a reference book, so you can find whatever you need *when* you need it.

The Table of Contents, which begins on page 13, lists all of the nondiseases in the order they occur in the book. On the left-hand side of the contents pages, you'll find descriptions of the conditions as they appear to you or to your doctor. Next to each of these descriptions is the medical term for that particular nondisease. You'll find these two distinct but coordinating labels repeated at the head of each listing in the text.

Your most important tool, however, is the index in the back of the book. The index lists each condition alphabetically, both by its everyday description and by its medical name. If, for example, your doctor informs you that you can't take your newborn home from the hospital because he has yellow skin, you can look up yellow skin in the index and turn to the page listed, where you'll find the section on physiologic jaundice, which is the medical term for the yellowing skin common to at least half of all newborns. If, conversely, the pediatrician tells you that your infant has physiologic jaundice, you can look up that term and find it just as well. In the index, some symptoms— vomiting, for example—are followed by several page references. In this case, you can turn to the appropriate pages one by one and very quickly discover which of them applies to your child. If you want to read still further, references to the medical literature are cited by number at the end of each section; these numbers refer to the list of references beginning on page 335.

The Parent's Pediatric Companion is designed to fully explain every growing pain your child may develop. It will also show you how healthy your child really is and help you gain the relaxed confidence that will bring you all the joy in each other you both deserve.

PART ONE

The Newborn—

From Birth to Six Months

Physical Conditions

1. Skin, Hair, Nails

BIRTHMARKS *(Nevi)*
Blue-Green or Blue-Gray Patch: Mongolian Spot

The Mongolian spot is a bluish splash like an ink stain with irregular borders that fade gradually into the surrounding skin. The mark was dubbed Mongolian because it was first noticed on Oriental babies. Actually, any baby with the tiniest degree of pigmentation in his ancestry can have Mongolian spots.

These birthmarks vary in size from a small dot to several centimeters in diameter. They're usually blue-green or, less often, blue-gray, and though they're most likely to appear on the baby's buttocks, sometimes we see them on the shoulder, the lower back, over the tailbone, or, for that matter, just about anyplace else. For no reason that we know of, they're more likely to appear on the left side than the right, and on the back of the arm or leg than the front.

In a recent study of more than 400 consecutively born babies, every one of the Oriental newborns had a Mongolian spot. Virtually all of the black babies, almost half of the Hispanic babies, and 9 percent of the Caucasian babies also had them. The percentage of Caucasian babies with these birthmarks undoubtedly would have been higher if more of the babies had had Italian, Greek, or Sephardic Jewish parents; the percentage would have been lower if more parents had been of German or Scandinavian origin.

The Mongolian spot is a true birthmark since it's always obvious from the moment of birth. It usually disappears completely by the time the child has reached two or three years of age. Only about 1 in 25 persists into adulthood.

Occasionally, a parent mistakes this birthmark for a bruise and suspects the obstetrician of dropping the baby in the delivery room. But the difference between the two is soon apparent. Bruises quickly change to a greenish-yellow color and vanish in a few weeks. The Mongolian spot, on the other hand, usually lasts a year or two. Perhaps its only importance is that it provides visible proof of the pigmented heritage we all share. (See p. 335, **Ref. 2**; see p. 335, **Ref. 11**.)

Flat Salmon Patch *(Nevus Simplex)*

The flat salmon patch is another extremely common birthmark. It's a salmon-red speck or patch that brightens to a scarlet red when the baby cries. This mark represents a cluster of an extra number of normally formed fetal capillaries. It has been discussed in the medical literature since 1880, but we still don't know what causes it.

Because salmon patches are most often found on the nape of the neck, they're frequently referred to as stork bites, which is as good a description as any. They can also appear at the root of the nose (the glabella) and on the forehead, the eyelids, and the upper lip. When they appear in these areas, people often call them angel's kisses, again, as good an explanation as any.

In contrast to the Mongolian spot (see p. 39), the salmon patch is the routine birthmark of the light-complexioned newborn. Girls are slightly more likely to have them than boys. They fade quickly and are usually gone by the end of the first year. Those on the back of the neck have a 50-50 chance of lasting into adulthood, but since they're covered with hair, who really cares?

Though the salmon patch itself has no medical significance, it can be confused with another flat capillary birthmark, the port wine stain (nevus flammeus). This birthmark is red to purple in color and can cover large areas of the body. Unlike the salmon patch, the port wine stain won't lose its color when you push on it, and, most importantly, this birthmark is permanent and is often associated with problems in the eyes and nervous system. So, for both cosmetic and medical reasons, it's important to determine whether the baby has a salmon patch or a port wine stain. (See p. 335, **Ref. 3**; see p. 335, **Ref. 4**; see p. 335, **Ref. 11.**)

Red-Purple Bumps: Strawberry Mark *(Cavernous Hemangioma)*

Like the flat salmon patch (see p. 40), this mark is the result of a clustering of extra capillaries, but it differs in many other aspects. In the first place, strawberry marks aren't present at birth. They begin to develop during the third to fourth week, and only 10 percent appear after one month. At first, the marks are either tiny, bright specks or threadlike streaks and are often surrounded by a zone of pale skin. During the next six months, they grow rapidly into sharply defined, raised, dark red or purple, rough-surfaced swellings that look for all the world like the outside slice of a slightly overripe strawberry. Tiny streaks of capillaries can be seen around the swellings. Pushing on them will partially, but not completely, blanch them.

Strawberry marks seem to follow a standard course. They stop growing by the time the baby is eight months old or, at the latest, the first birthday. During the second year of life, they begin their disappearing act. Half of the strawberries are gone by five years of age, 70 percent by seven, and 90 percent by nine. They fade away by developing grayish streaks on the surface, usually at the center of the swelling. The gray areas gradually come together, until the entire swelling becomes pink-gray. Eventually, the mark totally vanishes, leaving no traces except, in rare instances, an area of slightly puckered skin.

Roughly 8 to 10 percent of children under one year old have strawberry marks. Like other capillary-derived birthmarks, they're seen more often in girls than boys and somewhat more often in prematurely born babies. They're usually single marks, though about one fifth of children with strawberries have a bunch. They can occur anywhere on the body, but their favorite location is the head and neck area, with the trunk playing second fiddle.

Because of their frequent appearance on the head and their habit of early and rapid growth, strawberry marks can generate a lot of worry. This is the perfect moment for you to follow my favorite dictum: *Don't just do something, stand there.* If you feel that some action is called for, take pictures. When it comes to treating strawberry marks, no one can equal the success rate of Mother Nature. Treating strawberry marks by surgery, dry ice, and so on produces ten times the complication rate of those left to nature's curative powers, and the results are not so good! Of course, if the mark triples or quadruples in size within a few weeks, or if its location is particularly bothersome, such as over an eye or in the voice box, or if its location is causing it to bleed a lot or get infected, then some form of active treatment will be considered by your doctor. Otherwise, leave it alone. (See p. 335, **Ref. 4**; see p. 335, **Ref. 5**; see p. 335, **Ref. 11**.)

SCALY SKIN *(Physiologic Epidermal Desquamation)*

The normal full-term newborn is delivered with a cheesy material covering his skin. This material, called vernix caseosa, is usually washed off or rubbed into the baby's skin by the nursery nurse, who would be wise to use it on her own hands since it's a terrific hand softener. It's also a terrific baby-skin softener, and for the next few hours the baby has velvety smooth skin. After a few hours of this velvety bliss, however, the baby's skin becomes dry and scaly. It begins to flake away. Cracks appear and, in short, the baby looks awful. The awfulness continues for a week or more, and then the scaling and flaking stop. It's a normal process called physiologic epidermal desquamation; normal, that is, unless it's seen at the moment of birth. Dry scaly skin at the moment of birth is a regularly seen feature of the baby who remained in the womb longer than he should have, and your doctor will be on the lookout for that. Black babies have scaly skin more often than white.

When the scales are on the scalp, they're sometimes mistaken for a common scalp condition popularly called cradle cap. The difference between the two is as follows: The scales of cradle cap are yellow-orange and greasy, like the residue at the bottom of the potato chip bag; normal baby flakes are white and delicate and look more like snowflakes. Cradle cap often needs to be treated; scaly skin can be left alone. (See p. 335, **Ref. 6**.)

RASHES

Tiny Yellowish Bumps *(Milia)*

Have you noticed that many of the words we use to describe physical conditions are, in fact, the names of foods? *Milia* is one of them. It refers to a rash made up of tiny bumps the size of millet seeds that's seen on 40 percent of all newborns. I must confess that I've never laid eyes on a millet seed, but I've seen enough milia to make up for that shortcoming. Almost half of all newborns have it, usually on the cheeks, nose, chin, and forehead, but occasionally on the upper chest. The bumps are monotonously uniform in size, measuring only 1 to 2 millimeters in diameter. Their color is pearly-white to yellow, and the skin surrounding them appears entirely normal. They result from the accumulation of the cheesy material formed by the oil glands in the skin, which explains why they're only seen in the oily parts of the body. The eruptions usually disappear after the first month, but some of the stubborn cysts last into the third month.

Because there's no accompanying redness, milia is seldom taken very seriously by either parents or doctors. (I sometimes suspect that its only function is to remind us of the existence of millet seeds.) (See p. 335, **Ref. 7**; see p. 335, **Ref. 11.**)

Pimples or Dark Freckles Surrounded by Collar of Flaky Skin *(Transient Neonatal Pustular Melanosis)*

This rash rarely appears on white newborns and is seen in only 4 or 5 percent of black newborns. It's usually present at the moment of birth and consists of very superficial, fragile, small pimples that readily break open and disappear the first time the baby is bathed. When the pimples are scrubbed away, they often leave small dark spots. The little leftover freckles are usually surrounded by thin, white, flaky rings at the base, sometimes called collarettes or little collars. The spots generally cluster around the baby's forehead, chin, and neck, but they can pop up anywhere on the body, including the lower back and legs. The white rings disappear very quickly, and the pigmented spots fade away within three months. Black babies who have neonatal pustular melanosis often develop erythema toxicum (see below) as a follow-up.

Since the blisters of neonatal pustular melanosis only last until the first bath, this is a very easy rash to miss. The most conspicuous part of the rash is the freckle, and when that fades away at three months, who would really miss it? (See p. 335, **Ref. 5.**)

Yellow-White Pimples on Splotchy Skin (*Erythema Toxicum*)

This rash is so common that it's often called newborn rash. It consists of red spots varying in size from several millimeters to several centimeters in diameter. Neighboring spots often get together to form a diffuse red area, and then turn into firm yellow-white bumps or, occasionally, little blisters. All in all, erythema toxicum can be a mess. The eruptions cause the child to look as if he'd been attacked by a bunch of fleas, and parents often describe the baby's rash this way.

Newborn rash can be present at the moment of birth or, more often, make its appearance sometime during the first three days of life (just when the first wave of visitors shows up to admire the baby!).

Erythema toxicum can consist of a couple of spots or several hundred. It can appear anywhere on the baby's body except the palms and soles. Each individual spot usually lasts only two days but new ones can appear on and off during the first month. After that, they completely disappear.

This rash has no racial or sexual preferences. It never affects prematures, but up to 70 percent of full-termers have it.

Parents sometimes mistake erythema toxicum for a skin infection. Skin infections, however, grow in size hour by hour. Erythema toxicum does not. Your doctor can also differentiate this rash from an infection simply by opening up the bump and examining the material inside it on a slide. If the bump represents an infection, the physician will see bacteria and white blood cells of the inflammatory type. The erythema toxicum pustule scraping contains no bacteria. Instead, it's filled with cells that are normally seen only in allergic states. This doesn't mean that we regard this rash as an allergic reaction. It probably represents the newborn's immature response to irritative stimuli.

Erythema toxicum is most often mistaken for a milk allergy. When this mistake is made, the baby's formula is changed needlessly and repeatedly until the rash goes away. I've seen breast-fed babies switched to cow's milk because the parents thought the child was allergic to its mother's milk. If you're being advised to change the baby's milk because of this rash, you should have the rash looked at by the doctor. If the physician is in doubt, she can do a scraping and that should put the matter to rest. (See p. 335, **Ref. 5**; see p. 335, **Ref. 11**.)

Tiny, Uniform-Sized Bumps: Heat Rash or Sweat Blisters (*Miliaria*)

Miliaria is commonly known as heat rash. It's the result of a blockage of the baby's perspiration in the sweat glands, and the moisture's subsequent failure to make its way to the surface of the skin. When this blockage occurs, either one of the two following situations can develop:

One: The retained sweat can form tiny, pinpoint, water-filled blisters that are surrounded by completely normal skin. This condition is called miliaria sudamina or miliaria crystallina. It can be seen on the first day of life.

Two: The sweat can burst out of the sweat gland and into the tissues of the skin. Since sweat belongs on the skin, not in it, the skin around the blister reacts by becoming inflamed. This is called miliaria rubra, and usually begins after the first week of life. This sweat retention rash is the well-known prickly heat, most intense on the face, neck, and upper chest, and in the bends of the arms and legs. It consists of small, discrete, red-colored raised areas, many of which contain tiny, pinpoint blisters.

Almost all summer babies develop one or the other form of this rash, but even winter babies, if too bundled up, can get prickly heat. Since the tendency to blockage of the sweat ducts is greatest during the first two weeks of life, this is the time when heat rashes are most likely to occur.

As with erythema toxicum (see p. 44), the usual error is in mistaking this rash for a milk allergy. All that needs to be done is to take off the wraps and turn on the cool. (See p. 335, **Ref. 5**; see p. 335, **Ref. 8**.)

Swollen Pink Pimples (*Acne Neonatorum*)

This is the same acne that we came to know during our wonderful teenage years, and it has the same cause—stimulation of the oil glands by the male sex hormone, testosterone. It's more common in baby boys than girls.

Before birth, the baby received the hormone from the mother, and created his or her own as well. The fetal adrenal gland produces testosterone; so does the fetal testis. Since the baby boy has this extra source of the hormone, it's no wonder that he's more likely to have acne than the baby girl.

The acne eruption may be present at the moment of birth or it may appear early in infancy. It's recognizable as the familiar "zit" or, less often, the blackhead. The pimples are usually confined to the facial area, especially the cheeks. The chin and forehead are occasionally involved but, in contrast to adolescent acne, acne neonatorum always spares the chest and back. (See p. 335, **Ref. 5.**)

YELLOW BABY

Newborn Jaundice (*Physiologic Jaundice or Physiologic Hyperbilirubinemia*)

Even if the pregnancy, labor, and delivery went magnificently well, and the fruit of your labor is as perfect as can be, the odds are still 50-50 that your newborn's peachy skin will be a banana-yellow for several days. The term applied to this condition is *jaundice,* derived from the French *jaune,* meaning yellow.

Jaundice is so common in normal, healthy newborns that its occurrence during the first week of life is considered natural or "physiologic." The color comes from the buildup of a yellow-red pigment called bilirubin (pronounced *billy-roo-bin*) in the baby's blood. Bilirubin is a normal ingredient of all human blood, but it's usually present at levels too low to produce a yellow color. Virtually *every* newborn will develop levels of the pigment that, when measured, show slight elevations, but only half of all babies will develop levels high enough to cause the skin to appear yellow.

But if your yellow baby is perfectly normal, why is the doctor watching her bilirubin level so closely, and why is this common pigment talked about so much these days?

The answer is, in part, that bilirubin has a long and circuitous history.

Thirty years ago, when medical science was first exploring the consequences of Rh factor disease, we learned that babies with very high bilirubin levels were at risk of suffering a type of brain injury called kernicterus, and that, conversely, the risk of kernicterus in full-termers was extremely low if we could keep the bilirubin counts below 20 milligrams/100 milliliters. That was the beginning of "bilirubin watching" and the "20 phobia." Since those early lessons, however, the sanctity of "20" has fallen on hard times. We have seen premies get kernicterus at levels below 20 milligrams, and full-termers tolerate levels above 20 without suffering this type of brain injury. (Nevertheless, we continue to watch bilirubin levels for reasons that I'll explain further on in this section.)

Furthermore, physicians began talking to parents about bilirubin levels when it became a financial necessity for mothers and babies to go home from the hospital on day two or three, instead of day five. Back in the days when hospital costs were low, doctors were able to satisfy themselves on the subject of the baby's bilirubin count by the time mother and baby went home. The baby's bilirubin count would, in its normal manner, creep up slowly, and the baby would appear yellow on the third day. The doctor would check the level on the following days and see that it wasn't going to be a problem; then, on the fifth day, Mother and her slightly yellow baby would go home. Parents didn't need to know where the yellow went, or where it had been.

Today, because hospital costs are so high, mothers and babies are going home on day two or three—the very same day that bilirubin levels are going up. Sometimes mothers may go home but, at the doctor's request, leave their jaundiced babies in the nursery where the bilirubin level can be watched more closely. Some mothers take the babies home and return to the laboratory for additional bilirubin tests. For most babies, the level falls and the doctor stops testing. Sometimes, however, the level rises and the doctor will decide to readmit the baby to the hospital.

To understand why we're still so concerned about bilirubin, it helps to know how it's produced in the body, is processed in the liver, and finds its ultimate fate in the intestines. The production end involves the red blood cell (RBC), which delivers oxygen from the lung to the tissues. Within the RBC, the pigment hemoglobin actually carries the oxygen. The process is much like a truck delivering heating oil to your home. The RBC is the truck; the hemoglobin is the truck's storage tank; the oxygen is the heating oil.

After 100 days or so, the RBC grows old and is taken off its route, and new red blood cells arrive to take its place. In the process of dismantling the old RBC, the pigment hemoglobin is converted to the pigment bilirubin, which then enters the circulation. RBC destruction accounts for 75 to 80 percent of the bilirubin in the bloodstream. (The rest, called shunt bilirubin, comes from a number of other sources.)

The next step is to transfer the bilirubin to the processing center, the liver cell. Bilirubin travels to the liver cell bound to a carrier protein, albumin. Once it reaches its destination, a liver protein called Y plucks it out of the bloodstream, and another protein called Z slips it into the liver cell. Now the processing begins.

After the Z protein has positioned the bilirubin in the right spot in the liver cell, an enzyme comes along and combines glucuronic acid with the bilirubin, producing a new compound called conjugated bilirubin. Only conjugated bilirubin can be excreted by the liver, so this conjugating step is essential. Without it, the bilirubin would be condemned to remain in the liver cell forever.

Once the conjugated bilirubin has left the liver cell, it mixes with the bile and empties into the intestines. There it isn't reabsorbed, but is acted upon by the intestinal bacteria, and most of it is ultimately excreted. (This is what gives the stool its color.)

This would seem to take care of the bilirubin once and for all, but not quite. Because *some* of it isn't excreted. This leftover but still conjugated bilirubin gets stripped of its glucuronic acid by the bacteria, converted back into unconjugated bilirubin, and absorbed out of the intestine and into the bloodstream to make its way back to the liver for another go. At this point, it's in the same state as when it left the decrepit RBC. It, along with the new bilirubin, must make its way back to the liver to be conjugated, completing the last leg of what's called enterohepatic circulation (*entero* means intestine; *hepatic* means liver).

Before the baby was born, the only pathway of any importance was the one that connected it to the placenta. The placenta happily accepted all of the baby's unconjugated bilirubin and passed it on to the mother. The fetal liver got a free ride because the mother's liver was doing all the conjugating for it. Once detached from the placenta, though, baby is on his own, and his little liver has to work hard every step of the way.

In the first place, the baby's liver has had no practice conjugating bilirubin. In the second place, the newborn, with his large blood volume and high hemoglobin concentration, has many more RBCs per pound than the adult. Plus its RBCs don't last as long as the adult's. As a result, the newborn's daily production of bilirubin from hemoglobin is twice the adult's rate. And if this isn't tough enough, the baby has more shunt bilirubin and more bilirubin traveling along his enterohepatic circulation. The baby's body tasks are just beginning.

The bilirubin must get to the liver cell for processing. This requires a good circulation. Baby had one before he was born. The fetus's liver took its blood from the huge umbilical vein, one of the main vessels of the umbilical cord. But once the cord is tied, the baby's liver has to adjust to a brand-new, much smaller supply of blood. The net effect is a reduction in the amount of blood flowing into the liver. This doesn't help.

Furthermore, for the first five days of life, the liver cell is low on Y protein so it's less able to snare bilirubin out of the circulation. And once the bilirubin is in the immature liver cell, it runs into yet another, and most important, stumbling block. The liver cell doesn't have enough enzyme to go around. Without the glucuronyl transferase to conjugate the bilirubin, the whole process gets jammed up within the liver cell. In fact, even the conjugated bilirubin has a hard time making its way out of the immature, inexperienced cell. The newborn's liver cell is unaccustomed to conjugated bilirubin, and its ability to excrete it out of the cell isn't yet up to par.

So it happens that unconjugated bilirubin accumulates in the baby's liver cell, and eventually its concentration in the bloodstream rises, turning him yellowish. When an adult's level of bilirubin exceeds 2 milligrams / 100 milliliters, it's considered excessive. But for the newborn, as you've seen, it's pretty much par for the course. It's considered natural or "physiologic" for the bilirubin level to be above 2 milligrams / 100 milliliters from birth until the tenth day of life.

When the baby's bilirubin level reaches 5 to 7 milligrams / 100 milliliters, it becomes visible as a yellow color, and we say that the baby has jaundice. Half of the normal newborns and considerably more than half of premature infants have it, making it such a common occurrence that doctors are tempted to greet newborn jaundice with "What else is new?"

Yet, natural and normal as this condition is, doctors still ask a series of questions, beginning with "Is the jaundice physiologic or is something wrong with the baby?" As a rule, your doctor won't dismiss the jaundice as physiologic if it appeared in the first day of life, because physiologic jaundice never starts that early.

Also, if the total bilirubin level is rising by more than 5 milligrams /100 milliliters per day, it's going up too fast to be physiologic. If it has reached 13 milligrams /100 milliliters or higher, it's too high. If the yellow hasn't faded by a week for the full-termer, or two weeks for the premie, then, too, it's lasting too long to be dismissed as physiologic. Incidentally, once physiologic jaundice fades, it never returns. After the immature liver gets the hang of processing bilirubin, there are no other "natural" reasons for being jaundiced.

Finally, since the yellow from physiologic jaundice comes solely from the elevation of unconjugated bilirubin, any significant elevation of the conjugated bilirubin will be viewed with suspicion.

Only 5 to 15 percent of normal full-termers have elevations out of the range of physiologic jaundice. But for these babies, the doctor will run through his list of unnatural reasons for elevated bilirubin levels. He has a long list. At its head are the common causes of increased RBC destruction, such as mild blood-group incompatibilities, excessively high RBC counts, and excessive skin bruising. At its bottom are disorders more threatening to the baby's health. For the bottom's sake, the doctor will try to determine the cause for the excessive, non-physiologic jaundice.

The doctor will succeed in half the cases. He'll have no answer for the other half, but many of the unexplained cases will be associated with breast feeding. How this relates to the relatively rare condition of breast-milk jaundice (see p. 51) isn't yet understood.

We also don't know what the "critical" bilirubin level is for full-termers with unexplained nonphysiologic jaundice. Until that number is known, you can expect "20" to prevail. The proportion of jaundiced babies that are unexplained can be expected to decrease as our technology improves. Today's technology isn't sensitive enough to detect extremely slight increases in rates of RBC destruction or the reasons why some little livers are more laid back than others. For tomorrow's technology, these questions will appear too easy to bother with.

Meanwhile, unless your physician tells you otherwise, you can consider your yellowish baby perfectly normal. He'll be peachy-pink again in a couple of days. (See p. 335, **Ref. 1**; see p. 339, **Ref. 74**; see p. 339, **Ref. 75**.)

Breast-Milk Jaundice

This condition has been widely discussed lately, despite the fact that only 1 to 2 percent of all breast-feeding infants develop it. Babies with breast-milk jaundice show normal bilirubin levels (see p. 46) for the first three days, but on the fourth day of life their unconjugated bilirubin levels start to rise. If breast feeding is continued, the level can reach 30 milligrams / 100 milliliters. The levels remain high for four to ten days, and then gradually decline to normal by the time the babies are one to three months old.

No one knows the precise cause of breast-milk jaundice, but we do know that the breast milk from the mothers shows unusually high levels of lipase, an enzyme that increases the fatty acids in the baby's blood. These fatty acids apparently interfere with the liver's uptake and conjugation of bilirubin. There's also some evidence linking a certain factor in the mother's milk with an increase in enterohepatic circulation.

The elevated bilirubin levels of babies with breast-milk jaundice is not related to any weight loss that breast-feeding infants may have in their first week. Still, if a diagnosis of breast-milk jaundice is made, your doctor will ask you to temporarily suspend breast feeding. Even though the breast feeding isn't hurting the baby in any way, the elevated bilirubin level, if it gets over 20 milligrams / 100 milliliters, might do so. Within 48 hours, the baby's bilirubin level should drop significantly. At that point, your physician will suggest that you resume nursing. Your baby's bilirubin level may rise slightly; then it will slowly decline, eventually reaching normal levels even while the breast feeding is going on.

There's no good reason for a baby with breast-milk jaundice to be taken off breast feeding for more than 48 hours. (See p. 339, **Ref.** 74.)

TRAUMA

Bruises and Burst Capillaries (Ecchymoses and Petechiae)

The escape of blood from a burst vein causes the familiar bruise (ecchymosis). The escape of blood from a tiny capillary causes a tiny pinpoint bruise (petechia). If the thin wall of either type of blood vessel is stretched by a very tight compression upstream, it can burst and the blood can seep into the skin. This is a very common occurrence in the process of delivery and many babies arrive in the world with a few of these bruises.

If the squeeze on the newborn came from the umbilical cord around the baby's neck, only the blood vessels above the neck will be distended. If the squeeze was around the baby's waist, as the baby was trying to work his way through a tight birth canal, all the petechiae or ecchymoses will be above the waist.

Once the baby has passed through the birth canal and the tight umbilical cord is removed from his neck, there's no longer any reason for skin bleeding based on vessel distension. Any additional skin bleeding is never normal and must have another explanation. This is why many doctors draw circles around the ecchymoses and petechiae seen at birth and come back to check that no new skin bleeding occurs.

Bruises and burst capillaries are no threat to the skin, but as the blood is degraded in the skin, its hemoglobin is converted to the pigment bilirubin (see p. 46). Small petechiae make no real impact on the body pool of bilirubin, but large bruises certainly do. For this reason, your doctor will watch your baby's bilirubin count more closely if your baby happens to have large bruises. (See p. 335, **Ref. 9.**)

Redness and Scrapes (Erythema and Contusions)

We used to think that scrapes on a newborn's body were always the result of rough handling that the baby received during the delivery, either from forceful tugging or from the application of forceps. We now know that babies can get banged up to the same extent before they're born. This is especially true for very large babies or normal-sized babies who have to make it through a very tight birth canal.

Hard, Purplish Areas over Bones *(Subcutaneous Fat Necrosis)*

If the baby's fat gets caught between a bone and another hard place (either the mother's bone or the doctor's forceps), it can get crushed. Crushed fat crystallizes under the skin and forms sharply defined, extremely hard, purplish areas. The lumps are neither tender nor warm, and are always over that part of the baby's bone that did its share of the crushing. Common locations are the cheeks, back, buttocks, arms, and thighs.

Areas of subcutaneous fat necrosis are usually first noticed sometime during the first week of life, and last for about a month. They may be tiny lumps or they may be large plaques measuring several centimeters in diameter. Most of the time, the lumps disappear on their own, but sometimes their centers liquify and need to be drained.

Babies with subcutaneous fat necrosis look and are perfectly healthy. The hardness of these lumps and the fact that they aren't noticed for several days after the injury occurred combine to make these minor blemishes seem much more important than they actually are. (See p. 335, **Ref. 10**; see p. 335, **Ref. 11**.)

Sucking Blisters

Babies do a lot of sucking while still in the womb, focusing on whatever comes within reach of their mouths. If the sucking lasts for any length of time, a blister or a purple "hickey" is produced. At birth, you may see the blister itself or, if the blister roof ruptures at or before birth, you may see a very puzzling oval or round raw area with the remains of the blister roof. It's easy to recognize a sucking blister by noting whether or not the area involved is very accessible to the baby's mouth—the thumb, for instance. Unless the baby is a contortionist, there's no way that he'll be able to put a sucking blister on his head, face, or back. (See p. 335, **Ref. 8**.)

Pressure Sores

Pressure sores are found over the areas not padded by fat that were squeezed against the mother's bones. Most often, this means the scalp. The sore begins to develop after several days as a red swollen area, may go on to ulcerate, then gradually scabs over and heals. (See p. 335, **Ref. 8.**)

CIRCULATION

Faint Purplish Mottling (Cutis Marmorata)

When the baby gets chilled, from either changing or bathing, a light-purple marbled pattern appears on the skin. This pattern is the result of the dilation of the small veins and capillaries of the skin. It's an immature response to chilling. When the baby reaches three months or older, her body will react to cold by constricting the small blood vessels, thus producing a whitening of the skin.

You can eliminate the mottling promptly simply by warming her up. (See p. 335, **Ref. 5.**)

Red Color Shifting from Side to Side as Baby Changes Position
  (Harlequin Color Change)

This phenomenon is occasionally seen in full-term babies, but is mainly a specialty of the prematurely born infant. When the premies are placed on their sides, up to 10 percent of them undergo a strikingly bizarre color change. For 30 seconds to 20 minutes, the side that's lower becomes bright red, and the side on top becomes pale white. A sharply drawn line divides the baby into the two halves. If the "attack" is only partial, the color change will be brief and may not include either the baby's face or his genitals. Furthermore, if the baby begins to cry, the color change stops immediately.

Harlequin color changes occur most often between the second and fifth day of life but they've been seen as late as three weeks. Like cutis marmorata (see p. 54), they're the result of the baby's immature regulation of his skin circulation.

If you see this one, grab a camera. (See p. 335, **Ref. 5.**)

Blue Hands and Feet *(Acrocyanosis)*

This blue color change occurs in the glove and stocking parts of the baby when he's chilled. It results from the pooling of blood in the veins, which slows its flow. With the blood flow slowed, the tissues have more time to extract the oxygen from the blood, thus turning the blood more blue and less red.

This temperature effect, like cutis marmorata (see p. 54), can be quickly undone by warming the baby.

True *cyanosis,* as opposed to acrocyanosis, results from a heart or lung problem; it's a more serious condition that's visible all over the baby and doesn't go away when the baby is warmed. (See p. 335, **Ref. 11.**)

Ruddiness *(Plethora)*

Most babies have ruddy complexions at birth and look more like Peruvian Indians than like the kid next door. Once upon a time, we thought that the reason for this resemblance was that both the Inca and the fetus lived in an environment extremely low in oxygen. Although we haven't changed our minds about the Inca's home high atop the Andes, we have changed our thinking about the fetus's environment. Current research simply doesn't confirm our earlier thinking that the artery to the placenta carried blood that was extra low in oxygen. At any rate, for reasons not fully understood, most newborns have more than 5 million red blood cells in every cubic millimeter of blood, giving them a hemoglobin concentration of 17 to 19 grams per 100 milliliters and, therefore, a ruddy complexion. By way of contrast, the average three-month-old baby has 4 million red cells per cubic millimeter and a hemoglobin concentration of only 11 grams per 100 milliliters.

SHORT NAILS EMBEDDED IN SURROUNDING SKIN

Because newborns tend to have soft, flexible nails and fat, fleshy feet, they often appear to have "ingrown toenails"; that is, the nails seem to be growing right into the skin.

But nails don't become ingrown in this age group, even those that seem to be headed for the most trouble. Perhaps it's the softness of the nail that allows it to bend over the mound of skin, but whatever the reason, what appears to be an obstruction of skin doesn't present a problem for the newborn toenail. (See p. 335, **Ref. 12.**)

HAIR

The fetus begins to grow hair sometime between the 8th and 12th week of the pregnancy, and she continues to make hair throughout the pregnancy. This fetal hair, called lanugo, is fine, fair, and furry and it covers the entire baby. Lanugo is normally shed during the seventh to eighth month of the pregnancy and therefore isn't seen in full-termers. If the baby is born one to two months early, she may appear with lanugo hairs covering her face, trunk, and limbs.

Many newborns have a substantial crop of mature hair on their heads from the moment of birth. Don't be fooled. It may have the thick, coarse texture and dark color of mature hair, and in fact it *is* mature or "terminal" hair, as it's called, but it doesn't *behave* in a mature fashion. An adult's mature hair lasts an average of three years on the head. In babies, the scalp terminal hairs begin to shed within the first few weeks of life. Sometimes they fall out all at once; sometimes they fall out gradually. Either way, the first batch of terminal hair is usually replaced by a new crop by the time the baby is six months of age. This explains how little David can be born with long, black hair but by the time he reaches five months old have hair that's thick and blond.

Some newborns are born with coarse terminal hair covering areas not known for their hairiness, such as the forehead and the space between the temples and eyebrows. Don't despair. During the next 12 months, these hairs will lose their coarseness and will come to resemble the fine, pale fuzz (vellus hair) that sometimes covers the arms, legs, and faces of women and children. (See p. 335, **Ref. 12.**)

2. Head

TRAUMA

Long, Narrow Head *(Molding)*

In the normal course of events at birth, the baby's head being the advancing end, a great deal of molding of the head may occur. This is especially true if the baby is large or firstborn, if the labor is prolonged, or if the mother has a narrow pelvis or a rigid cervix.

As the baby's head is squeezed through the cervix, it's narrowed on both sides and gets higher in the back. With pressure from the cervix, the base of the skull swings inward and the forehead does the same. The result is a head narrow from side to side and front to back, but elongated and somewhat pointed at the rear. A dunce cap wouldn't fit badly.

As the bones shift under this pressure, spaces between them may be temporarily obliterated, and it may be impossible to determine whether or not the fontanels (see p. 61) are of normal size. As a result of the distortion of the shape of the skull, it may also be impossible to get an accurate measurement of the baby's head circumference. At this point, most head measurements are falsely low. On the other hand, because the back of the baby's head is pushed up and back, measurements of his entire length will be falsely high. If you ever wanted a tall baby, now is the time to measure his length. He may lose several centimeters by the next sunrise.

Within a few short hours, most of the baby's head molding disappears. By six days, his head has shifted back to its unmolded shape.

Upsetting as it may be to see your beloved baby arrive resembling a Conehead, think of the alternatives and consider what problems the baby would have if his head weren't moldable: it would probably break or transfer the tremendous compression to the brain itself. "Better the shell should mold than the yolk get scrambled." As for the "lucky" babies without molding, they're the ones whose heads never went one-on-one with a pelvis. This group includes babies delivered by Cesarean section, babies delivered from a breech presentation, and babies whose heads are abnormally small. Wouldn't you settle for a bit of molding? (See p. 335, **Ref.** 11; see p. 335, **Ref.** 13.)

Soft Swelling over Skull (Caput Succedaneum)

The scalp overlying the advancing part of the baby's skull may develop a diffuse, mushy swelling that often includes bruises. Since the swelling is the result of tissue fluid and blood in the scalp over the bones, its borders won't be restricted to any individual bone of the skull. The swelling will cross over the borders of bones and may cross over the midline.

This swelling is present at birth, and practically every baby has at least some of it. Caput succedaneum is usually gone by the second day of life, although the associated bruise may last a bit longer. (See p. 335, **Ref.** 11; see p. 335, **Ref.** 13.)

Sharply Demarcated, Balloonlike Swelling of Head (Cephalohematoma)

If bleeding occurs under the membrane surrounding one of the bones of the skull, the swelling that results is referred to as a cephalo- (head) hematoma (collection of blood). This type of swelling feels very different from caput succedaneum (see p. 58). Rather than mushy and diffuse, the cephalohematoma is balloonlike and springy and its borders don't extend beyond the edges of the bone that it covers.

Cephalohematomas occur in 0.5 to 2.5 percent of births and are associated with difficulties in delivery such as largeness of the baby, firstborns, the mother's small pelvis, and so on. They're more common in baby boys (they have bigger heads), and appear on the right side of the head three times more often than the left.

Typically cephalohematomas aren't seen in the delivery room. They're usually noticed during the first 24 hours of life, and they grow larger day by day for two to five days. Over the next few weeks to months, the borders of the swelling elevate and the center sinks in, creating a crater. Gradually thicker bone develops in the border area, and after one to two months the swelling is completely gone, leaving no traces.

At one time, doctors thought that all babies with cephalohematomas should have X rays of their skulls to see if there was a fracture underneath the swelling. We now know that only 5 percent or so actually have fractures, and unless there was considerable trauma connected with the delivery, such as very prolonged labor, vigorous application of forceps, or a very big baby, most doctors will opt not to take the X ray.

Another thing that babies with cephalohematomas are spared these days is being stuck with a needle to draw out the blood. Inserting a needle in a cephalohematoma is asking for trouble since it introduces the risk of infecting the swelling.

A large cephalohematoma can become a significant source of additional bilirubin (see p. 46), and is often the reason for excessive jaundice in the newborn. Accordingly, your doctor might follow your baby's bilirubin count extra-closely if your baby has one of these swellings. (See p. 335, **Ref.** 11; see p. 335, **Ref.** 14; see p. 335, **Ref.** 15.)

Soft Spots That Feel Like Ping-Pong Balls (*Craniotabes*)

When pressure is applied to a bone for a long time, the bone softens. If the bone happens to be the skull, the condition is called craniotabes (cranium means skull; tabes is wasting). It's usually limited to the precise spot on the baby's head that was jammed against the mother's bony pelvis while in the womb. For most babies, this means that the back of the skull, near the rear fontanel (see p. 61), will be softer than the rest of the skull. It feels like an old Ping-Pong ball when you push on it. After one or two months, the softness disappears.

Look for this condition if your baby's head was engaged in your pelvis, i.e., was "dropped" for a particularly long time. Craniotabes is harmless. We know of at least one baby whose entire head was softened but, after three months, hardened normally. (See p. 335, **Ref.** 13; see p. 336, **Ref.** 16.)

Scalp Scars from Fetal Monitoring Instruments

Sometimes your obstetrician will want to keep a very close watch on your baby during labor, and will monitor your baby's heart rate using wires that are clipped to the baby's scalp. This is called internal monitoring.

At the very least, the clips the physician applies will pinch the skin on the scalp and cause a small bruise. Sometimes a sore will develop, form a scab, and occasionally leave a small scar under the baby's hair. If the wires are forcefully removed, some hair may be yanked out, leaving a patch of baldness for a brief period. On very rare occasions, calcifications will develop in the healing sores and they'll be visible in the scalp if an X ray of the skull happens to be taken for some other reason. The calcifications are of no significance and eventually fade away. (See p. 335, **Ref. 13**; see p. 336, **Ref. 16**.)

BUMPS *(Prominences)*

Back of Head   *(External Occipital Protuberances)*

Your baby's head isn't a perfect sphere. It has bumps that existed from the earliest moments of its formation. You probably won't notice these bumps until the baby bangs her head and you feel all over to be certain that everything's all right.

Since most babies bump their heads when they fall backward, the bump most often discovered by parents is the one in the center of the back of the head. This normal bump is the external occipital protuberance, and can be felt on every baby's skull. Adults have them, too, but because babies lack the bulky neck and head muscles of the adult, there's less "meat" covering the infant's bumps, and they're easier to find.

Side of Head   *(Parietal Bossing)*

Besides the bump on the back of the head (see p. 60), babies have two other types of normal bumps, which are situated on either side of the top of the head. These are the parietal tubers (*parietal* means wall; *tuber* equals swelling) and they can vary greatly in size from person to person. Some babies have tiny parietal tubers that are barely noticeable; others have such prominent swellings that they're called parietal horns. (See p. 336, **Ref. 22.**)

NORMAL FONTANEL

The infant skull has two soft spots that you usually can feel with your fingers. The one in the back—the posterior fontanel—is sometimes too small to feel, but that particular fontanel is of no importance. The important fontanel—the anterior—is the one situated where the two bones of the forehead and the two bones of the side of the head meet. Molding of the skull (see p. 57) can temporarily cover up the anterior fontanel, but once the molding has subsided, it should be very easy to feel.

The anterior fontanel is diamond-shaped and, if you watch it closely, you'll see it pulse with each heartbeat. This pulsing action is responsible for the name *fontanel,* which actually means little fountain.

The anterior fontanels are extremely variable in size and shape and the point in time when they, like the posterior fontanel, close up. The length and width of the anteriors range from about 0.6 to 3.6 centimeters, but they usually measure about 2.1 centimeters.

Unusually large or small fontanels are sometimes related to certain diseases, which is why doctors measure them so carefully. When the baby has a normal head circumference, shape, and feel, and is otherwise normal, there should be no concern if the fontanels vary a bit above or below the average. (See p. 336, **Ref. 23.**)

LONG, NARROW PREMIE HEAD SHAPE

Most babies who were born prematurely will develop long, narrow heads. This is because premies usually lie on their sides in the nursery. Since their heads are relatively soft, and since they're likely to remain in one position for a longer time than the full-term infant, premies tend to flatten out their skulls. In time, their heads remodel to a great extent, but a trained observer can usually recognize the telltale shape that gives away their premature origins.

3. Face

LOPSIDED *(Asymmetric Molding)*

If the fetus is packed tightly in the womb, all sorts of temporary facial changes can come about as a result of the compression of the bones. These changes are called deformations simply because the change occurred in a part of the face that was originally entirely normal. If the part had been "wrong" from the start, the abnormality would have been called a malformation. Deformations will improve in time; malformations will not.

Temporary deformations include the following:

If the fetal chin was pressed for a long time against the chest, a small, Andy Gump–like chin can develop. Sometimes a dent will form in the upper chest at the spot where the chin was pushing in.

Similarly, if the shoulder was shoved up against the jaw, the baby will have an uneven jaw line, often with an indentation corresponding to the round shape of his shoulder.

Later on, after the baby has spent some time out of the tight squeeze of the birth canal, there will be catch-up growth of the small bones, and an evening out of all the bony irregularities. (See p. 335, **Ref. 11**; see p. 335, **Ref. 13**.)

DROOPING FEATURES *(Weakness of Facial Nerve)*

The nerve that directs most of the muscles of the face is the seventh cranial nerve, called, appropriately enough, the facial nerve. It originates deep in the brain (explaining why it's also called a cranial nerve) and has a bony protection just in front of the ear. Branches of the facial nerve extend to the forehead, across to the eyelids, and down to the mouth. Any or all of these branches can be damaged by pressure, either from the mother's pelvis before birth or from the doctor's forceps, a condition seen most often in large babies. When it happens, a corresponding muscle appears weak. The baby's eye may not close tightly, or her mouth might droop.

Most nerve compression occurs late in pregnancy, and the later it happens, the greater the chances for full recovery. Electrical studies on the compressed nerve can predict the likelihood that the problem will disappear. If the studies reveal a normal nerve or one that's damaged but improving, the baby's face will fully recover in several weeks or, at the latest, several months. (See p. 335, **Ref. 13.**)

4. Eyes

SWOLLEN LIDS *(Edema)*

Most parents, when seeing their baby for the first time, are especially eager to get a look at her eyes. Unfortunately, they seldom get a very good look. In the first place, most babies keep their eyes closed most of the time. In the second, babies are very sensitive to light and promptly close their eyes when they're exposed to bright light. What parents see instead of eyes are the baby's swollen eyelids. The lids are swollen from the physical trauma of birth, especially when the face was the "presenting" part. This swelling may take weeks to subside, but rest assured, it will do so. And be forewarned: Any attempt to forcibly open the baby's eyes will be met by marked resistance from the baby. (See p. 335, **Ref. 11.**)

BLOOD SPOT ON WHITE OF EYE *(Subconjunctival Hemorrhage)*

As the baby is squeezed out of the birth canal, the blood vessels of the face distend with blood. If the pressure in the distended vessel exceeds the strength of the vessel, the wall will rupture and bleeding will occur. This commonly happens in the eye.

Forty percent of newborns have blood spots on the white of their eyes. If the bleeding is near the pigmented iris of the eye, the spot is crescent-shaped. If the bleeding is farther away from the iris, the spot can take any shape at all. Examinations with an ophthalmoscope reveal hemorrhages of this type in the back portion of the eyeball in 25 percent of all newborn babies.

These blood spots are absorbed in one to two weeks and are nothing to worry about. (See p. 335, **Ref. 11.**)

RED EYES WITH DISCHARGE *(Chemical Conjunctivitis)*

Many states require nursery personnel to drop a silver nitrate solution into the newborn's eyes to prevent a serious eye infection caused by gonococcus bacteria. This solution, however, is highly irritating and the irritation occurs even when the silver nitrate is promptly rinsed out of the eyes with sterile salt water.

Ninety percent of treated babies show red, swollen, discharging eyes within three to six hours after receiving the drops. Almost all babies will recover from this reaction within forty-eight hours. Often parents mistake the red irritation for bacterial infection, but such infections are rarely seen during the first day of life in otherwise healthy babies. If any doubt exists, appropriate laboratory tests can be done. Any discharge, especially a copious discharge developing two or three days after birth, requires medical attention.

Eye contact is sometimes considered important in the initial bonding process between parents and baby, and if this form of communication is important to you, you might request some family time with your baby before the drops are put into his eyes. You might still be unable to look him in the eye, since most babies keep their eyes closed, but you're sure to enjoy the skin contact. (See p. 335, **Ref. 11**; see p. 336, **Ref. 17**.)

PUPILS THAT RHYTHMICALLY OPEN AND CLOSE *(Hippus)*

The newborn's pupils, the black centers of the eyes, are frequently tiny, measuring only 2 millimeters in diameter. If they rhythmically open and close to admit light, the phenomenon is called hippus. It's of no concern and is just another example of an immature nervous system. (See p. 336, **Ref. 18**.)

WHITE OF EYE LOOKS BLUE *(Blue Sclera)*

The sclera is the firm, opaque, white coat of the eye. The layer directly beneath the sclera is the choroid, which has a rich blood supply and many pigment cells. Since the newborn's sclera is relatively thin, it allows the color of the choroid to show through and, as a result, most babies have slightly bluish sclera.

While we're on the subject of eye color, I might mention that most white infants have irises that are blue-gray, while most black infants have brown-gray irises. During the first year, all irises gradually darken, and the final eye color is usually reached by the first birthday. (See p. 335, **Ref. 11**; see p. 336, **Ref. 18**.)

WHITE SPOTS ON IRIS *(Brushfield Spots)*

Twenty percent of all babies have salt-and-pepper speckling around the outer third of the iris. These white spots are called Brushfield spots. They're most striking in children with Down's syndrome, 80 percent of whom show Brushfield spots in their eyes. If your baby has them, it does *not* mean he has Down's syndrome. This condition is simply one of many that are shared by entirely normal children and those with Down's syndrome. (See p. 336, **Ref. 19.**)

ABSENCE OF EMOTIONAL TEARS

An upset, crying baby doesn't produce tears before three weeks of age. This doesn't mean that she isn't genuinely unhappy; it's simply the result of an underdeveloped tear-production apparatus. By three months of age, most babies do produce tears when they cry.

Despite the absence of emotional tearing, babies can and do produce the necessary tears for the cleansing and moistening of the eyes. (See p. 336, **Ref. 18.**)

TEARS AND MUCUS DRAINING FROM EYE
(Blocked Nasolacrimal Duct)

Don't be surprised if one or both of your newborn's eyes look wetter than they should and, at times, moisture flows down her cheeks. This overflowing of newborn's tears is called epiphora (Greek for sudden burst) and is usually the result of a blockage of the tube that's supposed to carry the tears from the eye to the nose.

This tube, the nasolacrimal (*naso* means nose; *lacrimae* are tears) duct, like most internal tubes, spends part of its fetal life as a solid cord, then hollows out by the time of birth. In the case of the nasolacrimal duct, this process of hollowing out, called canalization, begins at the eye and progresses downward. Many newborns still have a delicate membrane at the nose end of the tube that separates it from the nasal cavity, and some have even more canalizing to do after they're born. These babies account for most of those born with epiphora. (The other common cause of a baby's persistent tearing is something such as an eyelash stuck in her eyelid.)

Obstructed nasolacrimal ducts usually open up on their own during the first few weeks of life. In the meantime, you can help the tears along by massaging the inner corner of the eye with a cotton ball soaked with warm water. This will also help to keep the baby's eye uninfected while you're waiting for the duct to finish canalizing. If the tearing persists, the accumulated tears may well become infected, which will thicken the tears and cause swelling of the duct. This condition must be treated, or the obstruction will worsen. If the nasolacrimal duct isn't open within a year, you can bet that it isn't going to open by itself, and an outpatient probing of the duct by an ophthalmologist will be needed. Chances are good, though, that your newborn's excess tearing is temporary and will cease in a few weeks. (See p. 336, **Ref. 29**; see p. 337, **Ref. 38**.)

FAKE CROSSED EYES *(Epicanthic Fold)*

The upper lids of newborns often have a fold of skin that runs toward the nose, then curves out and attaches to the lower lid. In so doing, it manages to cover a part of the sclera (white of the eye). This fold, in combination with the flat, wide nasal bridge of most newborns, creates the illusion that the eye is actually turned inward. If you pinch the baby's skin over the bridge of the nose, you will, by so doing, uncover the hidden white of the eye and dispel the illusion. Or, if the doctor shines a bright light from a distance, aiming at the middle of the bridge of the nose, the reflected light will be centered symmetrically in pupils of the baby's eyes, proving that they're lined up correctly.

Because this skin fold over the inside portion of the eye creates an illusion, that is, fake crossed eyes, it's often called pseudostrabismus or pseudosquint. It's one of the most common newborn diagnoses. When I see this situation, I tell parents, "Your baby's eyes are straight; it's the face that's crossed." It is particularly noticeable when looking at photographs of the baby. (See p. 335, **Ref. 11**; see p. 336, **Ref. 18**.)

TRUE CROSSED EYES *(Strabismus)*

Once the baby opens his eyes, you may find that they aren't well aligned. One or both may truly turn inward when the baby appears to be looking straight ahead. Less often, one or both may turn outward. This condition is called strabismus, from the Greek word meaning squint. While strabismus is common in the immediate newborn period, only 3 percent of children still have it by the time they reach three months old. Half of the babies with persistent strabismus have a family history of weak eye muscles, or a lazy eye.

If your one-month-old baby is crossing his eyes, and if there's no family history of strabismus, it would be wise to wait a few more months to see if the eyes straighten out on their own. It is also helpful to know that babies getting medicine for colic may have difficulty focusing and may appear cross-eyed. If there's a family history of crossed eyes, or if the baby is three months old and still showing unbalanced eye movements, an ophthalmologist should be consulted for a complete examination.

Nowadays, doctors perform surgery on babies who are six months old to obtain the best binocular vision for the child. Waiting until the child reaches school age, and hoping that the eyes will straighten out spontaneously, may cause a loss of vision in one of the eyes (the one that was unconsciously suppressed by the child as he tried to avoid double vision). In other words, if surgery is delayed until school age, the only gain will be cosmetic.

Most babies whose eyes appear to turn in have pseudostrabismus (see p. 67), and some babies with true strabismus straighten out by three months of age. Only those whose eyes aren't straight at three months need to be treated. Certainly by six months of age, it is imperative to seek the help of an ophthalmologist, or a pediatric ophthalmologist if available. (See p. 335, **Ref. 11**; see p. 336, **Ref. 20**.)

SWINGING EYES *(Nystagmus)*

Nystagmus is the term for the involuntary swinging back and forth of the eyes that occurs when the eyes are trying to fix on an object. The oscillations can be horizontal, vertical, or circular. There are several circumstances in which these jerky eye movements are normal:

If you watch a series of objects, such as cars in a passing railroad train, move across your field of vision, your eyes try to follow one of the objects for as long as it's comfortable to do so. When it's no longer possible to continue the gaze, the eyes jerk in the opposite direction rapidly, trying to locate the next item in the sequence. This type of slow tracking eye movement is called opticokinetic nystagmus and is entirely normal. If your doctor wants to be certain that your child has vision, he may test for the presence of opticokinetic nystagmus; this eye movement proves that your child can see.

When you're trying very hard to stay with an object that has moved to the limit of your peripheral vision, your eyes may jerk in the direction of the gaze. This is called end-position nystagmus and can happen to anyone, especially if he's tired.

The third type of normal nystagmus occurs when infants are rotated or swung in one direction. Babies' eyes jerk in the direction that they're being swung, and even after the swinging stops, infants under six months will have jerking eyes. This is called rotational nystagmus.

Nystagmus that occurs in situations other than those described above is abnormal and needs to be evaluated by a specialist. If it's seen at birth or shortly thereafter, it's considered congenital, and there's a variety in this group that runs in certain families. I include this condition in this book for one reason: It tends to lessen with age. I've seen several babies with congenital hereditary nystagmus outgrow the condition entirely. One can't assume that this will happen, or that there isn't a more serious reason for the eye movements, and therefore the baby with nystagmus that isn't rotational, opticokinetic, or end position must be examined by a specialist. (See p. 336, **Ref. 20;** see p. 336, **Ref. 29.**)

5. Nose

THICKNESS AT ROOT OF NOSE *(Prominent Procerus Muscle)*

The procerus muscle attaches the root of the nose to the lower forehead, and occupies the space between the eyebrows. When the baby scrunches her face, this muscle produces horizontal wrinkles at the root of the nose.

We believe that this muscle was once used to move the snout around for better sniffing, but since sniffing has become something of a lost art, the need for the procerus has shrunk. As the bridge of the baby's nose develops, the muscle, along with its very prominent vein, will become unnoticeable. (See p. 336, **Ref. 22.**)

PUG NOSE *(Hypoplastic Bridge)*

Babies always have pug noses. As they mature, the bridge of the nose develops, but until then, there's a flat space above the nostrils and between the eyes. As described in the section on fake crossed eyes (p. 67), this flat space on the nose helps to create an illusion of crossed eyes. Eventually, the nasal bones grow to a size that varies greatly from person to person.

Unfortunately, growth of the nasal bones continues through adulthood, even in those who never ever tell a lie.

DEFORMED NOSE

The three most common things that can happen to a baby's nose during delivery are: (1) It can be pushed to the side, (2) the septum can be twisted, or (3) the septum can be dislocated.

It's not at all rare for the newborn's nose to be pushed off to one side, and nothing needs to be done about that.

The septum, which is the partition that divides the nose into two sides, normally fits in a groove along the floor of the nose. About 17 percent of normal newborns have had their septa twisted out of shape, but not actually pushed out of the groove. Two percent of newborns have had their septa pushed out of the track.

Time will straighten out the pushed-to-the-side nose. The deformed but not dislocated septum requires a little manual repositioning. The dislocated septum can be relocated, but the procedure is more complicated and should be done by a specialist. (See p. 335, **Ref. 13.**)

6. Ears

FOLDING INWARD *(Positional Deformity)*

Everybody notices ears, and since minor variations from the "normal" are extremely common, you might like to learn about the normal ear.

The external ear, the auricle, projects from the side of the head at a slight angle, usually not more than 30 degrees. The rolled outer margin of the ear, the helix, is attached to the side of the face above the ear, and, after sweeping around its edge, ends at the earlobe. A second fold, the anthelix, parallels the helix and ends just above the earlobe, in a small protrusion of cartilage called the antitragus. The counterpart of the antitragus is the tragus, the cartilaginous protrusion just in front of the ear canal.

This elaborate ear structure begins its development in the sixth week of fetal life. It starts out as six tiny hillocks of tissue around the ear canal that grow and merge together. After 14 weeks of following a precise pattern, the fetal ear finally achieves the adult shape. When you consider the complexity of their formation, it's a small miracle that ears come out looking as good as they do.

During the last month of pregnancy, the ear becomes somewhat rigid and the folds begin to stand out more prominently, so that, in this sense, ear stiffness is a criterion of maturity.

The baby's ear is one third the length of the adult's, and by the age of six years, the child's ear is close to adult size.

Folding inward is simply a result of facial compression in a tightly packed womb. If your baby's ears are folded forward, they will soon unfold.

MISSING PARTS: PROTRUDING OR LOP EAR

Commonly, a part of the outer roll of the ear, the helix, appears to be absent and the ear looks as if someone ran an iron over it. This is especially common in premies and they tend to complete the helix as they mature. Likewise, babies whose ears were pressed against their heads by crowding will also improve with time.

If the anthelix (another fold paralleling the helix) is sparse, but not absent, the ear will protrude. Usually this trait runs in certain families. It helps you to recognize kin when you're approaching a crowd from behind.

If the anthelix is totally absent, the ear protrudes and has a smooth, cupped appearance called a lop ear. These two groups of ears, protruding and lop, don't improve with age. In rare muscle diseases, the ear-wiggling muscle is abnormally weak and the ear protrudes. The conscientious doctor will test the child's strength after seeing a protruding ear. If there's no weakness, if the ears are really outstanding, plastic surgery should be considered to spare the child any ridicule that may occur when he starts school.

Almost anything goes when it comes to minor variations of the normal ear. Earlobes can be totally absent, making wearing earrings a challenge, or they can be plastered against the side of the face instead of dangling. These traits also tend to run in families. (See p. 335, **Ref. 11.**)

EAR TAGS, DIMPLES, AND BUMPS *(Preauricular Tags and Sinuses)*

Remember the six tiny hillocks of tissue that developed into the outer ear, as described on page 71? Occasionally an extra hillock appears that has no role to play in the ear's formation. Such accessory hillocks end up as nubbins of skin, often with a core of cartilage, situated just in front of the tragus. If the rest of the ear looks entirely normal, nothing needs to be done. If the rest of the ear doesn't look quite right, then the tag represents one of the necessary hillocks that went awry and the attention of a specialist is needed.

Pits, sometimes called preauricular sinuses, are small skin folds that can also be seen in front of the ear, or even in the ear itself. These were once thought to represent leftovers from the gill slits present on every fetus up to the third month of pregnancy.

These pits are now believed to be sections of skin that were trapped during the fusion of the six hillocks that made up the outer ear. Ear pits seem to appear more often on the left side of the ear than on the right, and more in black infants than in white. They're twice as common in females as in males. Only one third of them occur on both sides of the head. Almost 1 person in 100 has an ear pit, and in some families half the offspring have them. Unless pits become infected, which is a possibility, they're of no importance.

A common, normal ear variant is the Darwinian tubercle, first described by Charles Darwin in 1871. It consists of a thick nodule along the back of the helix, near the top of the ear. It usually projects backward. Darwin thought it represented a vestige of the erect, pointed ear of our primitive past.

Another normal variation is the satyr tubercle, a nodule with a point projecting upward. Both Darwinian and satyr tubercles are traits found in certain families and not in others. None of these variants have any medical significance. (See p. 335, **Ref. 11**; see p. 336, **Ref. 19**; see p. 336, **Ref. 21**.)

7. Mouth

CYSTS ON PALATE *(Epstein's Pearls)*

At least 85 percent of all infants are born with small, round, smooth, yellow-white swellings on their gums or palates. Those on the gums are usually 2 to 3 millimeters in size and are called Bohn's pearls; those on the palate are twice as large and are called Epstein's pearls. When viewed under a microscope, both types of "pearls" consist of the same material that produces milia around the nose and chin (see p. 43), and it isn't surprising that all three of these conditions disappear at about the same time—by one to three months of age.

Those who imagine that only teeth belong on the gums may mistake Bohn's pearls for teeth, but if you feel the bumps carefully, you'll note that they aren't as hard or sharp as teeth.

Epstein's pearls can be mistaken for thrush, a common fungus infection of the mouth, but the white deposit of thrush is plastered against the mouth and can be removed. Epstein's pearls cannot. (See p. 335, **Ref. 5**.)

WHITE PATCHES IN MOUTH

Milk remaining in the mouth will curdle and stick to the baby's cheeks or tongue as a gray-white patch. It can be scraped off with ease, leaving behind a completely normal surface. If you're certain that the patch represents milk deposits, there's no need to do anything about it.

If you want to be sure the patch is not thrush, try to scrape it off. The chalky-white plaque of thrush is firmly stuck against the mouth, and when you finally manage to get some of it off, you'll see that the surface behind it is swollen and red, and bleeds easily. Thrush is a true infection and produces an inflamed response; milk deposits are just interior decorating.

SUCKING BLISTERS

People who work with their hands get blisters on their hands, and babies who work with their lips get blisters on their lips. Not all babies get them, but those who do, develop a single blister in the center of the upper lip. The blister may peel and re-form over and over again.

Sucking blisters are a very visible sign that the baby is an avid sucker (not that a nursing mother needs to be reminded). They're occasionally mistaken for the blister of herpes. Since babies with herpes have many blisters not confined to the upper lip, and aren't likely to be avid suckers, this worry should be easily retired.

PROTRUDING TONGUE

Many babies allow their mouths to open and their tongues to protrude, particularly when they're relaxed. Unless the baby's mouth is unusually small, or her tongue unusually big, a protruding tongue shouldn't cause concern. If you need to be certain, simply push the baby's tongue into her mouth and hold her lips closed. If the tongue fits, let the baby wear it.

The tongue of a baby with Down's syndrome sticks out of her mouth, but it can easily be distinguished from the tongue of a normal infant by its rhythmical in-and-out protrusion and retraction. Furthermore, the tongue usually doesn't fit very well in the baby's mouth. Most of the tongue-related worries I hear are really Down's syndrome worries. Your pediatrician will have no difficulty recognizing Down's syndrome and will be able to dispel such concerns quickly.

TONGUE-TIE *(Lingual Frenulum)*

A fold of varying thickness holds the undersurface of the tongue to the floor of the mouth. This fold, the frenulum, runs along the middle of the undersurface out to the tip of the tongue.

Once upon a time, midwives used a sharp fingernail to tear through this fold on all newborn children in the hope of preventing speech problems. Not so long ago, doctors, before leaving the delivery room, would pick up a pair of scissors and snip the fold for the very same reason.

Based on precise measurements, guidelines have been suggested to help us recognize which children need referral for this minor procedure. They are as follows:

1. If the tip of the tongue can't be raised to touch the upper gums
2. If the child can't move the protruded tongue from one corner of the mouth to the other

3. If the tip of the tongue notches when the tongue is protruded

4. If your child is unable to produce certain sounds that require tongue-to-tooth or tongue-to-gum contact, due to any of the above traits

In these cases, your physician may decide to snip the frenulum.

LOPSIDED MOUTH WHEN CRYING *(Hypoplastic Depressor Anguli Oris Muscle)*

Until very recently, asymmetry of facial movements in the newborn led the doctor to believe that some injury had occurred to the facial nerve. Forceps usually took the rap, but in unassisted deliveries, it was assumed that pressure against the mother's pelvic bones had "bruised" the nerve before birth.

During the past ten years, a relatively common, easily recognized minor abnormality has become associated with asymmetry of the face, especially when the baby is crying. We see this in babies who look fine until they start to cry. When these babies cry, one side of the mouth doesn't move downward and outward as well as the other. This is the result of the absence or underdevelopment of the muscle that's responsible for moving the corner of the mouth. In this situation, only this muscle, the depressor anguli oris muscle (DAOM), is weak; the other muscles in the face are entirely normal. Therefore, forehead wrinkling, eye closure, and so forth go on as usual. Even the mouth works well for all its other functions, such as feeding and smiling.

If your baby is showing this asymmetry when she cries, carefully feel the lower lip on the side that doesn't move. If you find that the lip thins out as it nears the corner of the mouth, the asymmetric crying is the result of an immature or absent muscle. If thinning isn't present and if the doctor isn't sure of the cause, he may have special electrical tests done on the facial nerve and the DAOM. As babies with asymmetrical crying mature, the problem lessens. Many doctors believe that older children avoid the movements that lead to very obvious asymmetry and that's why it appears that the condition has improved, but it's also very likely that other muscles "help out" the weak or absent DAOM.

Once the diagnosis is made, the doctor will do an extra-thorough examination of the baby's heart, since in these cases there's some chance of finding a congenital heart defect. This is particularly important if other minor abnormalities have been found, since the odds of finding a major abnormality increase with each additional minor one that's discovered. For this particular condition, right-sided weakness seems to carry a greater risk of an associated problem. (See p. 336, **Ref. 25**; see p. 336, **Ref. 30**.)

8. Neck

SHORT NECK

Babies' necks can look ridiculously short. Some babies can rest their chins on their chests without even trying, which makes you wonder if some parts are missing.

To determine whether or not your baby's neck is normal, all you have to do is see if it moves normally. Short necks that have some abnormality always have limited flexibility, whereas the normal newborn's neck can be turned 80 degrees to the right or left, can be bent 40 degrees toward either shoulder, and will allow the back of the head to be brought back until it touches the neck. If your baby's neck can do all that, it's normal; if it can't, X rays should be taken to see if all the vertebrae are formed normally.

Normal short necks present problems only for the physician. They make it something of a challenge to carefully examine all parts of the neck. (See p. 336, **Ref. 26**.)

TURNED OR TWISTED NECK *(Torticollis)*

Babies can be born with a wry neck for several reasons. At one time, the twist was thought to result from the sort of difficult delivery that involves a great deal of pulling and tugging on the neck. We now know that injury to the baby's neck is just as apt to occur before delivery as during it.

The injured part of the baby's neck is always the large muscle responsible for turning her head to the side, the sternocleidomastoid (SCM). Whether the SCM is injured by tearing or pressure, it heals by scarring, and as the scar contracts, the muscle shortens. As a result of this shortening, the baby's head can't turn toward the injured side or bend away from it. Her head is tilted toward the bad side and the chin is rotated toward the good side. She looks as if she were trying to face the sun coming over her shoulder.

If you feel the injured muscle right after birth, it will usually be tighter than the opposite one. Sometimes when the baby is about two weeks old, a walnut-sized swelling will appear in the middle of the injured SCM. This is scarred muscle and represents the healing phase of the injury. This swelling is commonly referred to as a tumor, but when a baby has torticollis, it isn't a worrisome growth and doesn't need to be biopsied.

Torticollis acquired while still in the womb is usually accompanied by one or more of the other features of crowding, such as oblique modeling of the head and face and distortion of the ears. Torticollis that results from trauma at delivery isn't accompanied by all these other features of being squeezed into too small a space.

The SCM "tumor" disappears in eight to ten weeks and, with gentle stretching and encouraging the baby to turn toward the affected side, most torticollis disappears by the time the baby is six months old. Releasing the tight muscle by surgical means generally isn't necessary, but if after several years stretching hasn't worked, you should consider surgery. (See p. 335, **Ref. 13**; see p. 336, **Ref. 26**.)

9. Chest

HOLLOW CHEST WALL *(Pectus Excavatum)*

Many babies, especially those prematurely born, have chests that seem perfectly normal until they take a deep breath. When such an infant breathes in, the middle of the chest is sucked inward, creating a hollow in the breastbone. When she exhales, the chest loses the temporary hollow. This happens because the newborn's chest is very pliable, and when the suction of the chest cavity during deep breathing is great, the chest wall is pulled inward. As the baby ages, the chest cage stiffens and this hollow no longer appears.

MOVABLE BREASTBONE *(Xiphoid Process)*

The breastbone (or sternum) extends down from the base of the neck to the top of the abdominal wall. The piece of bone that lies in the upper abdominal wall is called the xiphoid process. It's thinner than the main part of the breastbone, and you can feel a depression if you run your finger down the breastbone. (This depression is commonly known as the "pit" of the stomach.) The xiphoid process is shaped like the end of a spear with the sharp end pointing downward. It's loosely hinged to the main part of the sternum and moves up and down easily.

Whenever the abdomen is full, the xiphoid—which sits on the abdominal wall—is pushed forward. This causes the free lower end of the xiphoid to stick out from the upper abdomen. Sometimes a baby's xiphoid is so movable that the physician can hold it between his thumb and forefinger and shift it back and forth. One baby of my acquaintance made a popping sound, like a champagne bottle cork, whenever he took a deep breath. Sure enough, I was able to pop his cork by grabbing the bottom of his xiphoid and letting it snap back. His mother was relieved to learn that her charming son wasn't extraterrestrial, and that the process was quite normal and down to earth. (See p. 336, **Ref. 22.**)

ASYMMETRIC CHEST WALL

Some degree of asymmetry of the chest is extremely common. There may be seven ribs reaching the breastbone on one side and eight on the other side. The lower ribs may flare out on one side and be perfectly flat on the other. There's no importance to minor asymmetry. Nobody's perfect.

BREASTS

Too Many Nipples (*Polythelia*)

Sit down for this one. Between 1 and 5 percent of us are born with an extra breast. Usually, this extra breast is represented by nothing more than a nipple. It's generally quite small and is mistaken for a mole. Actually, this extra breast is a leftover from the embryo days when a line of nipples ran from each armpit down to the upper thigh. All mammal embryos have this line of nipples. By the time they're born, the unnecessary ones have disappeared and each species ends up with its own appropriate number of breasts. What Mother Nature forgets to erase, remains. About 60 to 65 percent of individuals with poly- (many) thelia (nipples) have one extra. Thirty to 35 percent have a spare pair, and less than 5 percent have more than two extra nipples. In all but 5 percent, the extra nipple is located just below one of the normal ones.

A baby's extra nipple is easy to recognize. It's a light brown, flat, round, dime-sized spot, and if you gently pinch the skin around it, a dimple or horizontal crease will appear in its center.

Don't expect this spare nipple to go away. It will stay forever, but it won't grow larger unless glandular breast tissue is present as well. It should be viewed as a minor abnormality, one of many that commonly occur, and in itself has no medical or cosmetic significance. A single minor abnormality such as polythelia is generally found in 14 percent of all newborn babies and doesn't increase the baby's chances of having an important abnormality. But if the doctor finds two minor abnormalities, as occurs in 0.8 percent of babies, the baby's chances of having a major problem are five times greater than the general group of newborns. Only 0.5 percent of babies have three or more minor abnormalities, but 90 percent of them have one or more major defects as well.

This is the only importance of these trivial defects in development. They serve as an indicator that something else might have gone wrong— the more minor abnormalities a baby has, the greater the likelihood that the doctor will find some problem of significance. Remember, though, the presence of just one minor abnormality does absolutely nothing to increase the odds. (See p. 336, **Ref. 27**; see p. 336, **Ref. 31**; see p. 336, **Ref. 32**.)

Swollen Breasts *(Engorgement)*

The great majority of babies, boys and girls alike, are born with breast tissue. It appears before the baby is born, after the 13th week of the pregnancy, and it gradually enlarges, reaching a diameter of about 8 millimeters by the time the baby is 37 to 40 weeks old.

These baby breasts actually work. They produce real milk, and by the fifth day of life, milk can be expressed from their breasts. Take my word for it on this one. Don't squeeze the breast yourself. Expressing milk from your baby's breasts will only serve to stimulate the production of more of it and the manipulation might cause an infection, so I'm sure your baby would appreciate it if you didn't do it.

We used to believe that the mother's hormones were totally responsible for stimulating the baby's breasts, but we now know that the infant's own hormones are involved as well. Almost half of all premies, born without breast tissue, develop breasts during the first nine weeks of life. Premies' breasts don't grow as large as the full-termers', but it's clear that the breasts are developing without the help of their mother's hormones.

Contrary to popular belief, babies' swollen breasts don't disappear right after birth. After their initial engorgement during the first few weeks, they decrease in size until they reach about 10 millimeters in diameter. They remain at that size for four to six months, then begin to fade away during the second half of the first year. The breasts remain for a longer time on girls than on boys.

You may notice a firm white plug filling the tip of the baby's nipple. It consists of a tough, horny tissue called keratin, and will fall out one day without any help.

NEWBORN HEART MURMURS

Have you ever listened to the sound produced when you suddenly open and then close a faucet? This happens 100 times a minute in the heart and it, too, produces noise. Normally, the noise consists of two sounds that can be heard only with a stethoscope. The first is produced by the normal closing of the valves between the chambers of the heart, and the second by the closure of the valves where the blood flows out of the heart. Doctors generally refer to the two valve-closure sounds as basic heart sounds.

Rapidly flowing streams also make noise in and of themselves. Brooks babble, waves crash, electricity hums, and wind howls. Put your ear to a water pipe when the faucets are wide open and listen to the water flow. Better still, put your ear to a garden hose when the water is going full blast and hear the buzz.

Like the water pipe, the heart produces flow and the flow produces sound. Sounds in the heart that are produced by flow are called murmurs. Most flow is normal and, therefore, most murmurs are normal. Murmurs resulting from normal flow are called innocent murmurs. When the flow is abnormal, the sounds produced represent disease and are called organic murmurs.

The newborn heart produces these same normal sounds with a few variations. To understand why the newborn heart sounds different from that of an adult, you need to know how a mature heart functions.

The heart is a fist-sized organ situated slightly to the left of the chest's midline. Its function is to pump blood through two separate but contiguous routes, one to the lungs and the other to the rest of the body. In order to keep these two routes separate, the heart is divided into two halves by a vertical wall, called the septum. Each half of the heart is horizontally divided in half, creating an upper chamber, the atrium, and a lower chamber, the ventricle, making four chambers in all—two atria and two ventricles.

Blood enters the right atrium after completing its delivery of oxygen to the body. This dark, used blood is emptied into the right ventricle to be pumped through the pulmonary arteries (that is, arteries that lead to the lungs). While the dark, used blood flows through the lungs, it unloads its carbon dioxide and picks up a fresh supply of oxygen to become bright red once again. This red, rejuvenated blood returns through the pulmonary veins to the left atrium of the heart. From the left atrium it empties into the left ventricle, and from there it's pumped out via the great artery, the aorta, to nourish the body. For efficiency's sake, the heart is equipped with strategically positioned valves designed to open to allow forward flow, and shut to prevent backward flow. The valves ensure that all of the blood leaving the left ventricle, for example, heads out of the aorta, instead of paying another visit to the left atrium.

This is the circulation pattern that your baby's heart is aiming for. In the beginning, however, his little heart has some brand-new routes to learn. Here's why:

Because the unborn infant doesn't breathe, there's no need for his blood to circulate through his lungs. Actually, the fetal lungs are completely collapsed and it would take a great deal of pressure to force blood through the collapsed pulmonary circulation. Because the lungs aren't in use before birth, fetal circulation goes on by means of shortcuts that route the blood to the left, "systemic" side of the circulation.

The first fetal shortcut, or shunt, as we call it, runs between the two atria. Some of the blood that has arrived in the right atrium flows directly across to the left atrium through a special, temporary opening in the septum. The rest of the blood flows from the right atrium directly downward into the right ventricle, and from there, out the main pulmonary artery. But instead of going to the lungs, which aren't yet in use, the blood is shunted via a short channel into the aorta. This second shunt, the ductus arteriosus, exists for this diversion only, and self-destructs once it's no longer needed.

At the moment of birth, however, the ductus arteriosus is wide open and functioning as a shunt.

Now comes the action: newborn murmur number one. As soon as the baby takes his first breath and starts using his lungs, he no longer needs the shunt. In fact, the ductus arteriosus becomes a liability, since it prevents some of the used blood from reaching the lungs to be rejuvenated. Mother Nature to the rescue! In response to the now improving oxygenation, the body sends a chemical message to the ductus arteriosus to get lost. (It's the old story: What have you done for me lately?) The obsolete ductus begins to thicken its muscular wall and obliterate its channel.

While this old friend of the fetus is self-destructing, however, blood continues to flow through its ever narrowing opening. The narrower the opening, the more rapid the stream and the more noise it produces. In this way, a desirable change takes place in the baby and the audible proof of this is the special sound of the newborn murmur.

The process itself occurs in all normal newborns, but not every newborn will produce the musical accompaniment. Depending on the number of examinations, the noise level, and the level of the baby's activity, as many as one third of normal newborns will produce a murmur generated by the ductus arteriosus. It can be heard immediately after birth and can persist for several hours, several days, or more.

Of course, since the stimulus for closure of the ductus comes from the functioning of the newborn's lungs, the ductus may stay open for an abnormally long time if there's a problem with the baby's lungs. This is particularly apt to occur with premies who have respiratory difficulties.

Newborn murmur number two, which is heard in the hearts of as many as 55 percent of normal newborns, is also one of the most frequently heard innocent murmurs of later childhood. It's usually first heard during the first few days of life, but because it also occurs in older children, it's described in detail on p. 187 (pulmonary ejection murmur).

The third common newborn murmur results from the structure of the pulmonary artery in early infancy. At birth, and for several weeks after, the main pulmonary artery, as it exits from the right ventricle, is disproportionately wider than its two branches, the right and left pulmonary arteries. Furthermore, the two branches veer off at very sharp angles from the main trunk. As a result of these structural conditions, a great deal of turbulence is created as the blood flows from the main pulmonary artery to its two branches. This turbulence sets up vibrations along the arteries going to the lungs, which can be heard as a murmur all over the baby's back.

This third murmur is called physiologic (healthy) peripheral (away from the center) pulmonic stenosis (narrowing). It's short-lived. As the right and left lungs develop, the branch arteries that lead to them widen. The arteries also widen their angle of departure from the main trunk. The turbulence decreases, and usually by three months of age this murmur can no longer be heard.

The fourth innocent murmur—the ventricular septal defect (VSD)— represents a striking example of an abnormal situation correcting itself and becoming normal. This is the murmur produced by blood flow through a defect, that is, a "hole" in the wall dividing the ventricles.

The VSD is purely and simply abnormal. Fewer than 5 percent of babies are born with it and, in rare cases, it does create problems. Most often, however, these holes, which are sometimes large enough to strain a baby's heart, close up completely. Not by the hand of a surgeon. They do it entirely on their own.

We don't know exactly how often large VSDs close spontaneously, but we do know about the small VSD. By closely following babies with small VSDs, we've found that 65 percent of the holes situated in the thick muscular part of the septum spontaneously close. In the less common situation, where the defect occurs in the thin, membranous, upper part of the septum, only 25 percent close on their own. The overall spontaneous closure rate, which includes those babies whose defect position couldn't be determined, is 58 percent.

The proportion of closures may, in fact, be even greater than 58 percent. We very seldom find small VSDs in adults, so it's a fair guess that virtually all of them eventually close. We know, too, that even defects in the membranous part of the septum have better than one-in-four odds of closing on their own. (See p. 336, **Ref. 33**; see p. 337, **Ref. 34**; see p. 337, **Ref. 35**; see p. 337, **Ref. 36**; see p. 337, **Ref. 37**.)

10. Abdomen

BIG AND WIDE

Most babies have such round bellies that they look like overfed bull-frogs. In part, these big bellies are caused by their distended stomachs after they're filled with milk and air. The stomach, being on the left side, may give the belly a lopsided look.

Furthermore, babies have relatively large internal organs, such as the liver, that push out against the abdominal wall. Since the new-born's abdominal muscles are weak, they offer little resistance, and as a result, gravity determines the shape that the abdomen assumes. When the baby lies on his back, everything flows to the flanks and widens the shape. When the baby is upright, what's inside falls forward and gives the baby a beer belly.

Remember that the baby's torso is much larger proportionally than that of the older child. The trunk of the older child constitutes 67 percent of his body mass; for the newborn, it's 75 percent. (See p. 337, **Ref. 38.**)

HEALING NAVEL *(Umbilical Stump)*

After the umbilical cord is clamped and cut, the small length that remains begins to shrivel up and dry out. Skin bacteria aid in this process, and bacterial colonization of the umbilical stump is a basic part of the process. This healing can cause a mildly unpleasant odor that's pretty much par for the course. Unless there are signs of infection, such as redness, hardness, listlessness, and so on, the cord's odor alone is no cause for concern.

Nursery personnel routinely apply some form of antiseptic to the cord, which slows down the bacterial colonization. This isn't a bad idea since the best of hospital nurseries are likely to be home to certain bacteria that you wouldn't choose as colonists for your baby's belly button. Since bacterial colonization is slowed, so is the cord's separation. The more potent the antiseptic, the more delayed the separation.

Most cords separate during the second week of life. It's distinctly unusual for the cord to remain attached after four weeks. In some of these unusual situations, defects in the babies' immune systems have been found.

Don't blame the doctor for the way the navel looks after the cord separates. Remember, all the doctor did was to cut the cord; the way the stump separates is strictly between the baby and his stump. (See p. 337, **Ref. 39.**)

OOZING NAVEL *(Umbilical Granuloma)*

Navels ooze for a variety of reasons, but the most common one is the umbilical granuloma: a slowly growing pink mound of tissue rising from the center of the navel and producing a clear watery discharge. You may not see the pink mound until it grows out of the depression of the navel, but you'll see the discharge long before that.

Umbilical granulomas used to be treated with table salt and alcohol, but nowadays one or two applications of silver nitrate do the job. The silver reacts with the protein in the granuloma to form a scab that soon falls off. The fluid that oozes out as the silver nitrate is applied also contains silver, and it may leave a brown stain around the navel or on the doctor's thumb. Both will slowly fade away. The doctor shouldn't complain and neither should you.

If the navel ooze refuses to stop oozing, especially after two silver nitrate applications, other causes of this umbilical weeping should be considered. In rare instances, remnants of the primitive intestine or primitive bladder remain in the navel, and if they're present surgery is the only way to stop the oozing. (See p. 337, **Ref. 40.**)

UMBILICAL HERNIA

For a time very early in the pregnancy, your baby's intestines were so large they couldn't fit inside his abdomen. Where did they go? They went out for a while—through the opening of the navel. There they stayed until the abdominal cavity grew large enough to accommodate their entire length. When the intestines returned, their portal of exit from the abdomen, called the umbilical ring, was sealed by the merging of the midline abdominal muscles. If these muscles failed to meet, the ring remained open, and the contents of the abdomen were free to protrude. This protrusion is an umbilical hernia, a balloonlike painless swelling of the navel.

Slightly less than one fifth of all white newborns have umbilical hernias, as do slightly more than two fifths of black newborns. We also see them more often in prematures and in babies with extra-wide umbilical cords.

If the defect is small, say the size of your fingertip, it may only show up when the baby cries or strains, since both increase the pressure inside the abdomen. Since crying is so often followed by the belly button's bulging, some parents conclude that the hernia will disappear if they diligently respond to every whimper and prevent the baby from building up to a howl. Unfortunately, what they get instead is a spoiled baby with a hernia.

Large umbilical openings allow the intestines to protrude without effort, and when the baby stands up, a short, trunklike section may emerge through the defect. Often the baby will spend long periods pondering this appendage, wondering what pleasurable purpose it has.

As the baby gets older, the defect gradually closes. Most are closed within two years; 85 percent close by six years of age. Larger openings take more time to close than smaller ones, and a very small number never close. Since most umbilical hernias are harmless and heading for spontaneous closure, there's no need to rush the baby to the operating room. Nor is there any need to put tape across the navel, a binder around the abdomen, or tape or a coin over the hernia. The adhesive of the tape and the metal of the coin can easily irritate the skin. Since it's virtually impossible to securely bind the baby's midsection without compressing the lower rib cage in the back, belly binders can permanently deform the lower rib cage. All this for a condition that's trying its best to go away!

When must you repair umbilical hernias? Certainly when the loop of intestine that pokes out gets stuck and can't get back inside. Getting stuck is called incarceration, and if it injures the bowel, it's called strangulation. These conditions occur in only 2 to 5 percent of children with umbilical hernias, but once they happen, it's time to fix the hernia. There's little controversy on this point, but there are many opinions about when it's best to close the hernia that isn't causing trouble.

One approach to the question of when to take action on a trouble-free hernia is to base the decision on the size of the defect. This school of thought holds that umbilical hernias greater than 1.5 centimeters in diameter should be closed surgically in girls when they reach two years and boys when they reach four.

I don't favor this approach for several reasons. In the first place, umbilical hernias smaller than 1.5 centimeters are as likely to lead to incarceration as larger ones; and second, adults incarcerate their umbilical hernias at a rate 14 times greater than children. Therefore, it seems logical to leave the trouble-free umbilical hernia of any size alone during childhood. It almost invariably disappears on its own. (See p. 336, **Ref. 31**; see p. 337, **Ref. 41**; see p. 345, **Ref. 200**.)

11. Genitalia

LARGER GENITALS THAN EXPECTED

Many babies arrive with disproportionately large genitals. To a great extent, their genitalia are simply swollen from the trauma of birth, especially if the baby is delivered bottom (breech) first. Since both the girl's labia and the boy's scrotum consist of "loose," stretchable tissues, they're particularly likely to accumulate tissue fluid and swell up. This swelling rarely lasts more than one week.

In some cases, the labia actually grow larger because they were stimulated by hormones (primarily estrogen) that the mother produced to stimulate her own reproductive organs during pregnancy. Soon after the baby is born, and thus removed from the estrogen-rich environment, the estrogen effect wears off and the labia regress to normal size.

The estrogen-rich environment of the womb can also produce a temporary "feminization" of both little boys (breast enlargement) and little girls (breast and labial enlargement). These effects are completely normal and should be easy to live with for the short time that they last. On the other hand, you should never allow "masculinization" of either boys or girls to be accepted as normal or temporary. Enlargement of the clitoris or penis in the newborn is never normal, and if these conditions are present, prompt and expert attention is required.

PHYSIOLOGIC VAGINAL DISCHARGE

Most baby girls, especially full-termers, produce a white vaginal discharge at birth. This discharge is mucous, has no odor, and lasts for a week to ten days. It results from the estrogen-stimulated mucous glands that line the baby's cervix. As the estrogen level goes down, the glands gradually stop producing and the mucus either disappears completely or is gradually replaced by a pink to blood-red discharge.

Your baby girl's pink discharge represents the effect of estrogen withdrawal on her own uterus. Before birth, Mother's own estrogen thickens the lining of the fetal uterus. Afterward, when the baby is no longer drawing estrogen from Mother, her own uterine lining sloughs away, just like that of grown-ups who take birth control pills. As a result of this cutoff, your baby girl may have a three- to five-day "menstrual period."

As you're cleaning up your newborn daughter, think of the bright side of this discharge. She's demonstrating, in no uncertain terms, that she has a reproductive tract capable of responding to hormonal stimulation, and that the flow of its secretions isn't obstructed. In essence, this short period is a sneak preview of what your child can do once she starts producing her own hormones.

HYMEN PROTUBERANCES AND BANDS

Your baby girl's hymen participates very actively in the estrogen stimulation of her external genitalia. The borders of her hymen may well protrude through the opening of her vagina, and they may even be so prominent that you could mistake them for the labia minora.

Between 5 and 10 percent of baby girls have a hymenal tag, a slender, elongated stalk that projects from the inside border of the hymen. The length of these tags varies from the barely visible to 3 or 4 centimeters. Sometimes, a baby may have several tags. Most of them have tapered ends, and some end with a small yellow cyst. As the estrogen effect wanes, the tag shrinks away, disappearing entirely within a few weeks. If you can't wait the few weeks and are tempted to have it snipped off, my advice is to spare the blade and let nature do her own remodeling.

Hymen bands are less common than tags and, as far as we know, aren't the result of estrogen stimulation. The hymen band is a strand of tissue that crosses the opening of the hymen from one side to the other, dividing it into two parts. It's rarely mentioned in the abundant descriptions of the hymen found in fictional and nonfictional literature, and we see it in only 2 to 3 percent of baby girls. The band causes no problem for the baby, and thoughts of removing it should be deferred until adulthood, when it might conceivably interfere with sexual intercourse. (See p. 337, **Ref. 42.**)

NO APPARENT HYMEN OPENING

What happens if your baby's hymen has no opening? Where does all that mucus go?

Nowhere. It stays inside, filling and stretching the vagina, cervix, and uterus. The distended organs create a huge swelling in the baby's belly, and the straining, imperforate hymen becomes a visible bulge that protrudes through the widened vaginal opening. The doctor generally recognizes this scenario very quickly and promptly opens the hymen, and the baby lives happily ever after.

A more difficult question arises when the baby's hymen appears to have no opening, yet she shows no vaginal bulge or abdominal swelling. Where is the mucus going in this case?

This common situation can occur when either of two factors is present: first, if the amount of cervical mucus is too small to create a problem, and second, if the baby actually does have openings in her hymen, but they're pinpoint perforations too small to be seen. In either case, the baby stands a better than even chance of having a visible opening appear in her hymen before too long. If she doesn't, and if she begins to develop a bulge or a swollen belly, her hymen can be opened surgically at that time. Nothing has been lost by waiting. (See p. 337, **Ref. 43**; see p. 337, **Ref. 44.**)

CIRCUMCISION

There's no *medical* reason for circumcision, but if you decide to have your son circumcised, get ready to deal with the healing foreskin. Infections in this area are very rare, but freshly circumcised penises often look as if they were infected.

The circumcised penis appears ominous because, in the first place, the foreskin consists of "loose" tissue and can, therefore, swell massively whenever traumatized. Secondly, the healing skin is exposed to wet diaper irritation repeatedly. As a result, the cut edge heals slowly and often develops a soft, spongy puffiness around the wound, as well as a heavy, soggy, yellow-gray scab at the healing point. When the loose scab is dislodged by diaper changes, the healing tissues may ooze a thin, bloody fluid. All this is normal healing of a circumcision.

An abnormally healing circumcision is quite different. For starters, infected wounds are red, warm, hard, and painful, and the discharge is foul, yellow-green, and creamy. Fortunately, this is rare. What isn't rare is the suspicion of infection, since the freshly circumcised penis can look awful even when it's doing fine.

UNCIRCUMCISED FORESKIN *(Physiologic Phimosis)*

Practically all mothers of circumcised babies are given detailed instructions on the care of the penis. Practically all mothers of uncircumcised babies are given practically no instructions on the care of the baby's foreskin. To fill this void in doctor-patient communication, I'll tell you everything that you have to do. Don't do a blessed thing. Once it has been determined that the urinary opening on the head of your baby boy's penis, the meatus, is in the correct location, the foreskin should be left alone. You'll probably find that your newborn's foreskin is tightly plastered to the head of his penis. Only 6 percent of baby boys have foreskins that can be retracted from the head of the penis, called the glans. This foreskin covering your baby boy's glans is a good protection. Irritations of the urinary opening occur in an estimated 8 to 31 percent of circumcised boys, and virtually never in boys with intact foreskins.

In the past, doctors have maintained that circumcision makes hygienic care easier. This is certainly true. What's questionable is whether or not the baby gains anything by early hygienic care. (In my opinion, if there's no ritualistic or symbolic reason to uncover the glans, why do it?)

Is there any reason not to retract the baby's foreskin? Yes, indeed. Besides hurting your baby, you can produce dense scar tissue between the foreskin and the head that won't spontaneously loosen later on. The natural connection between the foreskin and the head loosens by itself. Baby boys start out in this world with tight foreskins, but only 8 percent of boys 6 to 7 years old, and only 1 percent of boys at 14, have foreskins that are too tight to be easily pulled back behind the head of the penis. The tightness of the newborn's foreskin is a natural condition and it loosens without any help from us. Which proves once again that nature is wonderful, especially when we don't look for ways to botch things up. (See p. 337, **Ref. 45;** see p. 337, **Ref. 56.**)

BLUE TIP OF PENIS

The head of the penis, or glans, consists of a very thin layer of skin covering a rich collection of veins that is, in turn, supported by a meshwork of spongy tissue. Since dark red blood in veins appears blue when seen through skin, the glans can also appear blue. The amount of blood and the thickness of the skin determine the depth of the blue color.

Do you suppose that this is why blue is the traditional color for boys? (See p. 336, **Ref. 22.**)

MONK'S HOOD FORESKIN *(Glandular Hypospadias)*

In the best of all possible worlds, the urinary opening (the meatus) is centered exactly at the tip of the penis's head (the glans). If the meatus doesn't make it to the bull's-eye, the condition is called hypospadias. Hypospadias tends to run in certain families, usually affecting the males to the same degree. In such families, some mothers identify their sons' penises with their husbands' and, mistakenly regarding both as normal, fail to get the necessary medical attention.

Hypospadias is very easy to recognize at birth, since even in mild conditions the foreskin looks abnormal—heaped up on top of the glans and too short on the bottom. This piling creates a "monk's hood" appearance and signals the presence of the hypospadias.

The most common type of hypospadias is the mildest form, called glandular, or first degree. In this situation, the opening is on the glans but displaced downward toward the underside. Since openings that are abnormally situated are often abnormally small as well, the doctor will check to see if the stream of urine is normal. If the urine flows properly, nothing need be done for the meatus. (A circumcision can still be performed, if you want it.) If the opening is abnormal, the opening can be made normal-sized by a urologist without too much trouble. This is a less common condition, but should be looked for.

There's some difference of opinion about the need to check the kidneys of boys with mild hypospadias. The odds of finding kidney malformations, such as a loss of kidney substance, are fairly low in this group, but they're still twice that of the general population. Since the stakes are so high, your doctor will probably decide that it's worthwhile to see if the kidneys are in jeopardy. Kidney malformations can be accurately diagnosed by ultrasonography without exposing the child to the radiation of the kidney X ray. If there's still doubt, a kidney X ray can be done. (See p. 337, **Ref. 46;** see p. 337, **Ref. 47.**)

SECRETIONS ENTRAPPED IN FORESKIN
(Smegma)

The cells on the outermost layer of skin are constantly shedding, a process called desquamation. When the surface of the head of the penis, the glans, desquamates, its skin cells can get trapped under the foreskin. The foreskin's own secretions then combine with the debris from the desquamated cells and produce a yellow-white, waxy, cheesy material called smegma.

If the inner layer of the foreskin is plastered against the outer layer of the glans, the smegma will be imprisoned. If the layer of foreskin covering the trapped smegma is thin, the cheesy material will be readily visible. If the layer of the foreskin is thick, only a lumpy outline of the hidden smegma will be visible. Your doctor can easily pull back the foreskin and remove the smegma, if he has a mind to. He can also leave it alone.

SOFT SCROTAL SWELLING *(Hydrocele)*

Testicles begin in the belly and end up in the scrotum. A brief discussion of their itinerary will help you understand how things can go wrong in the scrotum.

The testicle starts out resting against the rear wall of the abdomen, immediately behind the abdominal cavity's lining, the peritoneum. In time, the testicle, along with a small piece of the peritoneal lining, travels out of the abdominal wilderness by means of a band of contracting tissue, the gubernaculum. The gubernaculum pulls the testicle down and drags along with it the piece of peritoneum, creating a long tube, like a finger of a rubber glove, with its upper end opening into the abdominal cavity. Under ideal circumstances, the testicle reaches the bottom of the scrotum and the tube separates from the abdominal cavity. The upper part of the tube then dissolves, leaving at the bottom only a small piece that stays permanently wrapped around the testicle as a "protective water jacket." If all this goes smoothly, your baby boy arrives after a 40-week pregnancy with a bag containing two testicles, each wrapped with a small sack of peritoneal tissue, but none of the longer peritoneal tube.

Occasionally, however, the tube doesn't break off or dissolve. In this case, your baby may get either a hernia or a hydrocele. A hernia is the protrusion of a piece of fat or intestine from its peritoneal cavity through a defect (the open tube) in the wall of its cavity. A hydrocele is a collection of excess fluid accumulating in the "water jacket" around the testicle.

If the upper end of the tube doesn't break off from the abdominal cavity, what you have, in essence, is a continuation of the peritoneal lining out of the abdomen. This tissue then becomes an escape route for runaway abdominal organs. The escape route is referred to as the hernia sac, and the runaway, as the actual hernia of fat or intestine. In the groin, it is called an inguinal hernia.

Your physician will surgically correct this type of hernia as soon as she recognizes it. (Time doesn't work for the baby here the way it does in cases of umbilical hernia.)

If the upper end of the tube closes off while the lower end contains peritoneal fluid, the fluid gets trapped. When this happens, the baby is born with a round, fluid-filled sac in his scrotum that can range from the size of a marble, in which case it can be mistaken for the normal testicle, to that of a large egg, in which case Father may boast of his son's "virility." Alas for Dad, the hydrocele is only a water-filled sac. It may feel soft or tense, depending on the amount of fluid. Sometimes it has a slightly bluish color. It's called a physiologic hydrocele since it came about under the healthiest of circumstances. During the ensuing months, the lower part of the loop absorbs the fluid and self-destructs, and that's the end of the hydrocele.

Sometimes, too, the loop closes incompletely, so that fluid collects and gets trapped at various locations. If the fluid collects along the pathway of the spermatic cord, it's called a hydrocele of the cord. If it collects in a certain area of a baby girl's groin, known as the canal of Nuck, it is called a hydrocele of the canal of Nuck.

Physiologic hydroceles, as well as those of the cord and canal of Nuck, usually disappear by three months of age. Hydroceles that are still present at one year, and those that continue to grow, always have hernias associated with them and your doctor will treat them exactly like hernias. (See p. 337, **Ref. 40**).

UNDESCENDED TESTICLE *(Cryptorchidism)*

Fetal testicles usually descend from the abdomen by the 35th to 36th week of the pregnancy while the baby is still in the uterus. By the 40th week, they reach the bottom of the scrotum. A testicle is considered undescended, or cryptorchid, if its descent has been arrested along its usual route to the scrotum.

Doctors can feel about 85 percent of all undescended testicles in the groin, but they can't coax them into the scrotum. Another 10 percent of undescended testicles are still in the abdomen and can't be felt at all. Approximately 3 to 5 percent of hiding testicles are permanently missing in action, and probably were absent from the start.

Since testicles descend in the later weeks of pregnancy, a high percentage of infants born earlier than the 35th week have cryptorchidism. The incidence of undescended testicles in all premies is 30 percent. Not more than 2 to 4 percent of full-termers are cryptorchid.

What happens to the undescended testicle if it's left alone?

Most will descend by the age of three months. About one "high ball" in five will still be undescended by the infant's first birthday. From then on, spontaneous descent won't occur, so your doctor will take steps toward getting the testicle where it belongs. He'll choose not to allow a cryptorchid testicle to remain high in its perch for the following reasons:

In the first place, it doesn't look exactly right to have only one testicle in the scrotum, and at certain times in a young man's life, nothing matters unless he looks right in the locker room. Secondly, the undescended testicle can be damaged by the higher temperature of the abdomen and may be less fertile than its brother to the south. The undescended testicle is also at greater risk of being injured, getting twisted up, or developing cancer.

Do boys with cryptorchidism, like those with hypospadias (see p. 94), need to have their kidneys examined? No. Their risk of having a significant kidney malformation is no greater than that of the general population. (See p. 337, **Ref. 48**; see p. 337, **Ref. 49**; see p. 337, **Ref. 50**; see p. 337, **Ref. 51**.)

12. Bones and Joints

HIP APPEARS DISLOCATED *(Newborn Hip)*

The hip joint is a simple ball-in-socket arrangement, the ball being the end of the thighbone, and the socket being the cup-shaped part of the pelvis. Under normal circumstances, the ball is held firmly in place by ligaments and the fit is snug. If the ball is out of the socket, the hip is said to be dislocated; if the fit is not snug enough, the hip is said to be dislocatable.

It's extremely important to recognize either condition as early as possible since destructive and often irreversible changes in the hip joint can occur if the thighbone is out of its socket when the baby starts to walk and bear her weight. For this reason, your physician will examine your child's hips very carefully, looking for the subtlest signs of abnormality. He'll compare the baby's thigh creases and relative leg lengths, and he'll test the stability and range of motion of the hip joint. If he still isn't sure whether or not your baby's hip is out, he may want to get X rays.

Now here's the good news. Many of the time-honored signs of dislocation are now known to occur in children whose hips are completely normal.

For example, unmatched folds and creases in the thighs and buttocks used to be thought of as a sign that one of the thighs was out of joint. We've now learned that only half of all children under one year of age have symmetrical thigh creases; the other half have uneven creases or an extra crease. These uneven folds are probably just the result of the position of the baby in the womb. (Anything crowded into that small space would get a little wrinkled.)

Another "sign" that no longer automatically flags a hip dislocation is the apparent shortening of one of the thighs. You would certainly expect one thigh to appear shorter than the other if the hip was out of its socket. When the hip dislocates, the thigh gets pulled upward, which is why doctors look carefully at the height of the bent knees when the baby is lying flat and the hips are flexed. The knees should be exactly at the same height if the thighs are of equal length. We now know, however, that a thigh that appears shorter isn't automatically a sign of a dislocated hip. Surprisingly, the length discrepancies can disappear entirely the next time the child is examined. The wiggling infant once again defies all the rules!

Joint stability is another feature doctors always test. Four to 5 percent of all normal newborns have very mobile hip joints that sometimes even produce a click when the physician puts the hip through its range of motion. Sometimes a hip will click as it's turned, but will feel completely stable. Still, what do you think happens to the great majority of newborns with unstable hips?

You guessed it. They spontaneously improve. We now believe that extra-loose joints at birth are caused by a hormone called relaxin. The mother's body produces relaxin late in her pregnancy in order to soften up the supporting tissues around the joints. This hormone helps the mother's bony pelvis give a little more stretch when stretch is needed. Since relaxin passes through to the baby, his joints will be extra-loose until the hormone disappears from his circulation.

Another established test that produces "positive" results in half the normal children is the abduction (movement away from the midline) test. This, too, is a part of all the routine well-baby exams during the infant's first six months. It goes like this: While the baby is lying on his back, his thighs straight up and his knees bent, your physician gently spreads the thighs down toward the table. Doctors used to believe that anything less than a full 90-degree abduction was abnormal; we found fault with 80 degrees and tried our hardest to get the last 10 degrees out of the baby. We now know that we really didn't have to. In the first place, the pressure was uncomfortable for the baby, and even if it weren't, we could have settled for 60 to 70 degrees, since that's what 99 percent of normal babies can do. Abduction of 90 degrees is possible in less than half of normal infants, so we no longer have to lean on little babies who can't fight back.

How about X rays? They'll certainly show you and your doctor whether or not the thigh is out of its joint, and if there's still uncertainty about this point your physician may suggest an X ray. Do they help in recognizing the hip that might dislocate in the future? This is doubtful.

We now know that the range of normal thigh angles seen in an X ray is much greater than we thought, and that many abnormally high angles will come down with age.

Anyway, the crux of the issue is whether or not the thigh will dislocate as the baby becomes more active. X rays don't help much and physical findings may vary from examination to examination. It's no wonder that doctors now overdiagnose where we once underdiagnosed. It really isn't possible to predict which babies with unstable hips will need some form of treatment, so our extra precautions are probably for the best.

Many doctors advise double or even triple diapers for the baby with unstable hips, since this extra padding pins the baby's hips into a better alignment. Later on, if the hips are shown to be truly dislocated, more decisive treatment can be given. In the meantime, nothing is lost. (See p. 338, **Ref. 52;** see p. 338, **Ref. 53.**)

FEET

Foot Pushed Up Against Shin *(Calcaneovalgus Foot)*

This is another result of "no room in the womb." Crowding in the uterus can force your baby's heel down and the instep of her foot up against the outer side of her lower leg. She then looks as if she were trying to walk on her heels. You might also notice that there's less fat in the area of the baby's lower leg where it was compressed by the baby's foot, and very deep skin creases at the bend.

Pushed-up feet are especially common in breech deliveries and in large babies. They occur four times more often in girls than in boys, probably because of the greater degree of joint laxity in females. Your baby may have difficulty toe dancing for a few months, but ordinarily no treatment is needed, since the condition corrects itself on its own. Bracing, taping, or even casting can be considered if the return to normal is too slow for comfort.

Pushed-up feet are very different from what used to be called clubfoot. The bend of the clubfoot is down and in, instead of up and out, and instead of walking on his heels, a child with uncorrected clubfoot would walk on his insteps.

Foot Turned In *(Metatarsus Varus or Forefoot Adduction)*

Sometimes, the outside edge of a baby's foot is shaped like the letter C and his big toe is turned inward. This is usually caused by the pressure of one of the baby's legs' being crossed over the other late in the pregnancy. It's four times more common in boys than girls, possibly because boys are generally larger.

Your intoeing baby's foot is flexible, and if you can easily push the front part of it so that it makes a straight line with the hind part, nothing needs to be done for at least three to six months. Try to avoid letting the baby sleep on his tummy with his rump in the air and his legs tucked under him, because that position helps perpetuate the problem. If the baby insists on sleeping on his stomach and keeps tucking his feet in as fast as you pull them out, put him in a very warm sleeper. The warmth will encourage him to sprawl out.

Casting is reserved for feet that are too stiff to be passively straightened by hand. As long as the foot can be aligned easily, there's hope for success without casting.

Sometimes only the inner edge of the baby's foot is curved and the rest of the foot is pointing straight ahead. This happens when the baby uses his big toe as if it were a thumb. Then, instead of being parallel to the other four digits, his big toe is angled out like the independent, grasping toe of a monkey. Unless your baby spends all his growing years in a tree, this primitive reflex will be suppressed, and baby's big toe will fall in line with its peers. (See p. 335, **Ref.** 11; see p. 335, **Ref.** 13; see p. 338, **Ref.** 53; see p. 338, **Ref.** 54.)

Foot Turned Out

Outturned feet are common in grown-ups, but the exception in early infancy. When they do occur in an infant, for some inexplicable reason the right leg is turned out six times more often than the left.

Turning out is most apparent when the leg is dangling free, and becomes completely unnoticeable when the baby starts to walk. Turned-out feet cause no problem to anyone, and are best ignored. This is probably another effect of the baby's position in the womb. (See p. 338, **Ref. 55.**)

TWISTED LOWER LEG *(Tibial Torsion)*

This is the commonest reason for the feet to turn in, and the explanation rests not with the feet but with the tibia, the main bone of the lower leg. The condition results from the baby's being crowded in the womb in a cross-legged position with her feet turned inward. In this position, her tibia is twisted inward, swiveling the foot inward and the sole upward along with it. In severe cases, the baby looks as if she just stepped on something and is turning her foot in and up to see what she squashed. Extreme degrees of torsion occur in only 3 percent of newborns, but mild degrees occur so often that they're considered normal variations.

There's also a natural tendency for the tibia to rotate outward, especially when the child begins to walk. With time, mild torsions disappear, moderate ones become mild, and severe ones become moderate. Since this improvement occurs without treatment, most doctors leave tibial torsions alone, unless they feel that the torsion won't correct itself enough to be acceptable. Babies who sleep on their stomachs, resting their weight on their inturned feet, may be interfering with the natural untwisting of the tibia, so it seems reasonable to try to prevent this sleeping posture. If you want to help nature along you can flip the baby over on her back, pull her legs out from under, or tie her sleeper heels together.

Most specialists agree that nothing more "corrective" need be done for tibia torsion until the baby is 18 months of age. Some see very few reasons for correcting it at all.

Uncorrected tibial torsion that doesn't cause tripping has no functional consequences. Those of us old enough to have seen Jackie Robinson sprint around the bases with his pigeon-toed feet know that it didn't slow him down any. There's no evidence, either, that uncorrected tibial torsion can increase the arthritic degeneration of any of the joints in the legs. The reasons for correction that remain are: intoeing doesn't look graceful; intoeing causes shoes to wear out faster;

and intoeing may cause someone to cross his ski tips, which *may* make him fall and hurt himself.

If any of these reasons seem compelling, treatment can be started. It consists of putting the baby's feet in a pair of shoes fastened 6 to 8 inches apart, on a metal rod worn day and night.

Why don't you spend your money on a good dinner and show instead? (See p. 335, **Ref. 13**; see p. 338, **Ref. 53**; see p. 338, **Ref. 57**; see p. 338, **Ref. 58**.)

INFANTILE FLAT FEET *(Plantar Fat Pad)*

The ideal, romanticized foot has a long gentle arch that lifts the inner part of the foot off the ground. This type of foot is actually seen in some adults, few children, and no infants.

If the purpose of the two arches of the feet is to provide support for the standing body, then there's clearly no value in having an arch at birth. What babies have instead is a pad of fat filling the space. This is called the plantar fat pad.

We don't know the exact function of this fat pad, but it probably fills a protective role for the baby's still-tender feet. At any rate, if the shoe salesman serves up an arch support for your baby's first pair of shoes, don't bite. (See p. 338, **Ref. 53**; see p. 338, **Ref. 58**.)

TOES: OVERLAPPING, WEBBED, STUBBY

Rarely does the newborn have straight, even toes. Feet that are squeezed by crowding in the womb have long, deep creases on their soles, and toes that overlap. The third, fourth, and fifth toes tend to overlap toward the inner half of the foot. These toes will realign after birth and no treatment is needed.

If the skin between the baby's fingers or toes fails to separate completely, a connecting web of skin develops. This tendency to web is seen in certain families and not others. Webbing occurs most often between the third and fourth fingers, and between the second and third toes. I am sure that there's a very good reason for this, but I don't have it. Webbing does no harm.

There's also a tendency in certain families to have short, broad ends to the thumb and big toe. Stub thumbs are especially common in east European Jews. Since the size and shape of the nail is determined by the size and shape of the bone at the end of the digit, there's no need to X-ray the digit if there's concern about its stubbiness. If the digit looks stubby, so will its X ray. Needless to say, stubbiness does no harm. (See p. 335, **Ref. 13**; see p. 336, **Ref. 19**; see p. 336, **Ref. 21.**)

PALM CREASES

Palm creases result from the wrinkling of the skin at the line of bending. If there's no bending, there's no crease. If the baby's finger is very short and has only one bend, it gets only one crease. Since the thumb moves in many directions, it creates creases that diverge at many angles. Normally, the palm is long enough to generate two horizontal folds when the fist is clenched. The short palm, or the palm that has a very short fifth finger, may give rise to only a single crease.

One hand of 4 percent of normal newborns has a single palm crease. Only 1 percent of normal infants have single creases in each palm. For some obscure reason, single creases are twice as common in males as in females.

Because children with Down's syndrome are likely to have short, broad hands with short fifth fingers, they're particularly apt to have single palm creases. Nevertheless, 55 percent of children with Down's syndrome have the normal number of creases. One hundred percent of monkeys have a single crease, so it's now known, appropriately, as the simian crease. (See p. 336, **Ref. 19.**)

HEEL PUNCTURES

In all hospitals today, every newborn is tested for a certain disease that might cause mental retardation. This test consists of taking a few drops of blood from the baby's heel, collecting them on a piece of special paper, and then sending them to a central laboratory. This is why most babies go home with Band-Aids on their heels.

If your baby was jaundiced and had frequent serum bilirubin measurements (see p. 46) or if she had some other need for extra heel punctures, her heels might look pretty sore. Occasionally, the punctures will heal leaving a lump of scar tissue, which may calcify 4 to 12 months later. If, for some reason, the baby's foot is X-rayed, tiny white flecks will appear in the skin over the heel. They'll disappear by the time she's 18 to 30 months old. (See p. 338, **Ref. 59.**)

DIMPLES AT BASE OF SPINE *(Pilonidal Abnormalities)*

In the beginning, the embryonic nervous system consists of a gradually thickening band of tissue, called the neural plate, which extends up and down the middle of the back. As the embryo grows, the edges of the neural plate are pushed up, forming a groove that extends from the base of the spine all the way up and over the head to the bridge of the nose. The edges of this neural plate eventually meet and form a roof over the groove. This process begins in the neck and works its way up to the bridge of the nose and down to the base of the spine. By the embryo's third week of life, the neural groove has become a tube, sealed off at each end, and it eventually separates from the overlying skin. Sometimes, the skin over the embryo's back remains attached to the roof of this neural tube, but when it occurs at the base of the spine, the baby shows what we call a pilonidal abnormality.

In its simplest form, the pilonidal abnormality is nothing more than a shallow dimple at the base of the spine, or an extra-deep buttock crease. Over 4 percent of all newborn infants have them. They're considered normal variants and need no special attention.

Another 3 percent of newborns, however, have what are considered "significant" abnormalities at the base of the spine, and some of these bear closer watching.

There are three basic types:

1. Deeper skin depressions or dimples whose bottoms can only be seen with a lot of effort
2. Presumed sinus (meaning hollow) tracts whose bottoms can't be seen even with a lot of effort

3. Some form of protrusion, either a skin tag or a mound of skin surrounding a presumed sinus tract or deep dimple

The first type, the deep dimple, is a nuisance to keep clean. Various types of debris tend to accumulate there if you let them. If you wait long enough, however, the deep dimple will become a shallow dimple that needs no special care. Time also helps the presumed sinus tract. By the time babies reach six months of age, one presumed sinus tract out of five has graduated to deep-dimple status; that is, its bottom is evident.

The problem with the presumed sinus tract that doesn't become a harmless deep dimple after six months is that there's no way to tell whether it ends just outside the spinal cord or goes all the way to the cord. This is a major concern because the tract that enters the spine puts the baby at risk of developing infection and meningitis.

Two thirds of all sinus tracts end up in the spinal cord. The higher up they occur in the baby's back, the more likely they are to enter the spinal cord. For this reason, your surgeon will quickly excise any sinus tract that's situated over the spine and above the waist.

The situation is very different for the lower sinus tracts, especially those just above the buttock's cleft, because these rarely end in the spinal cord. This is not to say that they're completely innocent, but if these lower sinus tracts do get infected, the process is closer to the surface and doesn't lead to meningitis.

If your baby has this second type of pilonidal abnormality, and it's below the waist, your physician will probably recommend extra-careful cleaning of the area during his first six months, and hope that the bottom of the tract comes into view. If the tract happens to get infected during this time, he'll treat the infection thoroughly, then call for the surgeon to excise the tract. Infections produce scar tissue, making surgery more difficult, so doctors don't allow more than one infection to occur before excising the tract.

If no infections occur during the first six months in the lower pilonidal abnormality, and if the bottom of the tract still remains out of sight, it's time to make a decision. Your doctor can't get help in his decision making by doing tests. We used to inject dye into the tract and take X rays to see where the dye went, but since this test can introduce serious infections, it's no longer used. X rays without dye are less hazardous, but they don't give us particularly useful information. Perhaps new scanning techniques will help us in the future, but for now we have to choose between waiting to see if the sinus tract gets infected, and excising it before any infection can occur.

My vote, in this particular instance, is for early excision, at about six months, before any infection shows up. My reasons are: (1) In this area, infections are the rule, rather than the exception. (2) Infections tend to occur during adolescence or young adulthood, often coinciding with the appearance of hair in the area. (3) Pilonidal infections in this age group can be quite debilitating and costly. (4) Operating on the uninfected rather than the infected tract is fully effective much more often. (Incidentally, the association of hair and infection in this condition is the reason for the name *pilonidal*—*pilo* means hair; *nidal* equals nest.)

As for the third type of pilonidal abnormality, skin tags or mounds of skin, your doctor will leave them if they're small and remove them if they're large. (See p. 336, **Ref. 22**; see p. 337, **Ref. 40**; see p. 338, **Ref. 60**.)

1. Cardiovascular System

HEART RATE

The heart of a newborn baby beats quite a bit faster than it will at any other time in his life. The infant's heart is considered normal if it beats in a range from 90 to 150 times per minute. If the rate drops below 90 per minute and remains there, it's abnormally slow. It's also normal for the rate to drop by the time the child reaches two years old to between 85 and 125 per minute; by four years, between 75 and 115 per minute; by six years, between 65 and 100 per minute; and for the child over six, between 60 and 100 per minute.

To understand why younger children have faster heart rates than older ones, you must first understand why younger children also have faster metabolic rates. A hint: It has to do with their "size."

Doctors measure body size in two ways: weight and surface area. The two aren't exactly equivalent. A 10-pound child has one third of the surface area of a 50-pounder, not a fifth, as you would expect if the two were equivalent. Very small objects, be they newborns or snowflakes, have a lot more surface area than they have weight.

Surface area is more important than weight in determining the body's metabolic rate, that is, the rate at which the body burns fuel for heat and energy. On a per-pound basis, it costs more fuel to be small, since it means that you have relatively more surface area that needs to be warmed and energized.

The faster the body consumes fuel, the faster the heart must pump to deliver it and remove waste. Thus, heart rates are direct reflections of metabolic rates.

A good example is the water shrew, the smallest warm-blooded animal in the country. The 3-inch water shrew, when relaxing, has a heart rate of 700 per minute. When it's frightened, its heart speeds up to 1,200! As for high metabolic rates and energy requirements, these critters eat from one half to twice their body weight daily just to stay alive. Compared to the shrew, your baby's resting rate of 150 per minute seems nice and easy.

Not only does the newborn's heart beat at twice the rate of the adult heart, but the infant's chest wall is often so thin that you can actually see his little heart pumping away. If you can't see it, you can certainly feel it easily.

Both of these circumstances—the high rate and the thin chest wall—contribute to the mistaken notion that the newborn's heart is "racing." (See p. 338, **Ref. 61**; see p. 338, **Ref. 62**.)

HEART SOUNDS *(Embryocardia)*

The mature heart makes a basic sound something like *lub-dub*. The closing of the valves between the upper and lower chambers creates the *lub;* the *dub* comes from the closing of the valves of the great vessels where they exit from their respective ventricles (see p. 82). After the *dub,* there's a pause as the ventricles take time out to rest and refill with blood. This phase is called diastole, and it takes up about two thirds of the total beating cycle. This is why twice as much time elapses between *dub* and the next *lub* as between the *lub* and the *dub.*

This is not the case for the newborn. Your baby's refilling phase is no longer than her contracting phase. As a result, the time that elapses between the first and second sounds is the same as the time between the second sound and the first one of the next cycle. This is why her heart sounds more like the ticking of a clock, *tick-tack-tick-tack,* than the *lub-dub* of a mature heart.

This *tick-tack-tick-tack* is also the rhythm that you'll hear if your obstetrician has you listen to the fetal heart, either electronically or with a fetal stethoscope. Because it originates with the fetus (embryo), the rhythm is called embryocardia.

VARIATIONS FROM NORMAL HEARTBEAT
(Arrhythmias)

An arrhythmia is a variation from the "normal" rhythm. Unless you are personally monitoring your baby's heart rate, it is not likely that you will be the first person to notice that your baby has an arrhythmia. Your doctor may mention it to you and add that it is an extremely common condition, which it certainly is. Here's why:

Your baby's heart comes equipped with its own, built-in "pacemaker." This organic device consists of a knot of highly specialized cells in an area of the right atrium (see p. 82) known as the sinoauricular junction, or the sinus node. These cells tell the heart's muscle when to contract by rhythmically discharging electrical impulses through specialized fibers that conduct the impulse over the entire muscle.

If nothing interferes with sinus node's activity, this cellular pacemaker would simply fire away at regular intervals and there would be very little variation in her heart rate or rhythm. That would be about as exciting as having a metronome conduct the Philharmonic. It would work for the dull times, but it wouldn't allow for the necessary *andantes* and *allegros*.

Enter the nervous system, which in your newborn baby's case reads: Enter the *immature* nervous system.

Your newborn's sinus node is easily distracted. For example, breathing affects its activity. When the baby breathes in, the sinus slows down. When she exhales, her sinus and, therefore, her heart rate return to where they were. This pattern of varying rates that respond to the respiratory cycle is called sinus arrhythmia. It's normal in newborns. Some babies have it to a greater extent than others, but almost all will show some sinus arrhythmia. Incidentally, sinus arrhythmia appears throughout all of childhood. If it is found during a school examination by someone not accustomed to the normal workings of a child's heart, it can lead to a lot of unnecessary worry.

The sinus node also slows down, often dramatically, when the baby is engaged in certain activities. The heart rates of some babies drop in half when they're straining to move their bowels. Others will reduce their rates by 30 to 40 beats per minute when they yawn or hiccup.

This slowing of sinus activity is called sinus bradycardia (*brady* means slow).

Once these acts are completed, the baby's heart returns to its original rate. Though activities such as yawning or moving the bowels seem unrelated, they're actually tied together by the vagus nerve, the "vagabond" nerve of the vegetative or autonomic nervous system. When this nerve is stimulated by sensations from the organs of the chest and abdomen, it responds by sending out impulses that, among other things, slow the heart rate. Since the vagus nerve is a bit trigger happy early in infancy, sinus bradycardia is common during this time of life and the baby none the worse for it. (See p. 338, **Ref. 63**; see p. 338, **Ref. 64**.)

HYPERTENSION CAUSED BY OVER-THE-COUNTER MEDICATION

When an infant has high blood pressure, the cause is almost always in the kidneys or in a narrowing of the aorta. If your baby has an elevated blood pressure, your doctor will certainly take a thorough look at both areas. But she might or might not also ask you what medicines have been given to the baby.

A number of apparently harmless, over-the-counter medicines, especially those referred to as decongestants, contain chemicals that cause blood vessels to constrict. If your baby is given too high a dose, or for too long a period, high blood pressure can result.

In addition, eye drops and nose drops that constrict only the surface vessels of older children can be absorbed into an infant's bloodstream and cause widespread blood-vessel constriction, thus elevating the baby's blood pressure.

This doesn't happen very often, but when it does, it can lead a conscientious physician into an exhaustive, expensive, or invasive investigation. If your infant has high blood pressure, and if you've been giving him over-the-counter medicines, be sure to tell all to your doctor. She and your baby will be most grateful. (See p. 338, **Ref. 65**.)

2. Respiratory System

RAPID BREATHING

All the reasons that explain the newborn's rapid heart rate (see p. 108) also explain the newborn's rapid breathing rate. Remember the 3-inch shrew? Not only does its heart beat ten times faster than ours, it also has to breathe ten times faster.

The newborn breathes fast, but not that fast. His resting rate is 30 to 50 per minute. By the time he's 2 years old, the rate is down to 20 to 30 per minute, and by 15 years of age, his rate is the adult 15 to 20 per minute.

Newborns also breathe rapidly because of "dead space." This is the volume of air that moves in and out of the upper areas of the respiratory tract. In this twilight zone of the respiratory tract, air doesn't quite make it to the lungs. The effort involved in sucking it in and blowing it out is "wasted." The adult wastes one third of each breath moving air in and out of his dead space. The remaining two thirds of each breath reaches the lower, functioning area of the adult's lungs.

The newborn has proportionately more dead space than the adult, so two fifths of each breath doesn't reach his lungs. To get enough oxygen and carbon dioxide into and out of his lungs, your baby must work harder, i.e., breathe faster. (See p. 238, **Ref. 66**; see p. 238, **Ref. 67**.)

TEMPORARY RAPID BREATHING *(Transient Tachypnea)*

Sometimes babies breathe too fast, even for babies. If a baby is breathing faster than 60 times per minute, he could be suffering from a host of worrisome problems, such as pneumonia, heart failure, and so on. Often, however, the fast-breathing baby has nothing more than a harmless condition called transient tachypnea (*tachy* means fast; *pnoea* is breath).

Newborns with transient tachypnea are usually full-termers who huff and puff but don't appear to be laboring with each breath. The "attack" lasts three days at the most. Sometimes, doctors give the infants a little extra oxygen to keep them pink, but seldom in a concentration of more than 40 percent oxygen. Transient tachypnea tends to affect boys more than girls, and is common in babies who have had stressful deliveries, who have been accidentally chilled, or whose mothers were oversedated at the baby's birth.

A chest X ray will quickly reveal whether or not your baby has transient tachypnea. If she does, the X ray will show a mildly enlarged heart, distended blood vessels in her lungs, fluid in her chest, and overly inflated lungs. Fortunately, the baby won't look nearly as bad as the X ray. The whole affair blows over in a few days, which clearly explains the use of the word *transient* in the name of this condition.

If we study the hearts of babies with transient tachypnea carefully, we find that the quality of pumping of their left ventricles (see p. 82) is, for these few days, not up to standard. A little delay in clearing out the lung fluid that filled the baby's lungs before delivery also adds to the condition. And though it does seem reasonable that circumstances that might strain a baby's lungs, such as traumatic deliveries or excess drugs, would increase the infant's lung fluid surplus, we have no idea why little boys are more vulnerable to it than little girls.

One other brief period in a baby's life when his respirations can appear to be abnormal is immediately following his first breath. During the first half hour after delivery, most babies' breathing is somewhat irregular and shallow. Some babies' breaths appear labored and a grunting sound may accompany the expiration, especially if the baby's mouth, nose, or windpipe is filled with mucus.

After the mucus is suctioned out, the baby usually falls asleep and his breathing becomes regular, rapid, and somewhat shallow. At about three to six hours, there may be another burst of irregular breathing. This soon settles down to the regular breathing pattern of the newborn. (See p. 335, **Ref. 8**; see p. 338, **Ref. 61**; see p. 338, **Ref. 68**; see p. 338, **Ref. 69**.)

PERIODS OF BREATHLESSNESS DURING SLEEP *(Brief Sleep Apnea)*

How many of you have slipped into your baby's room to watch your blessed one sleep? When babies are deeply asleep, there can be no doubt about their heavenly origin. But if after a few minutes you dared to turn on the light, you may have noticed that your baby wasn't breathing evenly. Did you think your slumbering pussycat had forgotten to take his next breath? Did *you* remember to take *your* next breath? Or did you stop breathing out of sheer fear? Rest assured, all babies are "breathless" sometimes when they sleep. Here's why:

Your newborn's immature nervous system doesn't have the ability to fine-tune its rate of breathing to your baby's changing body chemistry. Instead of sensing tiny changes in the levels of carbon dioxide and oxygen, and sending out an "order" to breathe, your baby's respiratory headquarters requires more sizable changes before it responds. The less mature the baby, the less sensitive her respiratory headquarters.

In its typical form, a newborn baby's pattern of breathing is as follows:

She breathes rapidly (50 to 60 times per minute) for 10 to 15 seconds, then holds her breath for 2 or more seconds, and then starts to breathe rapidly again. If you could measure the depth of each breath, you would see that the first breath following the pause was quite shallow, but each breath that followed grew deeper and deeper.

Those moments when your baby's breathing suddenly stops and she's in her pause period can be very scary. Yet, as scary as it seems, at no time does the infant appear to turn a hair (assuming she has any to turn). Throughout your entire ordeal, your baby has remained pink and blissful.

The baby's cyclic respiratory pattern is called periodic breathing.

The pauses in this pattern are called periodic apnea. Some babies have pauses in their breathing even when the pattern is steady and not periodic; such breathlessness is called nonperiodic apnea. These pauses are not apneic spells, which *are* serious and extremely rare. Apneic spells last not 2 but more than 20 seconds, and they're accompanied by either a slowing of the heart or loss of color.

The brief periods of apnea that result from the immaturity of the newborn's respiratory regulation are harmless, and the more common of these is the nonperiodic type. Nonperiodic apnea almost always occurs when the baby is in a state of active or fretful sleep and it's usually very brief. During quiet or blissful sleep, apnea is much less common. When it does occur, it tends to be periodic and last a bit longer than the nonperiodic type.

We don't know how old most babies are when these episodes cease, if they ever actually do cease, or if they're related to sleep apnea of adults. We do know that apnea is common in babies, and as we develop better ways of observing sleeping babies and children, we'll be able to answer these questions. (See p. 338, **Ref. 68**; see p. 338, **Ref. 70**.)

MUCUS

It is important to realize that the "mucus" that newborns so often gag on is not the same mucus that drips from noses or is hawked out of bronchial trees. Newborn mucus isn't even really mucus. It doesn't come from mucous glands. Its chemical makeup is entirely different from the sort of mucus that discharges from the glands in our respiratory, intestinal, and reproductive tracts.

Newborn mucus is a unique fluid that's either secreted from the fetal lung alone or is a blend of amniotic fluid and fetal lung secretion. Before the baby takes his first breath, his lungs are filled with this juice. The full-termer arrives with about 80 to 100 milliliters of it in his lungs.

As soon as the baby is born, this mucus must make way for air. Most of it is absorbed into the baby's veins and the lymph channels of his lungs.

Up to 20 milliliters of the mucus is expressed through the baby's nose and mouth by the squeezing of his chest as he passes through the birth canal. This gets suctioned out while the baby is still in the delivery room, often before the baby is fully delivered.

The mucus that didn't get high enough to get suctioned, and didn't get absorbed into the lungs' veins, is eliminated during the first week of life. The lining of the baby's respiratory tree sweeps the mucus upward toward the mouth. Once it gets there, the infant swallows some, gags on some, and some ends up in your lap. Whatever the route of disposal, once it's gone, no more is produced and that's the end of the mucus. (See p. 339, **Ref. 71.**)

SQUEAKY BREATHING *(Congenital Stridor)*

Some babies squeak when they inhale. If that sound came from your car, you would probably reach for a can of oil. If it came from your baby, read on.

Doctors describe babies who produce a sound when they inhale as having congenital stridor (*congenital* means present at birth; *stridor* is harsh sound). Seventy-five percent of babies with congenital stridor also have laryngomalacia (the *larynx* is the voice box; *malacia* means softening). Doctors can recognize the great majority of laryngomalacia cases simply by the sound. Roughly one fifth aren't obvious until a specialist looks at the voice box.

Babies with laryngomalacia produce a high-pitched, fluttery, staccato sound as they inhale. It's loudest when the baby is excited, feeding, or lying on his back, and it may not happen with every breath.

Despite the squeak, a baby with laryngomalacia has a strong voice, his color is good, and he has no special feeding difficulties. If he catches a cold the mucus and swelling may aggravate things, and he needs to be watched a bit closer than the baby who doesn't squeak.

A baby's very first breath can produce a squeak, or the sound may not start until he's six months old. Squeaks usually stop before the second birthday, but some babies squeak until they're five. If a specialist looks at the baby's larynx, she will see an epiglottis that buckles when the baby breathes in, a thick wall of cartilage that caves in, or both. She'll tell you that, as the baby gets older, the voice box will become more rigid and the sounds will stop. She'll be right, of course. (See p. 339, **Ref. 72.**)

STUFFY NOSE *(Snorting Respiration)*

Your newborn doesn't breathe through his mouth unless he's crying. If his nose is blocked, he won't shift to mouth breathing as an adult would. Instead, he'll try harder to breathe through his nose. This not-too-bright behavior is called obligatory nose breathing, and it isn't the most comfortable obligation to have. Your baby's nostrils can be easily obstructed. Furthermore, a little bit of swelling goes a long way in narrowing his nasal passage. Both swelling and obstruction can greatly increase your baby's breathing work load. So, why did Mother Nature saddle babies with obligatory nose breathing?

One theoretical answer is based on evolution. It goes something like this:

Lower forms of mammals rely most heavily on their sense of smell to get by; i.e., they can never manage without their sniffers. Since the survival interests of these animals are best served if they can move all their air through their noses, nature equips them with wide nostrils and nasal passages that aren't easily obstructed. The newborn human arrives on the scene with primitive instincts based on the premise that his survival interests are also best served by routing every bit of air headed for his lungs through his nose. But by some fluke, he also comes equipped with a narrow nose and a tongue that practically fills his mouth. What a fix! Until the human baby catches on to the notion that nose breathing isn't helping him much, the baby breathes through his nose.

Believe it or not. Personally, I have my doubts. A more plausible theory puts the blame on the very high position that the baby's tongue occupies in his mouth, making mouth breathing more difficult. With maturation, the top of the tongue gradually moves away from the roof of the mouth, allowing more room for mouth breathing.

Regardless of the reason for the nose breathing, the results are quite clear. The rapid flow of air through the baby's nasal channels dries out the mucus that's normally produced. This forms crusts of mucus that encroach on his airway. This causes the baby to breathe harder, which further increases the rate of air flow. And so on and so on.

If the inhaled air is extra-dry from being overheated, the process is speeded up. The end result is a snorting baby trying to move air around and through his mucus crusts. The baby sounds like an elephant with a peanut stuck in its trunk.

Sooner or later, the crust begins to irritate the baby's nose, and a sneeze reflex occurs. If the crust isn't dislodged, another sneeze takes place. Now you have a sneezing, snorting, stuffed-up baby, and someone asks, "How long has your baby had his cold?"

Tell him, "Not so fast, buster. My baby doesn't have a cold." A cold is an infection, and babies with infections usually look and act sick. Your little snorter may sound awful, but he sure is acting all right. Furthermore, a baby with a cold produces a watery nasal discharge that flows from each nostril like the Nile. When he sneezes, the spray can be felt all over the room. Little snorters' sneezes are as dry as the Sahara. (See p. 339, **Ref. 73.**)

HICCUPS

All babies hiccup. By the time they get around to being born, they've been hiccuping for several months. Remember those little rhythmic "kicks" when your baby was *in utero?* They were hiccups.

The hiccup is the result of a sudden contraction of the diaphragm muscle. The vacuum produced by this contraction sucks air into the windpipe and, instead of passing all the way through to the lungs, the air is checked by the abrupt closing of the vocal cords. What comes out is a *hic.*

Because babies who feed ravenously, barracuda style, are more apt to hiccup, we believe that the air they swallow during feeding is involved in this process. It does make some sense to try to slow down the speed of the feeding, but I can imagine how much success you'll have trying to reason with a barracuda.

Members of the medical profession have been trying to stop hiccups since Hippocrates' time, but none of the countless techniques they engineered have withstood the test of time. I don't know what the fuss is all about, anyway. It doesn't embarrass the baby, and unless the hiccuping leads to spitting up, it's perfectly harmless and will eventually stop.

3. Digestive System

EARLY LACK OF INTEREST IN FEEDING

Some babies are eager feeders from the word *go.* They drain their first bottle dry or go to work on the breast as if they'd been coached while they were still in the womb. But the majority of newborns take their first few feedings with little or no interest. Some of them don't want to feed at all. They hang up the DO NOT DISTURB sign.

Don't take this personally.

Your baby doesn't *need* to feed. Every newborn's body is composed of 79 percent water. By the time the baby is ten days old, she's down to 74 percent water. We assume that she's simply using up the superabundance of water that nature provided to tide her over her first few days until Mother's breast milk comes in, or the formula delivery arrives, whichever the case may be.

If your full-term, healthy baby prefers to live off her surplus water for the first few days and is all right in every other regard, don't be discouraged. Don't try to stimulate her, pinch her heels, immerse her in ice water, or force-feed in any way. Let her sleep. How would you like it if somebody woke you up out of a deep sleep and decided that what you really wanted was a chicken burrito and an egg cream?

Use the time instead to count her fingers and toes. Take off her clothes, put her on your chest, and feed her with your love. When she gets hungry, she will want to be fed. Isn't she bright? (See p. 338, **Ref. 67**; see p. 339, **Ref. 76**.)

COLIC

Colic is the Tower of Babel in pediatrics. Every pediatric specialty speaking its own tongue has its own idea about what causes colic. Pediatric allergists believe that colic comes from cow milk allergy, while the endocrinologists suggest that it comes from the mother's hormones. Pediatric gastroenterologists contend an immaturity of the baby's intestines causes it, and pediatric psychiatrists that it's the baby's response to stress and tension. When the specialty of pediatric aerospace medicine is launched, I have no doubt that its practitioners will suggest that colic comes from outer space.

For the life of me, I don't know why every specialty claims to know what causes colic. None of them has an effective treatment, and you'd think that, given the lack of solid information or convincing arguments, they'd all keep quiet when the subject comes up.

Doctors don't even agree on what colic actually is. From its name, you would imagine that it had something to do with the colon. And, actually, when the term *colic* is used in its narrowest sense, it refers to the crampy, abdominal pain that some babies get while they eat. When used in a wider sense, it extends to excessive, cyclic crying of any type and from any cause; and finally, the term widens out to the horizons when the word *excessive* is scratched.

How can we recognize a "typical baby with colic"?

Charles Darwin described colic almost 100 years ago as "infants' . . . utter violent and prolonged screams. Whilst thus screaming, their eyes are firmly closed so that the skin round them is wrinkled and the forehead contracted into a frown. The mouth is widely opened . . . so as to assume a squarish form. The breath is inhaled spasmodically." That picture is still pretty good and can be completed by adding that the legs are either drawn up to the belly or forcefully stretched out, and the infant emits the sounds of passing wind. How often do we see this picture, and how often is the baby going through just regular cyclic fussing?

In the first place, since seven out of eight normal healthy babies have regular crying periods, you must assume that regular periods of crying are normal. Some people even suggest that crying serves a purpose, like blowing off steam.

How much do normal babies cry? During a baby's second week of life, the time spent crying ranges from one and one half to two and one half hours each day. The crying increases steadily, reaching its peak when the baby is six weeks old, at which point the time spent crying is one and three fourths to three and one half hours per day. As babies log more crying time, they also improve their sharpshooting, concentrating their crying between 6 and 11 P.M. Most babies' timing is exquisite. They know, uncannily, exactly when Father gets home from work, precisely when Mother is most physically and emotionally exhausted, when the grown-ups want their dinner, and when older siblings are in need of some solid help with the homework.

By 10 to 12 weeks, babies usually quiet down, perhaps because they're learning new tricks that enable them to blow off steam better. If that's what "normal crying" is like, what is it like to have a heavy-duty fusser—a "colicky baby"—in the house?

Roughly one baby in five is more than mildly "colicky." His crying is extra long, extra loud, and extra nerve-racking. Well over half of such babies are prime-time evening screamers. Contrary to popular belief, these babies aren't especially fast feeders, spitters, or more likely to have constipation or gassiness. Older mothers are just as likely to have colicky babies as younger mothers, and the family's allergic or stomach disorder background has nothing to do with the occurrence of colic. The baby's sex has nothing to do with colic, nor does intolerance to the protein or the sugar in cow's milk. If you think that breast feeding will lower the chances of having a colicky baby, you're wrong. Parents' emotional states and personalities have little to do with it as well. Mothers of colicky infants aren't more anxious, depressed, or unstable, or less "mothering" than mothers of infants without colic. They're just more unlucky.

If you're looking for suggestions for making colic less likely, here are a few.

Don't have a firstborn; they're more likely to develop colic. Instead, go right to a second-born. If this advice is too late, and you've already had a firstborn, make sure that he didn't have colic. If he did, that raises the odds for the second-born.

Also, be an unskilled laborer. Only 7 percent of babies of unskilled parents get colic. On the other hand, 16 percent of the offspring of skilled workers have it, and 23 percent of the children of professional parents. If the baby's father is a doctor, his chances of having colic double. They also double if Mother has had advanced education. (See "Education Can Get You Anything.")

If you find yourself with a colicky baby, you will, no doubt, be offered lots of advice. Well-meaning strangers and relatives will tell you that healthy babies never carry on like that unless something's wrong, "seriously wrong."

You'll be told that your baby feeds too quickly, the milk is too rich, and the baby is overfed. The next person to come along will tell you that your baby is hungry, the milk is too weak, and you should change to a different style of feeding. Use a pacifier! Stop using the pacifier! Give the baby water! Give the baby tea!

Give yourself a break. Don't listen to them. If you do, your nerves will shred, and you'll proceed to make any one or all of the following favorite mistakes:

You'll change whatever feeding method you're using. The changes don't have to make any sense, as long as a change is made. It doesn't matter that your baby is thriving and has no specific intestinal symptoms. You may abandon what is totally successful breast feeding because you're led to suspect that you aren't producing enough milk, or are producing a poor grade of milk. Your formula-fed baby may get to sample every formula ever sold, maybe all of them in less than three days. Goats, lambs, and soybeans will get milked dry. While the search for Mr. Good Bottle goes on, little things that seem to bring temporary comfort to Baby will be discovered. The baby will get picked up and walked and seem to be more content. The baby will be cuddled or swaddled and become still. But then, instead of continuing with what seems to be working, you'll respond to a new fear. You'll be afraid of "spoiling the baby."

Thousands of parents have been convinced that their baby is pretending to have colic because he wants to be walked. He's trying to trick them. When he screams for three hours at a time, he's testing their willpower. At three weeks of age, he has learned how to devise interpersonal strategy and is now engaged in the act of parental manipulation. As bizarre as these ideas may appear to you, the relaxed and rested reader, to the exhausted, frazzled, first-time mother, they're often accepted as sage advice.

The final misinterpretation is the worst. The mother of the fretful, inconsolable baby blames herself. She comes to believe that something is lacking in her mothering. If she has read that colic is the result of parental tension, transmitted to the baby, she responds by becoming tenser. If she has been told that her instinctive wish to pick up her screaming baby will cause irreparable spoilage, she learns to distrust her instincts. If she believes that she alone is responsible for her baby's colic, she's reluctant to burden anyone else with her problem. Wishing to spare those she's close to the punishment of spending time with a colicky baby, she refuses offers of help and companionship. She isolates herself.

Now, lonely and disappointed with both herself and her baby, she feels anger, resentment, and frustration; not the best foundation for motherly love. She experiences all these emotions because she believes that the colic comes from her, not the baby.

She's wrong.

Here's what the mother or, I would hope, the father of a colicky baby should do.

First, ascertain whether or not the baby is healthy, aside from being colicky. This involves seeing a pediatrician and sometimes a consultant or two. Every effort should be made to prove to yourself that your baby has colic and nothing more, because once the diagnosis of colic is accepted, the light at the end of the tunnel comes into view.

Colic has an end. Most colic ends by the third month. Some really severe cases often take another month, but even with these, the end *will* come. Once this fact is accepted, your focus can shift to short-term solutions. You can take the steps that will enable you to cope until the end is reached.

Here are some suggestions for coping:

Make contact with some knowledgeable person such as a pediatrician or a friend who has successfully coped with her own colicky infant. Accept advice only from your "colic connection." When others offer opinions, quickly take a nap and let them watch the baby while you doze.

Enlist all the help you can get. If anyone volunteers to help with any of your chores, accept. Sure, Superwoman never had to ask for help, but she never had a child with colic. Be supersmart instead, and get help. I especially like baby sitters and, as a rule, they'll accept lower wages than psychiatrists.

Do whatever seems to bring comfort to the baby. Practically everything will work, but not for very long. Any diversion is temporary, but better than nothing, and no diversion you come up with will spoil the baby. Carry him, cuddle him, swaddle him, swing him, sing to him, sleep with him, stand on your head with him as long as it comforts him.

The secret to successful coping is to remember that whatever is causing your child to have colic will go away by the time he reaches three or four months of age. The siege on your nerves will lift. Hang in there.

Before we leave this subject, I want to mention a particular type of crying that I call special-event crying.

The occasion can be the baby's first day home, his ritual circumcision, baptism, or any other exciting event. In its extreme form, the day goes like this: The proud parents pass their baby from one relative to the next. Flashbulbs pop. Likewise the champagne. Music is played. It's a party.

When the guests leave, the parents are exhausted, and the baby, overtired and overstimulated, begins to cry. Nothing helps. He cries until his strength is gone. Then he sleeps, and when he wakes up he's calm and contented, having totally forgotten about his "special event." All the parents had to do was pretty much the same thing I advise for colic: Hang in there. (See p. 338, **Ref.** 67; see p. 339, **Ref.** 77; see p. 339, **Ref.** 78; see p. 339, **Ref.** 79; see p. 339, **Ref.** 80; see p. 339, **Ref.** 81; see p. 339, **Ref.** 82.)

VOMITING

Overfeeding

Nearly every newborn will forcefully empty his stomach at one time or another. Babies vomit as a result of any one of a great number of diseases, but more than 95 percent of them vomit because of overdistension of their stomachs. Overdistension doesn't always mean overfeeding. The baby's stomach can just as easily overdistend with air.

Air enters a baby's stomach whenever she cries, sucks on a pacifier, gulps her milk, or makes an incomplete seal with the breast. If the air isn't promptly returned to the room via a burp, it warms up from room to body temperature. Being a gas, air expands as it's warmed, and the little gulps of it grow, distending the baby's stomach. This is called aerophagia (*aero* refers to air; *phagia* means eat).

Secondarily, milk can overdistend the baby's stomach. The average baby from ten days to six months old can hold in her stomach 30 milliliters of milk for every kilogram that she weighs. In other words, a 3-kilogram baby should be able to hold 90 milliliters in her stomach. But what if her stomach already holds 60 milliliters of air? In that case, putting another 90 milliliters of milk in will cause the same overdistension that feeding her 150 milliliters would produce. Whether milk or air, the result is the same. The baby's stomach muscle gets stretched and stretched, and when it reaches a critical level of tension, it contracts, emptying its contents.

If you could be sure how much air was in your baby's stomach at the start of feeding, you would know how much milk you could safely give without producing overdistension. Regrettably, there's no way of knowing, and that's why so many healthy, normal babies vomit.

What you might do to avoid vomiting is to try burping the baby just before you start to feed her. If she's a cooperative child, she'll oblige you by emptying the air from her stomach. If she's like most hungry babies, she'll cry until she gets what she wants. And she doesn't want to get burped. Still, the cause is worthy, and what do you have to lose?

Spitting Up and "Cheesing" (Reflux)

Regurgitating, spitting up, and *cheesing* are all terms for the nonforceful, partial emptying of the stomach. Sometimes just a trickle of milk flows out of the corner of the sleeping baby's mouth. Sometimes a burp carries an unexpected payload. Often, little more than chunks of sour, curdled milk ooze out of the baby's smiling mouth, staining and perfuming the baby's clothing, the baby, your rug, and you. The "cheese" of one of my children always landed in my shirt pocket, scoring a direct hit into a freshly opened pack of cigarettes. As you might imagine, this put a permanent end to my smoking habit.

Like vomiting, spitting can be a sign of any one of a long list of serious diseases, but in the overwhelming majority of cases, babies' spitting up is caused by reflux (*re* means backward; *flux* is flow) from the stomach back to the mouth. The primary culprit is the infant's immature esophagus.

The esophagus is the tube that carries fluids and solids from the mouth to the stomach. A ring of muscle fibers surrounds its end near the stomach. When the baby swallows, the muscle ring or sphincter relaxes, allowing the food to pass through. To keep the food from backing up, the sphincter then contracts, creating a zone of pressure higher than the stomach's. The difference in pressure keeps the flow of food from the esophagus moving in the direction of the stomach. If the pressure difference is reversed, gastro- (stomach) esophageal reflux (or GER) will occur.

GER occurs in infants with some regularity, especially right after feeding. Nursery staff members have been known to cringe as they watched the pediatrician examining a baby they'd just fed. Those who change baby's outfits are most keenly aware of what happens when she isn't handled extra-gently after a feeding. In Shakespeare's *As You Like It*, babies are described as "puking in the nurse's arms," the reason being reflux, methinks.

Infants who spit up occasionally just need gentle handling and small, frequent feeding with well-placed burps. If the spitting continues, the baby can be kept upright for 20 to 30 minutes after feeding. If this doesn't help, try keeping the baby in a vertical position for a longer period and thickening her milk with cereal. If the baby is healthy and thriving, you need do no more than this. Time solves most reflux, particularly the common, mild variety. For some reason, once the baby begins to walk, most reflux stops.

Reflux is talked about a lot these days, mainly because of its less common but more serious aspects. A few children who have it vomit so frequently that they lose weight. Another small percentage of refluxers bring up the stomach contents only as far as the lower esophagus but don't regurgitate at all. The latter often end up with their sensitive membranes inflamed by the acids of the stomach, a risk of blood loss, and sometimes scars that can narrow the esophagus significantly.

Lung infections and wheezing are two more rare complications that occur when some of the refluxed material is inhaled into the baby's lungs. This is more likely to happen when babies have nighttime GER.

All of these more serious manifestations of GER usually require more than just the passage of time to be cured, so, in these cases, doctors want a clear picture of just what's happening in the baby's esophagus.

In the past, the only way physicians could get a firsthand look at GER in action was X-ray examination while the baby swallowed barium. That test (the esophagram) presented lots of problems. Since GER doesn't occur continuously, the test often yielded normal results even when the problem existed. Also, very enthusiastic examiners, using very enthusiastic techniques, often got "positive" findings suggesting problems even in normal subjects. Eventually doctors began to consider minor degrees of reflux as normal, and only reflux that met certain criteria was considered significant. The catch here was in deciding on what was significant.

Technology to the rescue, by the way of tiny pressure transducers inside tubes that can be passed into the esophagus. These new transducers reveal whether or not the pressure in the baby's lower esophagus is too low to prevent GER. If your doctor wants to see if your baby's esophagus is inflamed by the stomach's acid, he can have a very narrow, illuminated, flexible tube passed directly into the gullet and see firsthand. Scanning over the esophagus and lungs after feeding the baby a radioactive compound is another space-age way of detecting GER.

These tests are wonderful, but luckily, most refluxers never need them because their health and weight remain normal, and, as for treatment, they respond to benign neglect. (See p. 339, **Ref. 83**; see p. 339, **Ref. 84**; see p. 339, **Ref. 85**.)

ELIMINATION

Soft Stools in Breast-Fed Baby (*Breast-Milk Stools*)

A healthy, breast-feeding baby can have bowel movements that give the distinct impression that something is wrong. The color and consistency of the feces can suggest diarrhea and the pattern of elimination can suggest constipation. Very often, mothers cease breast feeding on the basis of these mistaken impressions. This is doubly unfortunate, because the baby's stools look the way they do because the breast feeding was going so well, not because it was going badly.

The color of the breast-milk stool varies from a mustard-yellow to spinach-green. It usually contains little seedlike particles and has a slightly sour but not terribly unpleasant odor. It's surprisingly loose. In the earliest days of breast feeding, a small spot of stool may appear each time the baby feeds, but as he matures the stools become less frequent and larger. After a few months of faithful service, many babies decide to give their rectums a day off. Some babies extend the period a week or more. But when the long-awaited stool finally arrives, it's usually worth waiting for. If the daily stool weighs 30 to 45 grams, the stool after ten days will be 300 to 450 grams. Just like the rain in California; when it rains, it pours.

The stool of the formula-fed infant is much different, and using it as a standard against which to compare breast-milk stool is a too common error. Formula-fed stool is larger, harder, lighter in color, and stronger in odor. There's also more of it. These differences are entirely due to the differences in the chemical compositions of the two milks, especially the proteins.

Parents often think that their breast-feeding baby, whose stools are runny and wet, has diarrhea. Many happily nursing babies have been weaned for this reason. One way to avoid this mistake is to simply step back and look at the overall picture.

Infants who are breast feeding successfully are happy. They feed well, act well, and gain weight. Infants with diarrhea are sick. They feed poorly, act listless, and don't gain weight. Furthermore, if you take a good look at the stool of certain babies with diarrhea, you may see pus or mucus, or even blood. Even more striking is the difference in the stool's smell. With the incomplete digestion that results from the diarrhea, the baby's stool smells powerfully unpleasant and "sick."

The infrequent bowel movements of many normal, breast-feeding infants is commonly mistaken for constipation. But constipation refers to the passage of the stool, not the lapse of time between movements. If the stool is rock hard, bone dry, and difficult to expel, you will be correct if you say that the baby is constipated, regardless of how much time has passed since the last stool. Babies can deliver one of these pellets every hour and still be constipated.

On the other hand, if the nursing baby's "overdue" stool is like pea soup in consistency, voluminous, and easy to expel, you should say, "Hallelujah!" (See p. 338, **Ref.** 67; see p. 339, **Ref.** 76; see p. 339, **Ref.** 83; see p. 339, **Ref.** 86.)

Straining at Stool

Babies who are trying to move their bowels commonly turn red in the face, perspire, and grunt for a while. Some bear down so hard that a small rim of the baby's anus gets pushed out of the opening. This rim may ooze a pink, watery fluid at the peak of the baby's straining. Of course if the stool is hard and dry, the explanation is constipation. But what if the stool comes out soft and moist? Why was the baby working so hard to push out a soft, wet stool?

Using an old tradition, I'll answer that question by asking you another question. What happens when you squeeze the middle of a compressible tube that has two open ends, one larger than the other? You guessed it. The contents will squirt out the end having the larger opening. The larger outlet offers less resistance. This is exactly what goes on in the infant's large intestine when he attempts to empty his rectum. He squeezes his abdominal muscles, trying to increase the pressure within the lower bowel. Since the size of the baby's anal opening is smaller than the large intestine, the stool has an easier time going up than going down, and much of the baby's straining is unproductive.

What can the baby do? If he were a baby anything-other-than-human, he would get up on his haunches and push out his stool. Even baby hippopotamuses know that getting into a squatting position puts a crimp in the "tube" above the squeeze, changing the downward direction to the one of least resistance. All the baby human can do is look pitiful, and if someone hearing his grunts knows about emptying compressible tubes, the baby is in luck. By bending the baby's hips back and pushing his knees up against his chest, you'll be easing the baby into the position of squatting on his back and he'll have an easier time pushing out his stool. He'll be grateful.

Tight Anus

Many doctors routinely insert a pinkie into the baby's anus to determine its size. Since the anus contracts reflexively around the inserted finger, it now becomes very difficult to know if the anus was too tight to begin with.

Despite this difficulty, some doctors feel that a slight stricture (narrowing) of the rectum can be diagnosed in 25 to 40 percent of newborns. Of these, only one in four has any difficulty with bowel movements, and by three to six months of age virtually all of the "narrow anuses" become "normal" with no "treatment" ever applied.

All that means to me is that some normal newborns have narrower rectums than others. (See p. 336, **Ref. 31**.)

Blood in Vomit or Stool

Don't panic. This may not be as bad as it seems. The blood you see in your baby's vomit or stool may not even be his. It might be his mother's. There's still no reason to panic; she (or you) won't miss it.

Babies who swallowed tiny amounts of maternal blood can show bloody vomit or stools for hours. Your doctor can do a simple chemical test on the hemoglobin of the passed blood and determine whether it's the fetal type (coming from the baby) or the adult type (coming from the mother). Obviously, if the blood belongs to the baby, any further discussion doesn't belong in this book. If it's the mother's blood, there are only a few possibilities that can explain its presence in the baby's intestine.

If blood from Mother's placenta or cervix gets into the amniotic fluid, it will eventually be swallowed by the baby. Blood from the amniotic fluid is a common cause of bloody vomit and stool during the baby's first day and, despite its alarming nature, it's usually clear that the baby is well.

Swallowed maternal blood later on in the baby's life is less obvious, but can usually be traced to cracks in the mother's nipples. Mother's nipple sores may not look very impressive, but when the baby sucks on them, enough blood can be drawn out to produce bloody stools. The blood won't hurt the baby or his mother, and all that's needed is additional nipple care to heal the sores.

We have been taught that gastrointestinal bleeding is a sign of cancer. While this is true sometimes in adults, it is almost never true in infants or older children. (See p. 336, **Ref. 31**.)

4. Nervous System

JERKING MOVEMENTS

The normal newborn can pull a few quick moves on you that would be distinctly abnormal if he were a grown child. An infant's convulsive jerks and unexpected quivers are such standard procedure that their absence might be cause for concern. The immature nervous system functions so differently from the adult's that anyone unfamiliar with newborns might think that they were neurologically impaired. Even when your baby is resting blissfully, he'll move in certain ways that, if he were only a few months older, would be extremely worrisome.

For example, your newborn rests with his arms back, his elbows bent, and his hand held in a tight fist with the thumb tucked under the other fingers. If you try to uncrook his elbow, his arm will spring back to his "straphanger position" with so much force that he may punch himself in the head. You'll be equally unsuccessful if you try to pry his fist open and rearrange his thumb into a "normal" position. For the first 16 weeks of life, the straphanger is his only normal position; anything else would be abnormal.

If your resting newborn is startled by a sudden noise or a bang on his crib, or by some other disturbance, he'll shoot his arms and legs out to the sides, open his fists, then pull his extremities back in toward the midline in a series of movements that look like hugs. These hugging movements are called Moro's reflex, after the man who first described them. If any excavation is going on near the hospital, each blast of dynamite will elicit the reflex simultaneously in all the newborns in the nursery, which then looks like a baby exercise class. Once the baby is at home, Moro's reflex lasts for 16 weeks. It gradually fades away, and should be gone by six months.

At six months, your baby will begin to show the startle response, which is actually a "mature" Moro, without the elbow stiffening or fist opening. He may also produce another type of jerking movement during his early sleep. As some babies drift into sleep, they show a repetitive, symmetrical, synchronous jerking of their hands and feet. This is called benign neonatal sleep myoclonus (*myo* means muscle; *clonus* equals jerk), and is entirely normal as long as the baby is asleep, not awake. It's probably related to the sudden shuddering movement that many adults make as we fall asleep and proceed to knock our partners out of bed with our jerking. Mine usually gets a 5 on the Richter scale. (See p. 339, **Ref. 87.**)

JITTERY MOVEMENTS

During early infancy, it's normal for babies' arms and legs and chins to tremble slightly, especially when they cry. If you've ever seen a convulsion, you might think that you're seeing another one now. You're not. You're seeing the immature nervous system at work. Though these tremors might be confusing at first, there are several ways to distinguish them from convulsions.

In the first place, convulsions often produce abnormal eye movements. Newborn jitteriness doesn't. Second, convulsions are unexpected. They occur when they want to and not as a response to some external event or situation. Newborn jitters can be caused by handling, allowing the baby to cry, or any other type of stimulation. Just as convulsions are self-starting, they're also self-stopping. On the other hand, you can easily put a stop to newborn tremors simply by flexing the affected limb, or holding it still.

The last, and subtlest, way to distinguish between the convulsion and the normal jitter is to closely watch the movement. The convulsive movement goes through a fast phase, followed by a slow one. Tremors, or newborn jitters, have alternating movements that are of equal rate.

Once you've decided that the movement is a tremor and not a convulsion, the next step to take is to decide what kind of tremor it is. There are two kinds: ordinary (fine) and pronounced (coarse).

The ordinary tremor is fast (6 or more beats per second), and the movement is limited to 3 centimeters in either direction. The pronounced tremor is slower and the movement covers more than 3 centimeters. The ordinary tremor has no significance at all. If your baby has it, just chalk it up to the healthy but immature nervous system.

The pronounced tremor is sometimes associated with sick nervous systems, but if the baby has no serious infection, metabolic imbalance, or mother addicted to narcotics, the pronounced tremor alone isn't enough evidence to indict the entire nervous system.

The most that can be said about even the pronounced tremor is that it's frequently associated with difficult deliveries. It appears to be a nonspecific response to a stressful birth, but in the absence of other factors, the pronounced tremor is benign and is no sign of future problems. (See p. 339, **Ref. 88.**)

SLEEP-WAKE PERIODS

In my 20 years as a pediatrician, I've only heard one mother complain that her baby slept too much and I always worried about her. Ralph Waldo Emerson's practice must have been similar to mine since he said, "There never was a child so lovely but his mother was glad to get him asleep." There's no question that *mothers* need to have their babies sleep long hours, especially if they're the right hours. The question is: What do *babies* need?

The answer is: Not as much as we've all been led to believe. Not only were the old estimates of babies' sleep requirements way over the mark, but we now know that babies' sleep needs differ considerably one from another. From closely watching newborns in the hospital nursery, we've learned that newborns spend from 10.5 to 23 hours per day sleeping, the average being 16.6 hours per day. More time is spent asleep than awake during most of infancy, but exactly how the hours are divided varies tremendously from infant to infant. In this age of bottom lines, however, the bottom line for most parents is whether or not the baby is sleeping through the night. And if not, why not?

When you're evaluating your baby's sleeping habits, the first fact you should be aware of is this: It's always somebody else's baby who sleeps through, not only the first night home, but also every other night until the end of time. Accept this as a given and don't allow yourself to be disappointed by your baby so soon after she's born. There's time for that later.

We've learned by videotaping babies in their cribs at home that slightly *less* than half of all two-months-olds either sleep soundly or barely awaken through the night. The proportion of these solid sleepers increases to almost four fifths by the time they're nine months old. But here's the rub. According to parents, these figures are too low. When we add up the answers from parents who have completed questionnaires on the subject, we find that many more than half of their two-months-olds are sleeping through the night.

Why this discrepancy? The answer is probably either that pride makes parents exaggerate the quality of their babies' sleeping habits, or that fatigue prevents them from hearing their babies' cries and they truly think their babies sleep through the night. Either way, it doesn't really matter. No matter how we test babies' sleeping habits, we find that the distinctions between sleepers and nonsleepers disappear as half of the "good sleepers" become "bad sleepers" and vice versa before their first birthdays.

Not only does the amount of sleep change as an infant matures, but the quality of his sleep changes as well. We've come a long way from the sleep fairy in our understanding of the nature of sleep. We now recognize two distinct phases:

One phase, active sleep, is called REM (rapid eye movement) and quiet sleep is imaginatively called non-REM. Roughly 20 percent of the total sleeping time of adults is spent in REM sleep. The rest of their sleep time is non-REM. In the infant, 45 to 50 percent is REM, 35 to 45 percent is non-REM, and 10 to 15 percent is too disorganized to be classified and is called indeterminate sleep.

Most adult REM (active) sleep occurs during the last third of the sleep period. The infant's REM sleep happens throughout the night. (Some people believe that infants' extra REM sleep provides them with extra brain stimulation, which enhances their rapid brain growth.)

The adult's non-REM sleep is classified into four stages. He begins his non-REM sleep cycle with stage 1 (quiet) and progresses into a deeper and deeper sleep until he reaches stage 4. The adult then returns to stage 2, followed by a period of REM sleep. This is his time to have a sweet dream. After the period of REM, the adult reenters non-REM and starts a new sleep cycle. A typical night's sleep encompasses four to six of these cycles, each one lasting 90 to 100 minutes. Newborns have entirely different sleep cycles. They enter sleep via REM instead of non-REM, and the cycles are completed every 45 to 50 minutes. So, as you can see, your infant's sleep differs a great deal from your own. Many of the differences between adult and infant sleep begin to disappear when babies are about three months old, the age when most of them begin to assume better sleeping habits. At three months, infants enter sleep with prolonged non-REM, which has now, like adult sleep, become differentiated into four stages. Research may eventually show that infants need to be awake during the night, and only after this need is met will they sleep through.

Did you notice that I never once mentioned the role of solid foods in helping the infant sleep? That's because solid foods have nothing to do with the brain's maturation, and the brain's maturation has everything to do with your baby's sleeping through the night. (See p. 339, **Ref. 89**; see p. 340, **Ref. 90**; see p. 340, **Ref. 91**; see p. 340, **Ref. 92**.)

HEAD NODDING *(Spasmus Nutans)*

Spasmus nutans (*spasmus* means spasm; *nutans* is nodding) usually begins between the baby's 3rd and 12th months of life. Some cases have been reported in newborns, but since these reports have been coming in less often these days, I suspect that some of the cases diagnosed earlier may have really been something else, like congenital nystagmus.

In its full-blown version, spasmus nutans has three components. Most often, it begins with a rhythmic nodding of the head in the horizontal or lateral direction. When the baby is concentrating or asleep, the nodding doesn't occur at all.

The second component is torticollis (see p. 77). If the baby is trying to study an object, he tilts his head to the side and stares out of the corners of his eyes.

Third, we see horizontal jerking eye movements, or nystagmus (see p. 68). In the case of spasmus nutans, these jerking eye movements are often more prominent in one eye, and may even be limited to just one eye. You can cause the eye movements to increase by holding the baby's head still.

Well-behaved spasmus nutans disappears by the time the child is three years old. Severe nearsightedness and a tumor of the eye nerve cause similar nodding spasms, but these conditions don't disappear at three. Since the nodding spasms of both the harmless and the serious condition are so much alike, it's important to have an eye specialist examine all children with symptoms of spasmus nutans. Doctors used to believe that spasmus nutans was caused by poor lighting at home, emotional deprivation, or a disturbed mother-child relationship, and that children who had it might eventually show other behavioral problems, such as temper tantrums or shyness. But careful study of the families of children with spasmus nutans has shown that they're no different from families of normal children, so we can now say with full confidence that we have no idea what causes spasmus nutans. (See p. 340, **Ref. 93**; see p. 340, **Ref. 94.**)

TWISTING AND TURNING *(Paroxysmal Torticollis)*

Sometimes a baby awakens from sleep with his head tilted to the side. He may hold it there for a few hours or days before returning it to the center, and may turn it to the right one time, and the left the next. Some babies also throw their heads back and hold their trunks in a stiff posture during these episodes, which are called paroxysmal torticollis. Babies with paroxysmal torticollis usually act well in all other regards, though at times they appear to be dizzy or nauseated.

Episodes of paroxysmal torticollis can occur several times each month and stop completely when the child is three years old. Many of the mothers of these children have migraines, and some of the children develop their own migraines later on. Other than this condition, the episodes are harmless. (See p. 340, **Ref. 95**; see p. 340, **Ref. 96.**)

"BENIGN" CONVULSIONS

Convulsions cannot be regarded as benign. They represent abnormal brain activity and their cause should be ascertained as quickly as possible. When convulsions begin in early infancy, they may signal birth injury to the nervous system, or some chemical imbalance such as low blood sugar or calcium. When they occur repeatedly in the newborns of a particular family, some familial genetic disease could be creating a metabolic problem for the baby's nervous system.

But not all convulsions have such dire causes. When the convulsing newborn looks as good and acts as healthy as his nonconvulsing nursery roommates (when he isn't convulsing, that is); when he develops normally into a fine, healthy infant; when he stops having the convulsions by six to eight months of age; and when he has a bunch of relatives who grew up normally despite these same early episodes, you know you're dealing with a "benign" condition. Warning: You must still rule out the serious reasons for infant's convulsions. If that has been done, and if convulsions run in the family, what you're left with is little more than a family tradition that the family could do without. (See p. 340, **Ref. 97.**)

NERVE COMPRESSION WEAKNESS *(Peripheral Paresis)*

If a fetus's nerve gets caught between a fetal bone and a "hard place," and if the fetus is unable to change positions, the nerve can be injured. If the nerve compression occurs late in the pregnancy, you can expect a full return of strength within a few days after birth. The earlier in the pregnancy the nerve is injured, the later it will return to normal, and the more likely that the nerve function will be incomplete. The facial nerve (see p. 62), where it exits from the skull on either side of the ear, is the most frequent victim of this squeeze. In this case, the fetal skull is the bone, and the hard place is either the mother's pelvis or the doctor's forceps. Compression of the main trunk of the facial nerve produces weakness extending from the baby's forehead to her chin. If the compression is limited to one of the branches of the nerve, the weakness will be limited to whatever muscle is under the control of that particular branch. Most often, the branch compressed is the one that closes the baby's eyelid. When this happens, the baby will be unable to close his eyelid tightly.

Nerves that affect the extremities can be compressed as well. If the upper part of the fetal arm gets jammed against the rib cage, the radial nerve, which courses around the upper arm bone, the humerus, can be compressed. In this case, both the bone and the hard place belong to the fetus. When the radial nerve is compressed, the wrist droops.

Do you know what happens when the sciatic nerve is compressed? You got it: the foot droops.

In the vast majority of cases, unless the injury occurs early in the pregnancy, the nerve will return to normal function in a few weeks or months. (See p. 335, **Ref. 13**; see p. 340, **Ref. 98.**)

REPETITIVE, RHYTHMIC MOVEMENTS

Babies often use their mouths, lips, heads, trunks, and legs in repetitive, rhythmic ways. We still don't know if they do this to satisfy some primitive instinct, provide pleasure, release tension, drive you crazy, or actually promote development of the nervous system. For whatever reason, almost all normal babies do it.

The first of these activities is hand sucking. Ninety percent of all normal newborns suck their hands within the first two hours of life. The other 10 percent probably do it, too. We just didn't see them.

All babies have been engaged in this activity since they were in the womb. Kicking begins a few months later. Joyously happy newborns often show their ecstasy by rhythmically drawing their legs in and shooting them out. While this is going on, they may flap their arms up and down in time with their leg movements. These babies grow up and become older children who do a lot of foot dangling, especially when they're sitting on a fence. If you ever sat next to an adult nervously bouncing his foot up and down, you don't need to be told that rhythmic foot movements can persist for a long time.

Rhythmic movements are used by some babies to help them fall asleep. Some babies very slowly thump their leg against the mattress; some rhythmically scratch against the bed sheet with one finger (producing that eerie sound heard throughout the house at strange hours).

Children have several more rhythmic habit patterns that they generally start exercising at an older age. These patterns are described on p. 218. (See p. 340, **Ref. 99.**)

5. URINARY SYSTEM

THE FIRST VOIDING

The fetal kidney begins to create urine in the fourth month of the pregnancy, and at that point the fetal bladder empties it into the amniotic cavity in the womb. Without fetal urine, there would be considerably less amniotic fluid.

Ninety-three percent of newborns' first voidings take place within the first 24 hours after birth. Ninety percent of the rest urinate during the second day of life. Those babies who still haven't voided after the second—not the *first*—day should be evaluated.

Your baby's first few squirts are usually small amounts of dark, murky urine. This "sludge" appearance is the result of a high concentration of sodium urate crystals as well as certain proteins. The typical newborn urinates 16 to 24 times per day. Each voiding produces 15 to 25 milliliters, and the total amount of urine for the day is 45 to 70 percent of the baby's total fluid intake for the day. During his first six months of life, your infant will continue to void as often as he did the first days, but he'll increase the volume of the voiding to 20 to 35 milliliters.

The newborn's and infant's bladder is very different from the adult's. The adult bladder is dome-shaped and, unless it's very full, it stays within the pelvis. Your baby's bladder is spindle-shaped and extends up into the abdominal cavity, even when it's completely empty.

A baby's bladder also functions differently. The adult bladder empties when told to, leaving behind just enough urine to dampen its inside lining. No one can tell the newborn bladder when to empty, and when it does, enough is left behind to dampen anyone daringly standing directly in the way. Ask any pediatrician if this isn't so.

BRICK-DUST DIAPER STAIN *(Urate Crystals)*

Urine loaded with sodium urate—a compound normally excreted by infants—takes on a strange color. Depending on the urine's freshness and concentration, the color will be a brown-red or an orange-red.

If you've just joined the scores of parents who have been scared out of their wits by their baby's "blood-stained" diapers, stay calm for a few moments. Don't wrestle the diaper to the ground and rip it into shreds. Put it in a brown, unmarked bag and bring it and your baby to your pediatrician. Using simple methods, the doctor can test the "damned spot" for its hemoglobin content. If it flunks the test, it isn't blood; it's just ordinary brick-dust diaper stain. If, while you're sitting in the waiting room, the infamous diaper dries out, you'll see that the red spot has become a powdery collection of easily scraped-off "brick dust." You can laugh all the way home.

If, for some reason, your baby's reddish diaper has been destroyed, get a fresh urine sample from the baby and bring that to the doctor so she can examine it under the microscope. She'll quickly see if any red blood cells are present, or if, as is most likely the case, the red color came from urate crystals. In this case, nothing has to be done. With your nerves being the exception, no harm has been done.

6. Growth

UNEXPECTED SIZE

Doctors commonly compare a child's measurements—be they weight, head, or any other measurements—with those of other similar children, and express the comparison as a percentile. For example, if your baby's measurement is greater than that of 90 percent of similar children, we say that the child is in the 90th percentile with respect to that measurement. If he's smack in the middle, he's in the 50th percentile. According to this scheme, some children are at the extremes of percentiles, while most cluster around the middle. It has become customary to refer to the children whose measurements fall between the 3rd and 97th percentiles as normal, and those below the 3rd or above the 97th as abnormal.

Most of the time, human beings, like all other living things, breed true. Big parents tend to produce big babies. McIntosh apple trees tend to produce apples of the same name. But sometimes big parents produce small newborns, and sometimes large newborns end up as small adults. You can understand these apparent contradictions if you look at growth as a series of separate and distinct growing seasons rather than a single, continuous process. Actually, the adult's final size represents the end result of five separate "eras" of growth, each having its own set of influences. Your newborn's size is the outcome of only one growth era, the fetal period, and the factors that influence fetal growth determine his size. Some of these factors remain and continue to influence subsequent growth, while some are never heard from again.

Of all the factors influencing fetal growth, the most important one is the size of the mother, and if fathers think about it, they'll realize that this is only fair. When a Shetland pony mother has a foal with a full-sized father, the newborn horse is only one third the size of the offspring of a Shetland pony father and a full-sized mother. The mother must have the last word in influencing fetal size, since it's her body that the fetus grows in, and exits from. If this weren't so, can you imagine the consequences of a mating between a Great Dane father and a Chihuahua mother? Don't think about it too long.

Another factor influencing the fetus's growth is the fetal environment. Crowding in the womb restricts more than the fetus's movements; it also restricts growth. The opposite is also true; the more spacious the accommodations, the larger the baby. During the last two months of pregnancy, the fetus doubles in mass, growing to the limits of the inner wall of the womb. Twins grow at the normal rate for the first 30 weeks of pregnancy, but as soon as they fill up the womb their growth rate falls off, and for this reason twins tend to be small.

Uterine crowding also explains why firstborn infants tend to be smaller than second ones, that is, babies born of mothers who have had their wombs prefilled, and therefore prestretched. Also, since mothers' wombs are smaller in first pregnancies, firstborns fill the uterine cavity earlier and their growth rates decelerate earlier. Your baby's size is also affected by the other "member" of the womb, the placenta, which like uterine size ends its influence once the baby is born. Big placentas don't necessarily mean big babies, but if the pregnancy extends significantly beyond the normal 40 weeks, your baby may be on the slender side. This is because, after 40 weeks, placentas tend to run out of steam. Worn-out placentas don't adequately nourish babies, and typically "postmature" babies look as if they'd been dieting. If the placenta was damaged by the mother's elevated blood pressure, or cigarette smoking, the baby would tend to be small as well as skinny.

Another determinant of your baby's size is gender. Baby boys grow faster than girls during the last eight weeks of the pregnancy, and as a result boys are, on the average, 0.9 centimeter longer and 150 grams larger than baby girls. (See p. 340, **Ref. 100.**)

PART TWO

The Preschooler—

From Six Months to Six Years

Physical Conditions

1. Skin, Hair, Nails

YELLOW SKIN *(Carotenemia)*

This condition presents no problem for baby or parents until someone happens to notice that the baby is yellow, especially at the tip of the nose, palms, soles, and chin. At that point, considerable anxiety and money is often spent before a diagnosis of the harmless condition known as carotenemia is finally made. This is a shame because all that's needed for a correct diagnosis is to look the baby in the eye. If the whites of his eyes are white, the baby has carotenemia.

It's true, of course, that a baby's yellow skin can be an indication of a number of true diseases. But not if the whites of his eyes are white! This crucial point is sometimes overlooked, and I've seen several thriving, robust, white-eyed, yellow-beaked infants with carotenemia needlessly hospitalized for evaluation of suspected liver disease.

Carotenemia is simply the result of a carotene-rich diet. Carotene is the yellow pigment that gives carrots their color, and when babies eat large amounts of carrots or any other carotene-rich food, the serum level of carotene in their blood increases. When it exceeds a certain level (250 micrograms per deciliter), the thick outer layer of the baby's skin takes on the yellow color.

Contrary to all appearances, not only yellow vegetables are carotene rich. Other less obvious carotene-rich foods include asparagus, beans, broccoli, cucumbers, lettuce, mustard, and spinach. (The green pigment in these vegetables, chlorophyll, masks the yellow of the carotene.) Fruits rich in carotene include apricots, cantaloupes, mangoes, oranges, papayas, peaches, and prunes. And, surprisingly, butter, eggs, and milk contain plenty of the yellow pigment as well.

Some parents, under the assumption that every diagnosis has to have a treatment, change their carotenemic baby's diet to green vegetables, but they're usually disappointed with the results. A baby who's yellow from eating too much squash doesn't get any less yellow when he's switched to eating too many green beans.

On the other hand, some parents actually like carotenemia because it looks much like a tan. Skin-tanning products at the drugstore are actually carotenoid pigments and the people who use them are, happily, developing their own harmless carotenemia.

If you're inclined to fight carotenemia, you can do it without switching to green vegetables. Vegetables that have been pureed, mashed, and homogenized have their cell membranes ruptured, making their carotene more easily available for absorption. On the other hand, coarsely chopped vegetables of any kind don't produce this condition. Thus, by changing only the method of preparation—not the diet—you can eliminate your baby's carotenemia. The carotene in the coarsely chopped vegetables is still there, but less available for absorption.

Manufacturers of infant food usually include carrots in their meat-and-vegetable combination dinners, chicken and noodle dinners, as well as spaghetti dinners, so you can assume that any baby eating commercially prepared strained baby foods is getting a carotene-rich diet. (See p. 340, **Ref. 101**; see p. 340, **Ref. 102**.)

PALE SKIN *(Pallor)*

Depending on your point of view, light-colored skin is either "pale" or "fair." Fair skin is much appreciated in the world of literature. Writers use the word *fair* to describe the skin of damsels, maidens, Scandinavian beauties, Nordic heroes, and Erin colleens. On the other hand, parents, and particularly grandparents, don't favor that romantic adjective; to them, the baby's skin is "pale." Pale skin isn't popular with this group because it raises the specter of anemia, an unhealthy reduction in the amount of red blood cells. It's true that anemic children are pale, but most often pale children aren't anemic. Most of the time, the child's pallor is innocent, and the specter of anemia needn't have been raised. Here are a number of ways that you can put the specter down.

The most significant factor accounting for skin color is the density of the pigment melanin within the skin. This dark pigment is produced by special cells, the melanocytes (*melas* means black; *cyte* equals cell), which are scattered throughout the deeper layers of the skin. When these cells are stimulated by ultraviolet radiation, they make more pigment.

If your baby isn't getting much exposure to ultraviolet radiation, her pigment-producing cells won't get much stimulation and she'll appear pale. This happens when the sunshine is minimal, or when the child spends a lot of time indoors. Sometimes this situation can be corrected by taking your baby with you to Acapulco. On the other hand, sometimes it can't.

Some children are pale because their skin is sparsely endowed with melanocytes. No matter how much time they spend in the sun, they're still pale. These are the children of northern European ancestry, and when it comes to tanning, they should probably be considered lost causes. Acapulco won't help.

Another factor influencing skin color is the amount of blood coursing through the skin. Babies who are overheated by overactivity or overdressing have skin that's overcirculated. Their hot skin looks rosy-red, as does that of babies who are flushed with fever and babies just brought into a warm house after being out in the cold air.

The opposite happens when the skin's circulation is reduced. Babies who are assaulted by cold, pain, fatigue, or fear can pale before your eyes.

In short, skin color is seldom an accurate indicator of anemia. An anemic Hispanic baby who's tanned, overdressed, and feverish will have a deeper skin tone than a nonanemic light-skinned baby. Pale skin is usually best detected in areas that aren't normally pigmented or affected by changes in the skin's circulation, such as the eyelids, tongue, inside lip, and gums. If any of these areas isn't as red as your doctor would like, she'll take a blood count to see if anemia is present. If the physician finds your baby's pallor has no clinical significance, she can still make a diagnosis. The one that I make most often in this situation is "February." It goes away by itself.

BRUISES *(Ecchymoses)*

Many infants are born with ecchymoses, purple blotches that result from skin bleeding. Childbirth has its hard knocks, but once the newborn is no longer cramped into the bony confines of his mother's pelvis, and the bruises of birth trauma have faded, the infant enters a bruise-free period in his new sheltered, cushioned surroundings in the crib. Any bruising during this early period when your baby is stationary is cause for concern. Once he starts to get around, though, certain bruises become a part of the scenery. Pediatricians are so accustomed to seeing these familiar bruises that when a year-old infant doesn't have them, the doctor wonders if the baby is getting around enough.

For example, babies begin bruising their foreheads as soon as they start pulling up to a standing position. They take no exception to the rule that what goes up must eventually come down, often on surfaces hard enough to cause good-sized black-and-blue marks. Even more common are the bruises covering the toddler's shins from his ankles to his knees. Once children begin staggering and stumbling, their shins take on the familiar black-and-blue decor. Toddlers without decorated shins are either future Olympic medalists or aren't doing their share of toddling.

As a rule, ordinary bruises are found over bones and they have a reasonable explanation for being there. Problem bruises can appear anywhere and aren't necessarily caused by the baby's own activity. Sometimes the excuse for an ordinary bruise isn't immediately apparent, but when you question the child carefully about his habits, the explanation appears. Habitual head bangers, for example, habitually have bruised heads. Rocking-chair enthusiasts and break dancers have bruised backs, and children who lean their chins on the table when resting may have bruised chins. If enough force is applied to the skin, a bruise can appear anywhere. Often, parents bring their children to the doctor to be "exonerated" of supposed child abuse after some well-meaning neighbor "jokingly" asks how the bruises got there.

Some bruises leave behind a small nodule just beneath the skin. If this lump were examined under the microscope, you would see fibrous scar tissue growing into a collection of blood. This is one of the several methods by which the body deals with hematoma (*hemato* refers to blood;

oma is swelling) and the nodule gradually softens with time and disappears. This sort of bruise is called an organized hematoma.

Bruises inside the mouth are usually more serious, medically. On the other hand, I've seen a child with bruises on the roof of her mouth that disappeared as soon as she was persuaded to give up her habit of sucking on her tongue while pressing it up against her hard palate.

LUMP AFTER DPT INJECTION *(DPT Granuloma)*

By six months of age, most babies should have received three injections of the diphtheria-pertussis-tetanus vaccine (DPT). A fourth injection is usually given at 18 months and a fifth at 5 years. The last two shots are called boosters. These immunizations are usually injected into the outer half of the upper thigh muscle in the front, side, or back.

Roughly 60 percent of all babies develop mild local reactions consisting of redness, swelling, or tenderness at the site of the injection directly after the first three vaccinations. The other 40 percent get a more severe reaction consisting of some combination of redness, swelling, and tenderness. After the last two boosters, the ratio is exactly the reverse.

Sometimes, if the needle accidentally pierces a small vein on the way to the muscle, blood seeps out and accumulates under the skin. The bluish swelling that results is, again, a hematoma (see p. 148). Pressing on the swelling stops the ooze, and eventually there appears a bruise that's soon absorbed. If your baby has sustained one of these harmless hematomas, you may notice it while you're still in the doctor's office. Other DPT-related swellings may not appear for several days.

The most common delayed swelling is the DPT granuloma, which is caused by a low-key inflammatory reaction to some injected material that remains in the tissues of the baby's thigh. A DPT granuloma is a firm, painless lump under the skin, usually the size of a dime or quarter. If you pucker the skin around the lump, a dimple will appear precisely at the spot where the needle entered the skin. The lump can remain on the baby's thigh for weeks to months but it finally disappears. Parents seldom worry about DPT granulomas if they notice them immediately after the immunization. If they don't happen to see the lumps for a while, the connection with the immunization isn't so apparent and *can* become a mystery that someone with a scalpel might want to solve. If you're not sure what caused the lump on your child's thigh, take him back to the person who gave the injection and ask if the location of the lump is the same as that of immunization. If the answer is yes, your answer to the scalpel is no. You should, however, ask the person who gives your child his next DPT to apply it in a different area, deeper in the muscle, and to massage the area after giving the injection. Very few babies are severely irritated by DPT injections and develop an accumulation of pus, but those that do will need the attention of a physician.

LUMPS AND BUMPS *(Subcutaneous Masses)*

Most lumps and bumps on a child's body are discovered when a parent or grandparent is bathing the baby. If you find one or more of these, you will, of course, take the baby to your pediatrician to have her examined. The explanation that follows will help you understand how your doctor makes a diagnosis of the lump and why he draws certain conclusions about it.

Some lumps are no big mystery to doctors. Their location, appearance, or circumstance gives away their identity. For example, physicians know where normal lymph nodes occur in the body, and when we feel a lump in one of these places, and the lump has the characteristics of a lymph node, we conclude that it must indeed by a lymph node. Similarly, thyroid nodules, breast masses, and scrotal swellings all have their own features that make them recognizable. If we see a lump in the thigh in the exact area where a DPT injection has been given, we know that the lump is a DPT granuloma (see p. 149).

On the other hand, some lumps can't be immediately labeled. This makes them "unexplained lumps," and no one likes the unexplained, especially if it's a part of your very own baby. It's only natural that you'll worry. Your doctor will also worry if any of the five following risk factors are present:

The first is the age of the child. A lump appearing during the first month of life is worrisome. The second risk factor is growth, that is, a lump that's rapidly growing. The third: a lump that's deep in the tissue and appears to be cemented to it. Fourth, ulceration of the skin over the lump. Fifth, a lump that's hard and measures more than 3 centimeters at its greatest diameter.

If any of these factors are present, your doctor will have the lump promptly removed. Obviously, the greater number of these risk factors that are present, the faster the lump should become an ex-lump. Overall, only 6 to 7 percent of children's lumps have one or more of these characteristics, and research has shown that only one fifth of these are malignant.

What of the remaining unexplained lumps that don't have any of the five risk factors and, therefore, aren't speedily lopped out?

Six percent of these lumps don't need to be removed because they disappear in due time, or get "explained" by some means other than removal, and can then be left in place. Among these are benign rheumatoid nodules.

Children who are afflicted with rheumatoid arthritis often develop skin nodules, usually in front of the shins and over the instep. These firm, colorless lumps are painless and can vary in size from less than 1 centimeter to several centimeters. They may grow quickly, don't move much, and are fixed to the deeper but not overlying tissues.

A completely healthy child can develop identical lumps and these can be puzzling until they're biopsied. When microscopic examination shows them to be the same as the typical rheumatoid nodule, these lumps are called benign rheumatoid nodules. The lumps need no special attention. They may come and go for several years until they decide to leave for good. Children with benign rheumatoid nodules are normal and have no more tendency toward rheumatic diseases than those who don't have these nodules. (A diagnosis of benign rheumatoid nodules is usually made by a specialist.)

Also among the 6 percent of transient lumps are those that are regularly seen with certain skin disorders. Once the skin diagnosis is made, the lump can be judged by its cover.

What of the remaining 85 to 90 percent of superficial childhood lumps? Some slowly grow. Others slowly stick around. Since these lumps lack any of the five risk factors, your doctor's diagnosis that they're benign will be 99.7 percent accurate. The other side of that statement is that 3 in 1,000 will be malignant. For some reason, most parents identify themselves with the minority and are a lot happier after the surgeon goes ahead and performs his lumpectomy. For them—and for most doctors—the only good lump is the lump sitting in the pathologist's specimen tray after the operation.

Most lumpectomies are performed in some outpatient location at a convenient time. After it, the pathologist will make microscopic slides from the specimen, examine them, and give the lump its proper name. (See p. 340, **Ref. 104**; see p. 340, **Ref. 105**; see p. 343, **Ref. 151**.)

HAIR LOSS *(Alopecia)*

A certain amount of hair loss is normal. Adults lose up to 100 hairs every day. We don't know how much hair a child loses, but we think it's considerably less than 100 per day. If your child is losing a substantial amount of hair, and your physician tells you that the child doesn't have a disease that causes hair loss or a fungus infection of the scalp, the explanation is probably one of the following:

Alopecia areata is a benign condition in which skin suddenly appears where hair used to grow. The hair at the borders of these patches is loose, and the exposed scalp looks and feels entirely normal. If the patch is small, you can expect the hair to grow back within a year or two. If the skin is treated with medications, the hair will also grow back in a year or two. So I suggest you save the money. When the patches are extensive, or the baby is very young, the regrowth may be thin. Why these hairs should suddenly decide to fall out is a big mystery. We used to think that psychological stress had something to do with it, but most skin specialists have found no more stress in this group of children than in any other group.

Much hair is shed in the name of hair care. Trauma to the hair follicle can result from temperature, traction, or pressure. Hot combing, blow drying, and straightening all shake and bake the hair shaft, and before you know it hairs start to fall out, especially those by the hairline.

If too much tension is applied to the hair as a result of tight ponytails or barrettes, braids, or "corn rowing," hair may fall out around the periphery of the pulled tuft.

Black children often have this problem and the damage to the hair can be stopped simply by changing the severe styling to a more natural look.

Sometimes a child's hair loss is caused by trichotillomania (*tricho* means hair; *tillein* is pull; *mania* equals madness), the child's own nervous habit of pulling or playing with her hair. Some children pull or twirl their hair instead of biting their nails when they're tense or frustrated. If they only do it when they're falling asleep, their parents may be totally unaware of the habit. Hair loss caused by trichotillomania is irregular, and you can see short hairs that have managed to escape the grasp of the child's hand within the bald spot.

Spinning on one's head while break dancing breaks hairs off from the top of the head. Jogging while wearing heavy headphones causes its own unique pattern of baldness.

Continuous pressure on the scalp can also cause hair loss. Babies who spend too much time lying flat on their backs lose hair for this reason.

The last of the common causes of hair loss is called telogen effluvium. Following some major stress, such as a very high fever, a convulsion, a crash diet, or profound emotional stress, hairs that were formerly in the active growing phase are suddenly converted into the resting (telogen) phase. Two to four months later, these hairs begin to shed and continue to do so over a four- to six-week period. Unless the stressful event is repeated, all the hair returns. Telogen effluvium explains why so many mothers lose so much hair after childbirth. (Another reason is their babies' newly learned trick of opening their fists and grabbing things. What better thing to grab than their mothers' loose hair? (See p. 340, **Ref. 106.**)

2. Head

HEAD FLATTENING *(Positional Modeling)*

You may not notice that your child's head is flat in the back until you see her sitting up in the doctor's office. You may wonder then how it got that way.

Your baby's head undergoes its first remodeling as it gets squeezed through the birth canal. This reshaping is very temporary and doesn't last beyond the end of the first week. Her head can be subjected to molding once again, however, if it's once again subjected to pressure. Most often, this happens when her head rests in the same position for too long a period of time.

Uncorrected torticollis (see p. 77) subjects a baby's head to uneven pressure, which causes the back of her head to lose its roundness. If her twisted neck points her chin to the left, the right side of the back of her head is subjected to extra contact with the surface that she's lying on. This unequal pressure flattens out the right side of the head.

The same process occurs when your baby spends all of her time lying flat on her back. Babies who are left on their backs because they seem to like it better, and babies who are kept on their backs in the semiupright position to alleviate their spitting up, eventually flatten the backs of their heads. The sustained pressure that flattens these babies' heads also damages their hair, and they're usually bald where they're flat. If this positional flattening is caught early enough, their heads will remodel back to normal and their hair will return.

FOREHEAD RIDGE *(Metopic Ridge)*

You may have seen—or at least felt—a seam running down the middle of your baby's forehead. This is called the metopic ridge, and is the result of the following natural growth process:

The two halves of a child's forehead bone normally fuse together at six to ten years of age, after the skull has done most of its growing. If the bones fuse together while they're still actively growing, when they reach the meeting point they have no place to go but up. Like two giant plates of slowly moving land masses, the two frontal bones meet in the middle and create a ridge.

At least 8 percent of Caucasian adults have such a metopic (meaning forehead) ridge. It runs down the middle of the forehead from the front point of the anterior fontanel (see p. 61) and gradually flattens near its end at the bridge of the nose.

If this fusion occurs very early in infancy, the child's head will appear triangular and the distance between the eyes will be narrowed. Most often, the fusion is only slightly premature and the metopic ridge goes undetected. The parents usually examine their child's forehead for the first time only after his first three-point landing on it, and it is then that they may feel the ridge. It can help you stay calm if you're aware of the ridge before the first great fall. (See p. 336, **Ref. 22.**)

BIG HEAD *(Macrocephaly)*

All babies have relatively large heads for their bodies, so we aren't surprised if the baby's head looks big. To know if it's too big, doctors routinely measure the head circumference with a tape measure and compare the circumference with the measurements of other normal babies.

If a baby is born with a big or rapidly growing head, the cause can be: (1) too much brain water (hydrocephalus), (2) a brain tumor, (3) a thick skull, or (4) an entirely normal but large brain. The latter condition—an extra-large brain—is called primary megalencephaly (*mega* means large; *encephaly* refers to the brain), and it may well be an intellectual advantage. Byron, Bismarck, and Turgenev were all endowed with rare talents and massive heads.

The question is: What will your doctor do when he finds that your baby's head circumference is extra-large? During the years when the definitive big-head evaluation involved hospitalizing the baby to do some difficult and dangerous diagnostic procedures, most doctors, confronted with a seemingly normal but big-headed baby, usually settled for many serial measurements of the baby's head circumference, a skull X ray, and a lot of worrying. In these times, when all that's needed to evaluate a child's head is a simple, multimillion-dollar computerized mechanism (the CAT scanner), who needs to worry? On the other hand, if your doctor would like to help you avoid unnecessary, expensive investigations as well as unnecessary worry, he can do one thing before embarking on a CAT scan.

If your baby's head measures more than two standard deviations greater than the mean for the general population (a somewhat arbitrary statistical figure), the doctor can consider whether it's large for your family.

The doctor will then measure the circumference of your head and compare it to the standard table for adults. If the father isn't present, Mother might know if Father wears hats that are sold in the large or extra-large bin. Half of all big-headed children come from families with big heads, especially among the male members.

It should be no surprise that big heads and the male sex go together. At birth, the baby boy's head is bigger than the girl's by an average of 0.7 centimeter, and the male head remains larger than the female's from then on. Four fifths of all children with megalencephaly are boys. Again, no surprise. (See p. 340, **Ref. 107**; see p. 340, **Ref. 108.**)

SMALL HEAD *(Microcephaly)*

Doctors also worry when a child's head circumference is two standard deviations below the mean for his age and sex. This can happen when the skull bones fuse together too soon, preventing normal brain growth, or when the brain fails to grow at the normal rate. In the latter case, the microcephaly (*micro* means small; *cephaly* refers to the head) is really a result of microencephaly (*encephaly* refers to the brain). Since most microcephaly is found in institutions for the retarded, people often assume that microcephaly is synonymous with mental retardation. This assumption is unwarranted, but not totally surprising. People who go fishing in herring barrels catch herring. If they want to catch other kinds of fish, they have to do their fishing out in the ocean where the selection is greater. The same applies to determining the true incidence of mental retardation in microcephalic children. Most studies of such children are made in institutions for retarded children. If you look for microcephaly in institutions for retarded children, all the children found to have microcephaly will be retarded.

However, when microcephalics are looked for in open, noninstitutional waters, they turn up there as well. And their IQs are no different from those with heads of normal size—assuming, that is, that we define *microcephaly*, as we did in the beginning of this section, as two standard deviations smaller than the norm. If we define it as a head measurement 0.5 centimeter less than the two standard deviations, or three standard deviations below the norm, the chances of retardation are higher than normal. The greater the degree of microcephaly, the greater the likelihood of retardation.

Overall, up to 2 percent of normal schoolchildren have a head circumference two or more standard deviations below the average for their age and sex.

So if your doctor finds that your child's head measures smaller than the norm, remember this: Not every intellectual giant wears an extra-large hat, and some of the finest minds are found in the smallest packages. (See p. 341, **Ref. 109;** see p. 341, **Ref. 110.**)

3. Face

INJURY TO INSIDE OF CHEEK *(Popsicle Panniculitis)*

When your doctor surprises you by labeling what you thought was a skin infection inside your baby's mouth with the term *Popsicle panniculitis,* here's what he means:

Infants who love to suck on cold things, such as ice cubes or Popsicles, can develop cases of inside-the-mouth frostbite. Most infants don't seem to object to icy items remaining in contact with their cheeks, and after a while the cheek's fat pad can be injured by the cold. The result is called panniculitis (*pannulus* is a membrane of fat; *itis* refers to inflammation) and it looks just like an extensive skin infection.

If your baby has a panniculitis one or two days after the ice sucking, the skin over the cold, injured fat pad inside her cheek will grow hard, reddish purple, hot, and painful. The discolored area will spread out from the corners of her mouth and cover her cheeks. If nothing is done, the process will subside and the injury will heal within a few days.

If you bring your baby to the doctor with this skin condition, be sure to tell him about the Popsicle exposure. If you neglect to report it, the doctor might assume the problem is a bacterial infection and prescribe antibiotics. Antibiotics aren't needed for cold injury to the cheeks. All you have to do is avoid Popsicles or ice cubes until the baby is old enough to learn the proper sucking technique. (See p. 341, **Ref. 111.**)

4. Eyes

FARSIGHTEDNESS AND UNEQUAL PUPIL
SIZE *(Hyperopia and Anisocoria)*

If your toddler is diagnosed as being farsighted, this isn't necessarily an abnormal condition.

Most newborns are not only farsighted at birth, they also grow increasingly farsighted until they reach three years of age. Your far-sighted toddler adjusts to this condition by a process called accommodation, and he probably won't need to be treated for it. The average child doesn't have 20/20 vision in each eye until he's five years old, and mild farsightedness is still extremely common even in this age group. If all the five-year-olds who were still seeing 20/30 were put into one room, it would be a very noisy place.

Another common and equally harmless eye condition concerns the pupils, and you may notice this one yourself. Under certain conditions—if, for example, your child has received a blow on his head—your doctor may ask you to check for equality of pupil size. If the pupils aren't equal, neurologic injury might be suspected. But what if his pupils were unequal in size before the hit on the head? This means your child either hasn't completely recovered from his last neurologic injury, or he has some innocent form of anisocoria (*aniso* means unequal; *coria* is the pupil).

If the pupils are unequal, you may wonder which one is abnormal. As a rule, it will be the larger pupil if the unevenness is more striking in bright light; and if the anisocoria is maximal in dim light, it's usually the smaller.

Anisocoria is often familial, and the chances are good that if your baby has it, either his mother or father has it, too. It didn't hurt the parent and it won't hurt the baby. Babies with anisocoria who don't have a family history of it usually have the condition in a milder degree. Sometimes the baby's pupils take turns; one day the right one plays the large pupil and the next day the smaller one. This switching back and forth is called physiologic anisocoria, and it's usually outgrown.

Unequal pupil size can also be caused by unequal vision. In that case, the nearsighted eye has the larger pupil. For this reason, children with anisocoria should be seen by an ophthalmologist, just in case they need glasses to correct their visual problem.

Certain drugs taken internally occasionally cause the pupils to dilate, and one of them, Benadryl, dilates them unevenly. Eye drops unequally dropped into the eyes dilate the pupils unequally. (See p. 336, **Ref. 20**; see p. 336, **Ref. 29**.)

5. Ears

EARWAX *(Cerumen)*

I've never been able to understand why people make such a fuss about earwax. I happen to think that earwax has been getting a bad press for far too long. This protective coating of the outer ear is nothing more than desquamated cells from the skin of the ear canal combined with the oily secretions of the sebaceous glands and the pigmented, watery secretions of other specialized glands in the outer ear. This unique blend gives the wax or cerumen (*cera* means wax) its characteristic color and texture.

The ears of Caucasians and blacks produce a sticky, honey-colored wax, while Oriental ears tend to have a gray, dry, brittle wax that resembles rice bran. The nature of earwax is remarkably constant within the various ethnic groups, but there are, happily, easier ways to determine if a person is Japanese or Irish than by examining his cerumen.

Earwax, like most other body secretions, has several functions. Its sticky, greasy coating provides waterproofing for the outer third of the ear canal, and antibodies secreted into the wax help defend the ear against potential germs.

So why the aversion to earwax? Why the compulsion to enter the ear canal to get rid of it? When it comes to noses, we're content to wipe them when the need arises and feel no need to probe the nasal passages with cotton-tipped swabs. Every other "soiled" body opening settles for being wiped. Why the double standard when it comes to the ear?

I'm sure the answer stems from some mistaken association of earwax with ear dirt. As a result, we're convinced that it's not enough to have the wax that appears at the opening of the canal wiped away; the true "white gove" test is whether all the wax has been removed from the depths of the canal. Anything less than that is apparently a social disgrace. What mother doesn't hold her breath as the doctor examines her baby's ears, hoping against hope that the ears will be found "clean"? In the minds of most people, it seems, protective earwax is on a par with "ring around the collar."

To the rescue, the cotton-tipped swab! Inserting a Q-Tip into the ear has become a standard "hygienic" practice, and the waxy tip of the withdrawn swab sufficient proof of the need to rid the canal of its greasy debris. And what's the reward for this frenzied cleanliness?

For starters, a greatly increased rate of external ear infections, perforated eardrums, impacted wax, and hearing loss.

Hundreds of thousands of ears are injured every year by the insertion of cotton-tipped swabs. It's the number one cause of traumatic perforation of the eardrum. It's the most common reason for earwax getting impacted in the canal, because each and every time a swab is inserted, some wax gets rammed inward. After months of this ritual, the entire canal fills with impacted wax. If the canal's obstruction is complete, a significant hearing loss develops.

What happens if the earwax is left alone? Most of the time, the wax flows to the opening of the canal, where it's easily washed away. Occasionally, this normally discharging cerumen is mistaken for pus, especially when the flow of the wax is speeded up because the temperature in the ear has increased as a result of an ear infection or, for that matter, any infection producing a fever.

Roughly one child in seven has sufficient wax in the canal to make a thorough examination of the ear impossible. These children need to have their cerumen removed only if and when they need a thorough ear examination. The wax doesn't cause hearing loss unless someone impacts it by cotton-tipped swabbing.

I rest my case against the cotton-tipped swab in the ear. (See p. 341, **Ref. 112**; see p. 341, **Ref. 113**.)

6. Mouth

WIDE PINK BAND BETWEEN TWO UPPER FRONT TEETH *(Maxillary Frenum)*

You may notice this band if it bleeds or if someone suggests removing it. It's a vertical fold of mucous membrane that attaches the middle of the upper lip to the middle of the gum. At times the fold, or frenum (*frenum* means bridle), from the upper lip seems particularly wide and appears to take up a lot of space between the two front teeth. It's tempting to have this tissue removed before it causes a permanent, wide space between the teeth. Resist if you can.

An extra-thick frenum looks like a doubled-over, pink rubber band, and it may have a notch where it contacts the gum. Sometimes the frenum continues beyond the gum and attaches to the hard palate. When the primary front teeth erupt, this band creates a wide gap. This isn't the time to see the oral surgeon. Wait until all the front permanent teeth have erupted. The space tends to narrow as each permanent tooth appears, and the frenum usually shrinks from their pressure.

Besides creating the impression that it's going to space out the two front teeth, the frenum also tends to bleed a lot. If your baby falls on his face as he's turning, his upper lip tends to get pulled away from the gum, tearing the frenum. This is one of the "routine" injuries of childhood. If the injured frenum swells up from blood or tissue fluid, it can grow to sizable proportions. Under these circumstances, the frenum can look like a wedge of upper lip that got jammed in between the central incisors. Don't try to free it from the gum; it belongs there.

Cold compresses are all that's needed to shrink it down to size. (See p. 341, **Ref. 114;** see p. 341, **Ref. 115.**)

BREATH ODOR *(Halitosis)*

Offensive breath—halitosis (*halitus* means breath)—doesn't have the same significance for children as for adults. Disorders of the lungs and intestines affect the breath of an adult, but if a cause is identified for the child, it will be in the head and neck area.

Otherwise healthy children with "offensive" breath should have their teeth, gums, nose, and sinuses examined. If no foreign body is seen in the nasal passages and no food debris between the teeth, and if there are no signs of nasal allergy, gum infection, or sinusitis, I would advise less garlic and onions.

This problem tends to embarrass the parents more than the child, and if no medical cause is found, rather than drag the child from office to office, try breath fresheners until the problem blows over. (See p. 337, **Ref. 38.**)

TEETHING *(Dentition)*

Physicians and parents alike hate the unexplained symptom the way nature abhors the vacuum. We often hate it so much that we prefer to invent explanations, however shabby, and then convince ourselves of their truth, rather than allow the symptom to remain unexplained. This fable-for-fact switch gets perfected during the period of the baby's life when she's cutting her primary teeth.

Between 3 and 30 months of age, your baby will have unexplained instances of crying, rashes, fevers, sneezing, spitting, eating disturbances, sleeping disturbances, and too many other disturbances to mention. During this same span of time, teeth will appear in her mouth. Many folks connect this last event with any one or more of the previously mentioned disturbances and believe that the search for an explanation has come to an end.

If the symptom being explained away is trivial, no real harm will be done. In the long run, it doesn't matter much if excess drooling is attributed to overly active salivary glands or to "teething." But when significant symptoms are attributed to teething and real explanations are needed, we have a problem.

In one hospital, during one year, 50 children ranging in age from 3 to 30 months were hospitalized with symptoms of diseases that were attributed by their parents or their family doctor to the teething process. All but two were found to have a significant infection. One had spinal meningitis and 11 had convulsions. Attributing these symptoms to teething was dangerous but not terribly original. None other than Hippocrates himself taught physicians that teething children were prone to convulsions and, apparently, many of his disciples and their patients still believe him. When a large group of practicing pediatricians were recently surveyed about their ideas on teething, a surprising number of them reported their conviction that teething could cause fever, mucus, changes in bowel habits, and rashes. (As you can see, parents aren't alone in their misconceptions about teething.) When these same pediatricians were asked how they treated teething, almost all said they prescribed medications. The medicines used were generally pain-killers of varying strengths, sedatives, and local anesthetics. Fortunately, none were still practicing the ancient art of lancing the gum to ease the tooth through.

Virtually all parents assign some symptoms to teething. Furthermore, most doctors often agree with them, usually because the physicians find the parents' explanations correct or convenient. It's much easier to agree with a parent's harmless "explanation" than try to offer a new one that may require a lot of time and effort. On the other hand, doctors and dentists have been taught for years that teething bears no relation to real illness and that teething should be viewed as a natural and painless process.

So how did this incredibly pervasive teething myth get established so firmly in lay and professional minds? I believe that the answer can be found by looking at each of the myths and the coincidental event in the baby's development. To do this, we'll tackle these "unexplained" symptoms in the sequence that they occur.

The first symptom generally assigned to teething is drooling. It seems reasonable to associate saliva with teeth, since they both originate in the same area. In reality, however, the development of your baby's teeth and her saliva-producing glands proceed at very different rates. The saliva-producing glands grow steadily more active from birth onward, reaching the peak of their activity when the baby is three to four months of age. This high point precedes the eruption of the baby's first tooth by an average of three months. In fact, at three to four months, the baby's first tooth, usually the lower central incisor, is nowhere in sight or reach. The three- to four-month-old baby isn't drooling because he's teething, but because he hasn't yet gained control of the muscles of his mouth, and the surplus saliva dribbles out.

Another symptom often associated with teething is a baby's first infection. By three to four months of age, most babies have had enough contact with sick people to catch an infection. At this age, the protection a newborn normally receives from his mother's antibodies is at its lowest level, and the baby is most vulnerable. This inevitable first infection gets blamed on the inevitable first tooth, which often can't even be seen or felt. It's a bum rap. Careful studies of teething babies' temperatures have shown that teething doesn't elevate the temperature. If the baby is fretful and feverish, the only safe assumption to make is that he has an infection. Many is the innocent gum that has taken the heat for an infected ear.

While all this is going on, the baby's nervous system is making great strides. He learns how to open his fist and how to explore his mouth with his hand. His mouth, opened to allow the fist to enter, also permits the saliva to exit. Who, seeing this busy exchange, would question the assumption that the baby is teething?

Furthermore, after the age of six to eight months, by which time the first tooth has usually erupted, it becomes extremely convenient to blame the teeth for any excessive crying, especially at bedtime. Since crying babies put their fingers in their mouths whenever they cry, for whatever reason, it's easy to assume that the baby is crying because his mouth is bothering him. Not so. By six months of age, babies are fully aware of the fact that their crying can alter human behavior. It can cause people to notice them, pick them up, play with them, take them out of their cribs, and, in general, do what they want. So they cry. If it works, crying becomes the habitual way of manipulating the parents, who are still wondering when the blasted tooth is finally going to cut through. This is how bad habits get established around teething time. To avoid them, keep your eye on what's happening to your baby developmentally and away from what's happening to him dentally.

I always ask parents how their baby is teething because it gives me a chance to talk about some of the problems of normal development, such as separation anxiety, limit setting, consistency, and so on. Parents struggling with teething babies need counseling. What do their babies need?

The great majority need nothing. For most babies, the slow passage of a tooth through the gum is no more painful than the slow passage of a hair through the scalp. For others, it's an annoyance, but one that can be easily relieved by giving the baby a cold, hard item like a teething ring to bite on, or by massaging the gums with a loving, unmedicated finger.

There are several good reasons for ignoring the teething folklore. The first and most obvious one is that it may lead you to postpone getting medical attention for a child with a significant infection. Second, if you attribute all of the baby's behavior to his teething, you won't ask your pediatrician about that behavior or get the answers you ought to have. Finally, if you use medicine as the solution to this natural process so early in your parenting experience, you'll be starting out on the wrong foot. Wouldn't it be better to begin with some nonchemical method of coping with a difficult situation? (See p. 337, **Ref. 38**; see p. 341, **Ref. 116**; see p. 341, **Ref. 117**; see p. 341, **Ref. 118**; see p. 341, **Ref. 119**.)

TONSILS *(Palatine Tonsils)*

When I was 13 months old and had suffered my fourth throat infection, my worried parents took me to an important doctor on Eastern Parkway in Brooklyn. I left my tonsils there.

My father, a tax accountant but would-be doctor, administered the anesthesia. He dripped ether into a funnel that I was trying to breathe through. Miraculously, I lived. It may have been destiny (this book had to be written), but I still thank my lucky stars.

Certainly today, the millions of children who have their tonsils surgically removed receive a great deal more sophisticated care. Nevertheless, for every 16,000 children who have tonsillectomies, 1 doesn't live to come home. One child in 2,400 bleeds so heavily that more than four transfusions are necessary or further surgery is needed to tie off the bleeding artery. These aren't bad odds, but the high stakes make the risk considerable. Is it worth it?

One of the basic tenets of medicine is that treatment of any type should be administered only after carefully weighing all its risks and benefits. If the risk-to-benefit ratio is found to be favorable, treatment is recommended. A generation ago, experts judged the risk-to-benefit ratio for tonsillectomy to be favorable. Let me explain why.

During the Golden Age of the tonsillectomy, doctors believed that the tonsils served no purpose and were only a potential source of respiratory infections. During this preantibiotic era, infections were dreaded much more than they are today. Throat infections were often followed by rheumatic diseases and life-threatening abscesses. Furthermore, since the tonsils had no known function, it made good sense to remove them. As they grew larger and larger, the date for the inevitable tonsillectomy grew closer until eventually the child, and often for convenience' sake all of the siblings, underwent the surgery. After it, some children would show a dramatic drop in respiratory infections and their stories would be told over and over again. The majority would know no benefit other than relief at having gotten the inevitable operation over with.

Now, a generation later, we've learned how to subdue serious throat infections. We've become aware of the vital role that the tonsils play in the throat's fight against infection and we've come to understand that big tonsils are normal at certain ages.

Nevertheless, the controversy over the benefits of tonsillectomy continues, with strong feelings on both sides. Doctors who strongly recommend tonsillectomy today for children with frequent sore throats base their recommendation on personal opinion, parental pressure, or, heaven forbid, financial incentive. On the other hand, doctors who argue vehemently against tonsillectomy are also basing their decision on personal opinion and, heaven forbid, a prejudice against an overly performed procedure. I'll try to be objective.

When tonsillectomies are performed for serious, tonsil-related disease, such as frequent, well-documented strep throat, the likelihood for substantial benefit seems to be at its maximum. This has just been painstakingly proven after an 11-year study of children suffering repeated sore throats. It was concluded that, for these most frequently infected children, having a tonsillectomy will spare them one or two episodes of throat infection for each of the first two years following surgery. After that, surgery doesn't seem to make any difference. And on the other side of the coin is the fact that these children had one more operation and one more general anesthesia than the children not subjected to tonsillectomy. On my balance sheet, the benefits of tonsillectomy, even in the most severe group, are too trivial and brief to justify surgery.

How about size of the tonsils as the reason for removing them? Even today, the most common reason for performing a tonsillectomy is "enlarged tonsils." But before the size of the tonsils can be interpreted, your doctor must consider your child's age. Tonsils are tiny at birth, and usually remain quite small for the first two to three years. During the next three years they grow, and by the time the child is six years old they're adult-sized. Not being content with adult size, they continue their enlargement, and by age ten the average child has tonsils that are twice as large as her parents'. During adolescence, the tonsils gradually shrink to adult size. Anyone used to looking at adults' tonsils would be tempted to call children's tonsils enlarged and, in the old days, that was exactly what happened. Since *enlarged* meant abnormal, out they went. What wasn't recognized was that the tonsils' growth was a direct result of their function.

The tonsils function as a division of the lymphatic system, a great network of vessels and filtration stations. Except for the brain and spinal cord, this system exists everywhere in the body. It wears many hats, being an essential part of our circulatory, digestive, and defensive systems.

As part of the return side of the circulatory system, the lymphatic system's vessels return the fluid that regularly seeps out through the thin walls of the capillaries. In the digestive system, special lymphatic vessels called lacteals play a prominent role and are essential for the absorption of certain nutrients. The part of the lymphatic system that involves the tonsils is the department of defense.

The lymphatic system functions everywhere as the body's lint trap. Since the lint fights back, the trap has to have the capacity to eliminate as well as filter. It works like this: Lymph, the very same fluid that we find in blisters, flows through the lymphatic vessels until it reaches a lymph node. Whatever foreign particles are present get filtered out as the lymph percolates through strategically positioned collections of fighter cells within the lymph node (see p. 171).

As part of the lymphatic system, the tonsils work much the same way. The tonsils, together with the adenoids and the lymphatic tissue at the back of the tongue (the lingual tonsils), make up a deeply entrenched, formidable ring of lymphatic tissue guarding the entrances to the airway and digestive tracts. The adenoids, at the top of the ring, are located behind the nose on the back wall of the throat about 2 to 3 centimeters above the area normally visible when the mouth is open. The lingual tonsils, at the ring's bottom, are on the surface of the rear third of the tongue. This part normally faces the back of the throat and isn't seen unless the tongue is stuck out. If the out-thrust tongue belongs to a child six to ten years old, the back of it looks like it's studded with smooth pink pebbles.

The palatine tonsils (usually called just plain tonsils) make up the two sides of the ring, projecting inward toward the midline from the beds within the side walls of the throat. Tonsillar size is usually gauged by how close their inside surfaces come to touching each other. If they actually meet, they're tenderly referred to as kissing tonsils. However, tonsils also furrow forward, outward, or downward as they enlarge. Since the usual estimate is only based on one of the tonsils' dimensions, it's a poor guide to total size.

This brings us to the new wrinkle in the tonsillectomy question. As the tonsillectomy fell from the ranks of routine surgery to become almost universally condemned by practicing pediatricians, the number of children with massive tonsils grew and we began to see a new, related problem—breathing difficulties.

If the ring of lymphatic tissue surrounding the windpipe's entrance gets large enough, it encroaches upon the airway, increasing the resistance to the flow of air. This greatly increases the work of breathing and eventually strains the chest wall, heart, and lungs. We began to see desperately sick children with heart failure whose only problem was lymphatic obstruction of their upper airways, and who needed immediate, emergency tonsillectomies. As more of these children appeared, we learned to identify them earlier.

Children whose lymphatic tissues are beginning to encroach on their airways show problems with sleep early on. During sleep, especially if a child is lying on his back, his tongue and palate normally fall back, narrowing the upper airway. If his airway is already narrowed, this does it even more. These children snore loudly. Their breathing is irregular and labored, and there may be long pauses between breaths. They often assume strange sleep postures. Some prefer to sleep sitting up. Others keep a finger or two in their mouths, pulling their tongues forward. It's no wonder that, after nights like these, they often have morning headaches, are moody and very sleepy during the day, and do poorly in school. Their voices are nasal, they breathe with open mouths, and they talk as if they had a hot potato in the back of their throats.

Many children with massive tonsils have the daytime symptoms just mentioned without having any sleep disturbance at all. In these cases, we assume that something special is going on during sleep. Perhaps the sleeping brain's control of breathing and muscle tone is involved in this problem.

The relationship of tonsils to breathing problems has only recently been appreciated. At this point, it's still a difficult diagnosis to prove if the condition hasn't progressed to the point of straining the lungs and heart. Our methods of proving the connection between large tonsils and significant problems in the lungs and heart are cumbersome and expensive. I do know this much: Children are still growing pretty big tonsils, and parents who have been getting a deaf ear when they approach the pediatrician about a tonsillectomy may soon be getting a warmer reception from the pediatric cardiologist. (See p. 336, **Ref. 24**; see p. 341, **Ref. 120**; see p. 341, **Ref. 121**; see p. 341, **Ref. 122**; see p. 341, **Ref. 123**; see p. 345, **Ref. 201**.)

SPLIT PIECE OF FLESH AT BACK OF MOUTH *(Bifid Uvula)*

Dangling from the end of the soft palate is a short, cone-shaped structure called the uvula. It's split into two halves in 1 percent of Caucasians, 10 percent of Japanese and American Indians, and 20 percent of the siblings of people who have split or bifid (meaning cleft into two parts) uvulas.

A bifid uvula is actually a "touch of a cleft palate," since it represents a failure of the last section or the two halves of the palate to meet in the midline and fuse together. For this reason, your doctor will feel your child's hard palate with her finger, just to be certain that the bones have fused together. If the bones are fused and there's no gap beneath the covering, there's no need for any further concern. (See p. 336, **Ref. 21**.)

7. Neck

SWELLINGS ON CHIN OR NECK AFTER CONTACT WITH COLD *(Chin-Strap Buckle Panniculitis)*

This isn't a common problem for the Sun Belt crowd.

If exposed skin has prolonged contact with a very cold metal object such as a snap, zipper clasp, or chin-strap buckle, a localized frostbite reaction can occur. If the skin gets wet, it's exceptionally vulnerable. The area affected is usually the neck or the underside of the chin; the more chins the child has, the greater the risk.

You may notice this injury after your child comes in from the cold and gets warm. The cold-injured spot turns from a yellow-white numb area into a hard, swollen, tender, red area. The affected skin remains firm and sharply demarcated from the neighboring skin for several weeks; than it gradually softens.

If the injury is severe, blistering, crusting, and peeling can occur. Even in this case, new skin replaces the damaged skin and no treatment is needed.

The same type of injury can occur without any contact with cold metal if the child's skin has been in contact with ice or exposed to extremely cold air. In those situations, it's most often the cheek that's affected.

For some reason, perhaps related to the chemical makeup of their fat, children are more prone to this type of injury than adults. My personal belief is that it's related to their not knowing when, or being too busy, to come in from the cold.

People living in the Sun Belt are not without a buckle worry of their own. They have the opposite problem. They have to be on the lookout for car seat-belt buckles heating up from the sun's rays and causing severe burns on their babies' exposed skin. (See p. 341, **Ref. 124.**)

BALLOONING NECK *(Apical Lung Herniation and Venous Lake)*

The apex of the lungs normally extends upward out of the chest and into the lower neck. At their highest point, the lungs reach about 2 centimeters above the collarbone. Under most circumstances no one notices, but when some children cry, strain, cough, or forcefully exhale, they create a froglike ballooning in the lower neck. This disappears as soon as they relax. Under ordinary conditions, this ballooning (apical lung herniation) is prevented by the presence of a dense wrapping of gristly connective tissue around the dome of the lung, and we believe that the ballooning only happens to children whose gristly connective tissue is weak or absent from this area. It doesn't matter anyway. No treatment is called for.

The swellings in the necks of another group of children also fill the middle part of the lower neck. These children are also perfectly healthy. Their explanation rests with their veins, not their lungs, and this form of swelling is called a venous lake. It results from a slightly modified flow pattern to the veins of the neck, giving them a bit more difficulty in emptying under certain conditions, such as straining.

You can reproduce the venous lake swelling just by hanging these children upside down for a while, even if they're not straining. This simple maneuver establishes the fact that the swelling is venous, since lung swelling only happens during straining. It's treated the same way. Nothing needs to be done. (See p. 337, **Ref. 40**; see p. 341, **Ref. 125.**)

LUMPS ON NECK *(Enlarged Lymph Nodes or Reactive Lymphadenopathy)*

You may notice some bumps on your child's neck when you bathe or caress her, especially if the child is thin. If your baby is examined by your pediatrician, he may describe the bumps as enlarged lymph nodes. They occur in the following manner:

The lymphatic system, as you may have read in the section on tonsils (p. 105), functions as a part of the body's defense system. The lymphatic vessels are the channels through which foreign material in the lymph fluid, such as that in blisters, is carried to the lymph nodes. Special cells within the nodes trap and eliminate the enemy. The lymph nodes also provide the body with antibodies, and dispatch fighter cells, called lymphocytes, to other parts of the body.

In much the same way as the police department divides the city into precincts and the army divides military theaters into combat zones, the lymphatic system divides the body into lymph-sheds. Every part of the body, except the central nervous system, is defended by a regional network of lymphatic channels flowing toward a central cluster of regional lymph nodes, sometimes called lymph glands.

Like sentinels, these nodes are strategically positioned and poised for action. The action comes when the lymph percolating through the node contains a protein that's recognized as being "foreign." When a lymph node is called to action, among other things, it enlarges. Let us see how.

Foreign proteins, called antigens (*anti* equals against; *gen* means produced), turn on the lymphocyte in two ways. Both processes make the lymph node larger. The first response of the stimulated lymphocyte is to multiply by simple cell division. The node, having more cells than before, gets larger. The other response is an increase in large undifferentiated lymphocytes. This larger cell secretes antibodies, the body's chemical response to the antigen. It also secretes chemicals that recruit other, unexposed lymphocytes to behave as if they, too, had been turned on. Once recruited, the "bystander" lymphocytes undergo the same two processes that the exposed lymphocyte underwent, namely cell division and differentiation into lymphoblasts. The net result of all this activity is lymph node enlargement, and the process is called reactive hyperplasia.

Children's lymph nodes enlarge faster, get bigger, and stay that way longer than adults'. This is a characteristic of all childhood lymphatic tissue. The term *lymphatism* was applied to this characteristic by Dr. L. Emmett Holt, professor of diseases of children at Columbia University from 1901 to 1923. In 1899, he referred to the "exaggerated susceptibility of lymphoid tissue in children to respond to any inflammation by *hyperplasia* (growth) which may be out of proportion to the exciting cause, and which continues after the cause has ceased to operate." Lymphoid tissue hasn't changed since that statement was made. I like to explain the persistence of the lymphatic response after the threat has passed by comparing it to the peace-keeping force that remains behind after the battles have all been fought. They both seem to last a lot longer than would appear necessary.

The lymph nodes in the head and neck area are usually the first ones to be "discovered." The nodes receiving lymph from the scalp and back of the neck are situated at the base of the skull, just above the top of the collar. They're called occipital nodes because they sit over the occipital bone. Tiny BB-sized occipital nodes are easy to find in young, hairless infants. They can also be felt in roughly 5 percent of older children. These nodes are expected to enlarge whenever the scalp is irritated. The usual stimuli in this lymph-shed are cradle cap, heat rashes, insect bites, and eczema. Occipital node enlargement is sometimes an early feature of roseola, a common infant's disease. It may occur before the rash and can be a clue to the diagnosis. The enlargement in these cases is minor, though equally harmless massive enlargement does occur in this area with a heavy infestation of head lice and infected scratches.

The lymph from the eyelids and temples drains to the front of the ears, to the preauricular lymph nodes. There are no innocent causes for these nodes to enlarge.

The lymph from the outer ear and ear canal flows to the nodes behind the ears, the postauricular nodes, as well as forward to the nodes in front of the ears. Children commonly get minor infections in these areas, and pea-sized nodes are almost routinely felt here. Infected earlobes as a consequence of ear piercing will cause these nodes to enlarge.

The lymph from the nose, face, lips, and mouth drains to nodes running along the lower jaw, the submaxillary and the submental lymph nodes. As these are common areas of minor infections, these nodes are also frequently enlarged. They are especially noticeable in children who habitually bite their cheeks when they're nervous, in children who get a lot of canker sores, and in older children with infected acne. The only time that striking enlargement is usual is in cases of primary herpesvirus infections of the gums and mouth. In this condition, the nodes that enlarge are the ones directly under the chin, the submental cluster.

The lymph from the back of the tongue, tonsils, back of the throat, and voice box drains to the nodes of the neck, the cervical nodes. Most of these nodes lie under the major muscle of the neck, the sternocleidomastoid, the wide muscle running from the collarbone to the skull behind the ear. But there are also chains of nodes, like strings of pearls, running along each side of the muscle. These are the nodes that swell with colds, sore throats, laryngitis, and in general all upper respiratory infections. Only children born without lymph nodes, or raised in germ-free environments, will lack nodes in the neck. In other words, all normal children have lymph nodes that can be felt in the neck.

In this area, there are several popular scenarios for lymph node misinterpretation: In one, little Johnny, a perfectly healthy, skinny, active five-year-old, while turning his head to the side, causes a normal neck node to be silhouetted against the background. Even though it's about the size of a small marble, in the brief moment the parent discovers it, it becomes the size of Johnny and Johnny becomes marble-sized. Johnny, somewhat puzzled, is rushed to the doctor, who assures his parents that nothing's wrong; the node will go away. Johnny goes home, still puzzled, but his parents go home with the weight of the world just taken off their shoulders. A minor variation on this theme consists of the node discovery during the evening bath. The same set of responses occur.

Act Two: Healthy, active, skinny Johnny still has his node, agonizing days have passed since the reassuring visit to the doctor, and his parents are stooped over from the earth's weight once again. No one told them *when* the node would go away. Something must be wrong by now. Variations on the waiting-for-the-node-to-go-away theme occur whenever the doctor forgets to tell the parents that the node is likely to stay awhile.

The next common scenario consists of confusing an enlarged lymph node in the neck with mumps. Many are the parents who have brought their child to the office to confirm their suspicion that their child has mumps, only to be told that the swelling is a lymph node. Surprisingly, this happens even when the child has been immunized against mumps. It's usually quite easy to tell the two apart, although those children who are diagnosed as having mumps repeatedly during childhood are undoubtedly having repeated bouts of lymph node swelling. Ordinarily, when it comes to mumps, it's one to a customer.

Mumps is an infection of the parotid gland. This is the largest of the paired, saliva-producing glands, and most of the gland is situated above the jawline. It extends backward behind the ear, forward over the major chewing muscle, and as high up as the ear canal. If this area isn't involved in the swelling, it isn't mumps. Further, the swelling in mumps is on both sides in three fourths of the cases.

There's another way that your doctor can tell if the swelling is the parotid gland or not. He can look for the center of the swelling. The parotid gland is centered at the point where the earlobe attaches to the face. If he can put his finger between the front of the ear and the angle of the jaw and feel the mouth opening and closing, it isn't mumps. If the swelling is centered below the jawline, it's probably a lymph node.

The nodes in the armpit receive the lymph from the thumb's side of the hand, the arm, the upper chest wall, the upper flank, and part of the breast. They can be felt in 70 to 90 percent of children between 2 and 12. Armpit, or axillary, nodes are especially prominent in children with eczema and in children who have just been given an immunization in that shoulder.

The lymph from the pinky side of the hand and forearm drains to a small bunch of nodes near the "funny bone." These nodes, the epitrochlear, are only normally felt in nail biters. These children usually have continuous minor irritations around their nails, which serve as a continuous source of stimulation for the epitrochlear nodes. The only other common condition that causes these nodes to enlarge is infectious mononucleosis.

The last group of nodes are those in the groin, the inguinal nodes. These receive the lymph draining from the genitals, the anal area, the skin over the lower belly, and the legs. Since these nodes have no fat covering them, they're very easy to feel in virtually all children. They enlarge with such mundane conditions as diaper rashes and immunizations given in the thigh, and swell up with any infection in the foot or leg. Occasionally, other solid structures wind up in the groin, such as undescended or retractile testes. A quick testicle count should settle that issue. At times, inguinal lymph nodes have been mistaken for hernias or hydroceles (see p. 95).

If the lump in the groin pops back into the abdomen when you touch it, it was a hernia. If the lump swells before your eyes as you watch it, it's a hernia. If the lump is sausage-shaped, has a spongy rather than a rubbery, solid feel, and is larger than an almond, it's probably a hydrocele. Hernias and hydroceles are significant lumps. How can your doctor tell when the lymph node in this area, or any other area, is significant?

There are eight characteristics of lymph nodes that help determine how significant they are. Just like in real estate, the first is location. Although no group of lymph nodes can be said to be totally safe or totally dangerous, some are better than others. For example, cervical nodes high in the neck are less worrisome than those that are low. Nodes in the front part of the neck tend to be less serious than nodes at the back. Nodes just above the collarbone are likely to have a more serious cause. In contrast, enlargement of the epitrochlear nodes is virtually always of limited importance.

The second characteristic is duration. The longer the node has been around, especially without changing, the more likely it is to be free of serious disease. For this reason, nodes that are questionable the first time they're seen may be reexamined by your doctor to see what has happened with the passing of time. Questionable nodes that don't seem to be doing anything over periods of weeks or months lessen in importance. When a parent discovers a node in an otherwise healthy small child, I ask her to measure it and give her an appointment as far into the future as her nerves will tolerate. This gives the parent a second chance to measure it and to see what effect time has had.

The third trait is accountability. It's always comforting to know why things are happening, especially if the reason is innocent enough. When, for example, your doctor finds a scalp rash to explain a swollen occipital node, the discovery goes a long way to reduce the worry that the node might have caused. Seeing a lump from a previous DPT immunization in a thigh does the same for an inguinal node sighting.

Certain nodes are so routine, they need no accounting. For example, upper respiratory infections are so common, and the nodes persist for so long, that your doctor won't question the origins of high cervical nodes. They could be a response to last week's sore throat, or the cold of three months ago. He will, on the other hand, regard other large, unaccountable nodes more seriously.

Your physician will also want to know if the node is painful or not. The nerves that carry lymph node pain are located in the outer capsule that encases the node. Whenever this capsule gets stretched, the node gets sore. For this reason, we generally assume that painful nodes are actively growing, or have very recently been actively growing. Most tender lymph nodes result from an active infection, and if the doctor suspects that the infection is bacterial, he'll likely prescribe an antibiotic. Tender nodes aren't always the result of a bacterial infection. Viruses, such as German measles, can also tenderize lymph nodes.

The fifth characteristic your physician will look for is the node's mobility. Most lymph nodes, even the swollen ones, are readily movable. The skin slides over them without dimpling, and they can be rolled around over the muscles they rest on. Mobility is a good sign; it implies that the process that's enlarging the lymph node is still confined to the node itself. If the cause of the swelling—whether cells or germs—breaks through the capsule of the node and escapes into the surrounding structures, the node gets stuck and loses its mobility. Or, if one node gets matted to a neighboring node, it becomes impossible to feel the full outline of each one of the nodes. This last process is called fixation.

The sixth characteristic your doctor examines the node for is size. A node isn't abnormally large just because it can be felt, but once it gets larger than a lima bean size, it can be called big. Even big nodes deserve a chance to get smaller, so if size is the only worrisome characteristic, you can afford to wait a few weeks. Size is a pretty poor indicator of the cause of the node's enlargement.

The seventh factor is the node's texture. Practically all lymph nodes in children feel the same way, namely, like firm rubber. Hard lymph nodes are cause for concern, but even rubbery-feeling nodes can harbor serious disease.

The last, and perhaps most important factor, has to do with the child, not the node. Your doctor will check for weight loss and weakness. He'll want to know if your child is taking any medication that could increase the size of the lymph nodes, such as diphenylhydantoin (Dilantin). Does he have a medical condition that includes large glands, such as an overactive thyroid gland, or one of several types of anemia? Does he show any enlargement of internal organs, such as his liver or spleen? Are the nodes of only one region enlarged, or are the nodes generally enlarged?

There are individual and racial differences in reactivity of the lymph nodes. Experience shows that a slight, generalized enlargement of the lymph nodes is more common in black children than white. I've also seen children whose nodes typically overreact to the slightest provocation, and if I hadn't known from my experience with these particular children that this was their usual response, I might have been more concerned than necessary.

The key issue for your doctor is determining whether the node is large because it has reacted to a process that is now or will soon be over, or if the node is involved in an active, progressive process itself.

In the great majority of cases, the node will be a reactive one, but since the causes of enlarged nodes include a number of serious diseases, your physician will establish the precise diagnosis only after giving careful consideration to the eight lymph-node characteristics. (See p. 336, **Ref. 22**; see p. 341, **Ref. 126**; see p. 341, **Ref. 127**; see p. 342, **Ref. 128**; see p. 342, **Ref. 129**; see p. 342, **Ref. 130**; see p. 342, **Ref. 131**.)

8. Chest

BREASTS SWOLLEN SINCE BIRTH *(Persistent Infantile Hypertrophy)*

You may notice that some babies, especially girls, keep their enlarged breasts longer than the expected first six months (see p. 81). Sometimes, in fact, these little girls never part with their infantile hypertrophy and continue to have softly swollen breasts all through childhood. When puberty begins, these girls have a head start.

It is important to differentiate the "never lost it" girls from the "I found it" group. Those who never lost it need no special medical attention. On the other hand, toddlers who begin to grow breasts after their infantile breasts have faded away will be carefully examined by the physician. Usually, the doctor will want answers to two questions: First, where is the child getting her estrogen, the hormone responsible for her swollen breasts? Second, is the "feminization" limited to her breasts, or is the girl starting a full set of pubertal changes?

BREASTS SWELL AFTER BIRTH
Very Early Breast Development *(Premature Thelarche)*

The term used when breasts start to develop in little girls who show no other signs of sexual development, and who go no further with their pubertal changes, is premature thelarche (*thele* means nipple; *arche* equals beginning). Premature thelarche is harmless as long as the child remains childlike until the proper time for puberty to begin.

The first sign of premature thelarche is a firm, sometimes tender disc of tissue directly beneath one of the nipples of a completely normal child, usually one and a half to four years old. If this disc occurs on one side only, it could be misread as a chest lump rather than breast tissue, and assumed to be something as scary as a tumor. In the worst-case scenario, the doctor may feel compelled to take a piece of this so-called tumor to see what it is. This can be disastrous if too big a piece is taken and not enough breast tissue is left. A major no-no.

If, on the other hand, the tissue starts out under both breasts, or the other side quickly catches up, the swellings are almost always recognized as "breast buds." Now, however, the worry is shifted from "tumor" to "precocious sexual development."

Breast development in toddlers may indeed be the first sign of precocious sexual development. For this reason, doctors examine girls who show this early swelling several times a year, and watch for additional signs of sexual maturation.

The breasts of children with premature thelarche may grow quite large, but they seldom reach adult size, and, totally unlike the adult's, they don't develop pigmentation of the nipple and areola. Aside from their breasts, these girls have no other signs of maturation such as growth spurts, advanced bony maturation, sexual hair, or menstrual bleeding. When their blood and urine is tested, they're found to have the normal amounts of hormones for their age.

We don't know what causes some girls to develop premature thelarche. The most popular explanation offered used to be that girls with premature thelarche had breast tissue that's extra-sensitive to estrogenic stimulation from the normal minuscule amounts in the prepubertal child's blood, but this view is no longer held. We now suspect that premature thelarche is a result of the secretion of a small amount of estrogen from the child's ovary, especially from a small ovarian cyst.

More common than premature thelarche is what appears to be early breast development in obese girls. Despite the size and shape of some of these breasts, they're nothing more than accumulations of fat and will disappear with weight reduction. (See p. 342, **Ref. 132.**)

Puberty from Accidental Estrogen Intake (*Exogenous Estrogenization*)

There are a number of ways that children can accidentally receive the hormone estrogen. Eating meat from animals treated with large amounts of estrogen is one way, and it has occasionally produced "epidemics" of breast enlargement. Estrogen dust in the air and on the machinery in pharmaceutical plants has accidentally contaminated medicines taken by children. Estrogen administered in the form of a skin or vaginal cream has been absorbed into the bloodstream.

Regardless of how the estrogen gets into the child's body, once it's in, it can produce a host of developmental changes that mimic precocious puberty. Of course, if the child happens to be a boy, the changes in his body will be limited to his breasts since nothing else in his body will respond visibly to the estrogen. If a girl receives the hormone, not only will her breasts enlarge, but also her nipples and areolae will become heavily pigmented. In addition, her vaginal lining will mature and her uterus may develop to the point of producing menstrual bleeding. In short, she'll seem just like a teenager starting puberty, the only problem being that she may be only two years old at the time.

There are several simple ways your doctor can distinguish a girl who has been accidentally and unknowingly taking estrogen from one who is truly starting an abnormally early puberty. First, a girl who is embarking on a full-blown puberty will have a growth spurt, and an X ray will show signs of skeletal maturation, whereas one who has been briefly stimulated by "outside" estrogen will have no pubertal growth spurt or bone maturation; i.e., if she's three years old, her height and bone age will be that of a three-year-old. However, if the exposure to outside estrogen was more than transient, there may be a growth spurt.

The second way is by carefully and repeatedly measuring the level of gonadotropin in the blood. Gonadotropin is a hormone sent from the pituitary gland in them head down to the ovaries to direct them to produce estrogen. When the reason for feminization is exogenous (outside) estrogen, this control system is bypassed and the levels of gonadotropin are, in fact, lower than normal. If your doctor finds this low level of gonadotropin, he'll suspect that something fishy is going on. Either somebody is unintentionally giving the child estrogen, or more seriously, the child has a tumor that's secreting estrogen. The latter, although very rare, must be considered if no exogenous source of estrogen is found, or if the feminization appears to be permanent. If all the sexual changes disappear on their own, or after the removal of the source of outside estrogen, you can be sure that the false puberty was caused by estrogen intake. (See p. 342, **Ref. 133.**)

INNOCENT HEART MURMUR *(Functional Cardiac Murmur)*

Virtually every child will have an innocent heart murmur at one time or another. Innocent murmurs are called innocent because they're harmless, have nothing to do with disease, and, furthermore, never will. Children who have them need no medication or restriction of their activities. Having one is as much a sign of health as not having one. If your doctor tells you that your child has an innocent murmur, you should react as if he said that your child has a nose or a navel. But most parents don't. Most parents act as if they've just received bad news, and the diagnosis itself often causes immeasurable anxiety, confusion, and sometimes lasting psychological damage to children. I have yet to see the parent who felt happy after being told that her child had an innocent murmur.

But an innocent murmur isn't a blight on the health of the child! So why is the word *murmur* so frightening that even modifying it with the word *innocent* fails to remove its dreadfulness? I suspect that today's irrational fear of the innocent murmur has its roots in the last century, when murmurs were first heard.

The first stethoscope (created by René Laënnec in 1819) was probably capable of transmitting only those murmurs that were coming from obviously diseased hearts. Innocent murmurs were never heard, so if a murmur *was* heard, it was undoubtedly significant. Later, doctors came to recognize that some murmurs are heard in perfectly normal hearts, but this important fact wasn't widely disseminated.

The first campaign for widespread recognition of the innocent murmur was begun in 1925 by Sir James Mackenzie with words that *should* have been heard around the world: "Individuals may show heart murmurs and be in perfect health, and lead strenuous lives, and never show the slightest sign of heart failure. From this we can conclude that murmurs may be a physiologic and normal event, and indicate neither impairment of the heart's efficiency, nor foreshadow the oncoming of heart failure." Although Mackenzie was talking about adults, truer words were never spoken about children's hearts, because children's hearts are noisier than adults' and the noise is easier to hear. And yet, in spite of the efforts of many medical writers to lay the ghost of the innocent murmur to rest, it still stalks, perhaps because most people today hear the word *murmur* for the first time in connection with some child who needs a catheterization, operation, or heart transplant. It's as if the word *murmur* was too pejorative to be neutered. Some words are simply too tainted to pass. While I was writing this book, in fact, my own wife was upset by my partner's diagnosis during a routine checkup of our daughter, Helen. Helen, my wife was told, has an innocent murmur. I immediately explained to my wife everything that you'll read in this section, and after several hours of discussion I was satisfied that she'd totally accepted the normalcy and harmlessness of Helen's murmur. At least she said that she did. I was happy. But several minutes later, my once again worried wife looked at me and asked, "Do you think that David (our son) has one, too?"

If the term *innocent murmur* doesn't allay a parent's fears, is there a better one? No less than 121 terms have been proffered by doctors through the years, and we all know that we haven't yet found one that adequately conveys the true meaning. Yet it's absolutely imperative that parents have a full understanding, or else there may be unpleasant consequences for them and their child.

The worst are the psychological effects on the child. In their confusion, parents suddenly view the child as no longer having "health," but not as "diseased" either. It's like being arrested but not indicted; the child is definitely not guilty, but he's not entirely innocent, either. He's in limbo, in what's called, these days, nondisease.

There are two ways for a child to enter this limbo of cardiac nondisease. The first is by having an innocent murmur misdiagnosed as "significant." This is an extremely common event. In every children's cardiac clinic in the world, the biggest single group of children doctors see are those without heart disease. The proportion of children who are diagnosed as having heart disease but who are in fact completely normal, to those who do indeed have heart disease, varies from one out of every two children in Seattle, Washington, to four of every five in Shiraz, Iran. The number one misdiagnosis is rheumatic heart disease. Later on in this section, we'll see how this common mistake is made.

Once these children are "overdiagnosed," they're in danger of overtreatment. Most are treated with daily penicillin to prevent a "recurrence" of rheumatic fever. Some have their tonsils removed, again as a preventive measure. Many are put to bed for extraordinary lengths of time. Yet, all these children really need is intensive delabeling. They have no disease.

The second route to cardiac limbo is by way of a correctly diagnosed innocent murmur that the child's parents interpret to mean that something's wrong with the child's heart. These children, in contrast to the first group, aren't in danger of medical or surgical overkill, but they are in danger of having their life's activities needlessly restricted and curtailed. Some aren't allowed to go to school or take part in social or physical activities with their friends. Some are just prevented from overexertion. Others are allowed most activities, but are the recipients of a lot of worry, are viewed as unhealthy, and are therefore treated differently from children "without heart trouble." All in all, there are more children leading restricted lives for nonexistent heart disease than for real heart disease. Why this waste of good health?

Only part of the responsibility is the parent's; the rest is the doctor's. Half of this restricted group of children have been diagnosed as having rheumatic fever, and "limited activity" was what the doctor prescribed. The parents were only following doctor's orders. But for the others, the problem stems from faulty communication between doctor and parent, and widespread public misunderstanding of the meaning of innocent murmurs.

The less you understand about your child's condition, the more likely you are to restrict your child's activities. Uncertainty breeds anxiety, which, in turn, leads to overprotectiveness. To begin with, it will help you to understand the difference between adults' hearts and children's. Everyone knows that adults with heart disease are liable to have heart attacks that seem to come out of the blue. Many people wrongly suspect that children are subject to the same sort of sudden catastrophic events. With very rare exceptions, sudden severe symptoms never occur in children, even when they have heart disease. (Not being aware of this difference, many parents are tempted to "play it safe" and keep a tight rein on their children's activities.)

Now, here's what you should know about children's innocent heart murmurs:

1. How Common Are They?

It depends on who is listening and under what circumstances, and on what instrument is being used. Actually, since these murmurs result from the flow of blood, every beating heart can produce such a murmur, and indeed this is what you'll find if an electronically amplified stethoscope is used. When the examiner uses a simple, conventional stethoscope, he'll hear murmurs in the hearts of from 80 to close to 100 percent of all normal children. The number gets closer to 100 if the examiner listens to the child's heart more than once, if he exercises the child before he examines her, or if he's a skilled heart specialist with a trained, expert ear as well as a sensitive stethoscope.

2. What Does It Mean When Your Doctor Refers Your Child to a Specialist?

Most innocent murmurs are simple to recognize by their sounds alone. On occasion, the sounds may not be so easy to interpret, and the doctor may want to get more information before making a definite diagnosis. He may want to have an X ray or electrocardiogram taken, or he may want to send the child to a pediatric cardiologist.

Even in specialty clinics and specialists' offices where children who are suspected of having a significant heart murmur are examined, a high percentage turn out to be innocent. Of 1,702 children referred to such a clinic in St. Louis for suspected heart disease, 36 percent were found to have innocent murmurs. At the cardiology clinic of the National Naval Medical Center, the equivalent figure was 56 percent; in a Toronto cardiac registry, 61.5 percent; in the office of a pediatric cardiologist in Connecticut, 65 percent; and in England, 73 percent.

Don't assume that these figures reflect badly on the referring doctors. Each of these doctors, being uncertain at a time that demands certainty, did the right thing. Rather than hem and haw, the referring doctor directed the parents to the place where a firm diagnosis could be made, ending, he hoped, the parents' uncertainty and anxiety.

3. What Happens to Innocent Murmurs?

They go away. By age 14 years, 90 percent are gone. For the remaining 10 percent, it doesn't matter that they're still present. The murmurs didn't bother the children as toddlers, and they won't bother them as young adults. For people who still have them 20 years later, the diagnosis remains innocent murmur for all but 2 percent, making the diagnosis of innocent murmur in childhood accurate in 98 percent of cases. Not too shabby a batting average for the human ear.

4. *What Causes the Murmurs to Be Heard in the First Place?*

Ultimately, all sounds are started by vibrations. The vibrations responsible for the "regular" heart sounds are generated by the opening and closing of the heart's valves and the contracting and relaxing of the heart's muscle. In contrast, the vibrations that are heard as innocent murmurs come from the flow of blood. Just like any other slowly flowing stream, blood moves in parallel layers or sheets. This pattern is called laminar flow, and it creates very little turbulence within the stream. It doesn't make waves or murmurs until the flow speeds up.

High-velocity flow causes a spinning off of some blood, producing eddies that, in turn, produce vibrations within the chamber or vessel into which the flow is directed. (This is called the vortex-shedding theory.) The vibrations become sounds that travel through the chest wall, up the stethoscope, and into the listener's ear, where they're heard as murmurs. The faster the flow, the louder the murmur. This explains why murmurs are most likely to be heard when a child has a fever, or when the child is frightened, has recently exercised, or is anemic. In all of these situations, the flow rate is extremely rapid. (Knowing this, it's easy to understand how the innocent flow murmur of the frightened, feverish, aching child could be mistaken for the significant murmurs of rheumatic fever. Not knowing it led to the tremendous overdiagnosis of the past.)

Once the murmur is produced, the sound has to make its way out of the chest. Chests that are thickened with fat or muscle dampen the sounds, and thin chests pass the sounds through more easily. Sometimes, a child's murmur will "appear" as soon as his infant chest padding is shed. The reverse is also true. Some of the innocent murmurs heard in skinny ten-year-olds are never heard from once the teenager fills out.

5. *Why Didn't the Other Doctors Hear the Murmur Before?*

If the child's murmur is heard for the first time after a previous doctor didn't hear it, it usually means that previous circumstances concealed the sound. If the child is screaming, breathing loudly, fussing, squirming, and in general not giving the doctor a chance to get a good listen, the odds are good that the murmur won't be heard. If there's a conversation going on between the doctor and the parent, or if there are other children in the examining room carrying on, the murmur probably won't be heard, either. Just about any background noise can screen out the sound of the murmur and the problem isn't limited to the pediatrician's office. Hospitals can have noisy environments, too.

During the routine examination of a child in the pediatric-clinic examining room of a major medical school, the recorded noise level was 75 decibels. This wasn't much different from the boiler room of the same hospital, where the noise level was 100 decibels. For comparison's sake, the noise level inside a DC-6 airliner is 105 decibels, and the noise becomes painful at about 130 decibels. It follows from this that the best place to have your child's chest examined is in a quiet house in the country, where the noise level is a mere 30 decibels. Of course, if you're in the city at the time, your doctor will have to use a very long stethoscope.

Speaking of stethoscopes, they also vary a great deal in their ability to transmit undistorted sounds. They vary in length of tubing, as well as size and shape of the chest piece and earpieces. (The original stethoscope was an instrument for the protection of the patient's modesty, not for diagnosis, and was designed to avoid direct contact between the doctor's ears and the patient's chest.)

There are also differences in sensitivity from one listener to the next. When it comes to hearing soft sounds in noisy rooms, not all doctors are created equally. I can still remember listening to detailed descriptions of murmurs heard by my colleagues in medical school, and when it was my turn to listen to the same chest, all I heard was my own nervous heartbeat.

And what is heard in the ear must then be interpreted higher up. In this regard, too, two doctors are rarely alike.

Finally, it's the nature of certain types of innocent murmurs to come and go from one day to the next. Some murmurs are heard only when the child is sitting up. If the previous doctor examined the child while the patient was lying down, the doctor wouldn't have heard the murmur. This leads us to the next question.

6. *How Many Types of Innocent Murmurs Are There?*

There are five basic innocent murmurs and it's not uncommon for a child to have two or three of them at any given time. Furthermore, many children outgrow one type only to have another one take its place. Your doctor may provide you with the name of your child's innocent murmur, which is probably among the following:

The best-known innocent murmur is frequently called Still's murmur, after its discoverer, Dr. George Frederick Still. This is one of the most commonly heard murmurs, and can be instantly recognized by the quality of its sound. It's heard most often in preschool and early grade schoolchildren and sounds just like a plucked tuning fork. Its musical qualities have led to such descriptions as "fiddlestring," "buzzing," "vibratory," "twanging," or "groaning."

Once this murmur is heard, it's easy to diagnose; but it may not be heard if the examiner happens to place his stethoscope on a part of the chest that isn't transmitting it. The precise source of Still's murmur is still unknown. Most used to think that it arose from a vessel outside the heart, but the best evidence now is that this innocent murmur is caused by rapid blood flow across the chordae tendineae (see p. 282), the fine threadlike attachments from the inner lining of the ventricles to the tricuspid and mitral valves (see p. 82 for the structure of the heart).

The next murmur originates in the main pulmonary artery at the point where it receives its spurt of blood coming out of the right ventricle. For this reason, it's called the pulmonary ejection murmur. The pulmonary ejection murmur is closely tied to changes in flow rates. It may be very loud if the child is feverish, or barely audible if the child is well. For this reason, a murmur that's heard for the first time when the child has a fever often requires reexamination once the fever is gone. Recognizing this innocent murmur isn't as easy as pinpointing Still's murmur because its diagnosis depends on more than just the quality of the sound. Sometimes, the ears of a pediatric cardiologist need to be recruited to be certain about this diagnosis.

The third murmur, the cervical venous hum, is heard in the neck, originating in the jugular vein, the main vein of the neck. Its sound is a continuous, roaring, low-pitched hum. The turbulence causing this murmur is created by the blood returning to the heart from the brain. Two thirds of the brain's blood returns via the right jugular, and the cervical venous hum is usually heard on the right side.

The good news about this murmur is that it's a cinch to diagnose. The doctor can turn it on or off just by turning the child's head to the side, or by putting his finger over the vein, blocking the flow. If you see your doctor engaged in these practices, you can be sure that he's admiring your child's venous hum.

The next common innocent murmur is also heard up in the neck. When the left ventricle squirts its blood load into the aorta, the major vessel exiting the heart, it creates a noise that comes from a spot just above the collarbone. This sound is called the supraclavicular (above the clavicle bone) arterial bruit (*bruit* means noise in French), but since it can also be heard over the path of the neck's main artery, the carotid, it's sometimes called the carotid bruit. How common is this murmur? You might better ask: How common is it *not* to have this murmur? The answer: Only one child in eight under the age of four years does not have a supraclavicular arterial bruit or carotid bruit murmur.

The last of the common innocent murmurs probably isn't really a murmur at all, in that we don't believe that it comes from the flow of blood. It's called the cardiorespiratory (*cardio* refers to the heart; *respiratory* to the lungs) murmur, and is thought to come from the impact of the beating heart on the surrounding lung. It's by no means as common as the others, and your doctor may not immediately recognize it as an innocent sound. Its characteristics are so unique, however, that any doctor who has heard it before will have no trouble recognizing it again. Those who haven't heard this bizarre whistling, whooping, scratching sound usually refer the child to a pediatric cardiologist for diagnosis.

These are the five most common innocent murmurs of childhood. It would be very unlikely if your child didn't have one or more of them. Some children have them all. They're none the worse for it.

7. *Should Your Doctor Tell You Your Child Has an Innocent Murmur?*

If doctors could think of a good term that wouldn't automatically drive parents up the wall, this question wouldn't need to be asked. But things being as they are, it's virtually impossible for a physician to do a complete examination, tell a parent that the child has an innocent murmur, and still have enough time at the end of the visit to deal with all the anxiety that he just generated. Something has to be left out, and usually it's the full explanation. True, some parents readily accept the innocence of the diagnosis and calmly leave the office. Others appear to accept the diagnosis and remain cool all the way home until they share the news with their spouses. Then the phone calls start. Many parents don't bat an eyelash at the moment, but every time they return to the office with their children, they ask if "the murmur is still there." It doesn't add up to a hill of beans if the murmur is or isn't still there, I always insist. "I know," the parents answer, "but I'd still feel a lot better if it was gone, all the same." I grind my teeth and wonder where I went wrong in my explanation. I wonder if there is a right way. Perhaps it would be better if parents were informed of their child's murmur only when the doctor had questions about its innocence and special tests or referrals were needed. Perhaps when the doctor is fully confident that the murmur that he hears is an innocent one, he shouldn't bring it up and create needless anxiety. After all, when your doctor feels a normal liver edge, or sees a normal set of tonsils, his usual comment is "Everything seems all right."

Even this approach can cause lots of trouble. Sooner or later, someone will tell the parent that her child has a murmur. What often follows is (1) the first doctor is discredited, (2) the child is taken to a pediatric cardiologist, and (3) lots of worry, energy and dollars are spent. (See p. 342, **Ref. 134;** see p. 342, **Ref. 135;** see p. 342, **Ref. 136;** see p. 342, **Ref. 137;** see p. 342, **Ref. 138;** see p. 342, **Ref. 139;** see p. 342, **Ref. 140.**)

9. Abdomen

BULGING MIDSECTION *(Diastasis Rectus)*

You may have noticed that your toddler's belly bulges when she sits up from a lying position, or strains to move her bowels. Here's why:

On the sides of the belly's midline are parallel sets of straplike muscles, the recti *(rectus* means straight) abdominis. These muscles run down the front of the abdominal wall, reaching from the lower rib cage to the pubic bone. They're first formed in the back of the tiny fetus and have to migrate all the way around to the front. Most make it to the front by the end of the third month of the pregnancy.

The recti meet in the midline south of the navel, but above the navel they're separated by a band of connective tissue. The width of this band depends upon how close the muscles get. If the migration is complete, the band is narrow. But if the baby's rectus muscles are lazy, there will be a wide spread that can be several inches wide, called a diastasis (separation) rectus.

Since this band contains no muscle tissue, it isn't a terribly effective girdle. This explains why a smooth bulge sometimes appears in the middle of a baby's upper abdomen when she strains or tries to sit up. Aside from looking funny, it's of no concern, since there's no way for anything that bulged out to get stuck or trapped. As the baby's muscles grow and develop, the gap fills in, and the diastasis resolves. (See p. 336, **Ref. 31**; see p. 342, **Ref. 141**.)

10. Genitalia

VANISHING TESTICLE *(Retractile Testicle)*

If one side of your baby boy's scrotum looks bigger than the other, your doctor will have two things to consider. Either one side has too much, or one side has too little. The surplus items have already been discussed in the sections on hydroceles beginning on page 95, and the undescended testicle accounting for an empty scrotum on page 97. It's now time to discuss the *undecided* (or retractile) testicle, the yo-yo or migratory testicle that can't seem to make up its mind where it wants to be. This distinction is very important, because the undescended testicle should be treated while the undecided testicle can be left alone.

It's not hard to tell one from the other. Just by looking at the sac itself, your doctor will get a fairly good idea of which one your baby has. If the missing testicle never made it to its proper place, then its corresponding space in the scrotum will be underdeveloped and the ridge that normally runs down the middle of the scrotum will be over on the side of the missing testicle. On the other hand, if the missing testicle normally occupies its time in its proper place, then its half of the scrotum will be more normally developed and the ridge will appear in the middle. In this case you have a yo-yo, and the question is, if the testicle once descended to the scrotum and filled and stretched its proper space, why isn't it still there and where has it gone?

Many is the boy who has pondered this question, perhaps none with more imagination than Alex Portnoy in Philip Roth's *Portnoy's Complaint*. As Alex recounted, ". . . one of my testicles apparently decided it had enough of life down in the scrotum and began to make its way north. At the beginning, I could feel it bobbing uncertainly just at the rim of the pelvis and then, as though its moment of indecision had passed, entering the cavity of my body, like a survivor being dragged up out of the sea and over the hull of a life boat . . . alas, the voyager had struck off for regions unchartered and unknown. Where was it gone to! How high and how far before the journey would come to an end! Would I one day open my mouth to speak in class, only to discover my left nut out on the end of my tongue?"

What happened to Portnoy happens to the vast majority of young boys who have an empty scrotum. The culprit is a small bunch of abdominal muscle fibers that got looped around the testicle while it was en route from the abdomen to the scrotum. This loose arrangement of muscle fibers is called the cremaster (suspender) muscle. When it contracts, the testicle gets pulled upward, retracting out of the scrotum into a space in the groin just beneath the skin. In that location, it's easy to find. Less often, it makes a full retreat all the way back to the canal through which it originally descended.

The cremaster muscle contracts involuntarily whenever the inside of the thigh is stroked. Some boys have hair-trigger reflexes, and if the boy is cold, embarrassed, or frightened, or especially if the examiner's hand is cold, the testicle is likely to scamper off to loftier sites. Since none of the above are uncommon events in the ordinary examination, it isn't at all surprising that retractile testicles are commonly discovered by physicians. The doctor then must ascertain, by the method described above, whether the testicle is merely retractile or truly undescended. As soon as all parties concerned are convinced that the testicle is really all right, nothing more has to be done. With time, the cremasteric reflex gradually becomes less active and the boy less frightened, the mother reminds the doctor to warm his hands, and the testicle settles into its rightful niche. (See p. 342, **Ref. 142**; see p. 342, **Ref. 143**.)

SCROTAL SWELLING

Swollen Pink Scrotum (*Acute Scrotal Edema*)

Most often, the sudden swelling of the scrotum signifies that something serious is going on such as an infected or twisted testicle. However, it sometimes turns out to be an entirely innocent condition. The first is called acute scrotal edema.

In this condition, which usually occurs in boys three to nine years old, there's a sudden and often considerable accumulation of tissue fluid in one half of the scrotum, the penis, and the adjacent skin of the thigh or groin. The swelling is firm and painless, and the skin gets a bright pink color. It vanishes after 24 to 48 hours, often as suddenly as it came. We don't know if acute scrotal edema is an allergic reaction, or if it's caused by a blockage of the lymph channels in the groin. Whatever the causes, it disappears promptly without treatment, although sometimes it comes back for an encore.

Painful Lump on Scrotum (*Scrotal Panniculitis*)

The second harmless scrotal swelling starts out scary because it's painful, but it, too, has a happy ending because all the action takes place in the fatty tissue of the scrotum, not in the testicle.

This condition is characterized by the sudden appearance of a painful lump just beneath and behind one of the testicles of a prepubertal boy. If the doctor is sure that the swelling is completely separate from the testicle, he'll opt to leave it alone and watch as it goes away. If he isn't sure, he may have the lump removed, in which case it will be found to be an inflamed piece of fat. It is, in fact, the scrotum's equivalent to the face's Popsicle panniculitis (see p. 157). The cause of this condition is completely unknown. It doesn't require exposure to cold and it isn't connected with obesity. It only occurs in prepubertal boys since adult men don't have any fat in their scrota. (See p. 342, **Ref. 144**; see p. 342, **Ref. 145**.)

VANISHING PENIS *(Penis Embedded in Prepubic Fat)*

Many chubby little boys build up a big collection of fat in front of the pubic bone. Like a 3-foot fire hydrant in a 4-foot snowdrift, the penis gets buried under. Since the fat slowly accumulates around the shaft of the penis, it may not be obvious at first glance that the problem is the fat and not the penis.

There are two things to remember after the initial wave of panic has passed. First, think back to earlier days before your son was so chubby. If he had a penis then, believe me, he has one now.

People who do circumcisions are especially familiar with this phenomenon. The *mohel* who circumcised our son warned my wife and me about the possibility of the pubic fat's concealing David's penis if he happened to grow chubby later on. This wise *mohel* had no desire to be called back to search for the embedded penis six months later.

If you're still nervous about your son's vanished penis, ask your pediatrician to measure the length of the stretched penis from the tip to the pubic bone. By referring to a table with the statistical norms for boys of different ages, she should be able to reassure you that all is well.

The average stretched length for a two-year-old's penis is a bit less than 5 centimeters; for the six-year-old, it's close to 6 centimeters. And that's stretching the point. (See p. 343, **Ref. 148**.)

VANISHING VAGINA *(Labial Adhesion)*

You may discover this phenomenon while you're bathing your child. Where once there was an opening, there's now a membrane of cellophanelike skin sealing the vaginal slit shut. What has happened is quite common.

"Vanishing vagina" usually occurs in the two- to six-year-old girl. We believe that it follows a prolonged vaginal infection so mild that it may not have been noticed. As a result of this minor infection, the inner surfaces of the child's labia minora exude a discharge and the sides get plastered together. This process, called labial adhesion, and sometimes labial agglutination or fusion begins in the rear and works its way upward toward the urinary opening.

Although labial fusion may seem shocking, it has few consequences. Any interference with the escape of vaginal secretions may accentuate the vaginal infection that started the whole process, or if the fusion makes it all the way up to the urinary opening (the meatus), it can interfere with the flow of urine and produce a urinary infection. This is the only meaningful threat of the fused labia. If there's no obstruction to the urine's stream, the fusion is totally harmless and can be left alone.

If the labia need to be unfused, your doctor may suggest a vaginal cream containing estrogen for a period not exceeding two weeks. Since the estrogen will be absorbed, this treatment carries the risk of producing a temporary feminization (see p. 180). Your physician will undertake it only if there's a risk of urinary infection.

There's no justification for tearing the labia apart, no matter how gently. It never fails to hurt the child and the labia will invariably refuse during the healing process. Sometimes, paying more attention to vaginal hygiene helps, but labial fusion tends to be a "sticky" problem that often plagues the child until puberty. (See p. 343, **Ref. 149.**)

11. Bones and Joints

KNOCK-KNEES AND BOWLEGS *(Genu Valgum and Genu Varum)*

These conditions are grouped together because, for the most part, they represent different stages of the same set of knees. You can, in fact, think of your child's life as a progression through different "knee eras," instead of the usual infancy, early childhood, later childhood, and so on. In this historical scheme, the child starts out bowlegged, then passes through a brief period of being straight-legged, only to become knock-kneed. Ultimately, when the rest of her straightens out, so do her legs.

There are a number of reasons why an infant's legs resemble a set of parentheses. In the first place, the legs' position in the womb actually causes them to bow. In the popular Buddha style, the thighbones turn out from the hips, and the long bones of the lower legs twist internally. This produces a bowing at the knees as well as the intoeing described on page 102.

In the second place, an optical illusion is created by the uneven distribution of fat over the baby's legs. Since more fat covers the outside of the legs than the inside, the outer line of the lower leg is rounded, creating an extra appearance of bowing.

By the time the child is 18 months old, her legs should be fairly straight. The reasons for the unbowing are the reverse of the reasons for the bowing. As the baby begins to stand, the bones of her legs remodel into a straight line. As the muscles required for walking develop, the soft tissue pants rearrange themselves on either side of the leg, thus eliminating the added illusion of bowing.

Of course, if the bowing appears to worsen rather than improve, or if the legs haven't straightened out by the time the child is three years old, your physician will consider other causes.

When a normal child reaches the age of three to four years, she progresses to the knock-kneed stage. When she stands with the feet comfortably parted, her knees aren't. Here again, there are two explanations: a bony one and a fleshy one.

If you drew a line down the front of your child's thigh, and then one down her lower leg, the two lines would form an angle opening toward the outside. This is more pronounced in girls than boys, and is thought to be due to knees' loose-jointedness.

As with bowlegs, visual effects play a part here. Given the same angle, long-legged children tend to appear more knock-kneed than shorter children because the distance between their ankles is, perforce, greater. Also, children with very fat thighs appear knock-kneed because their knees are almost always touching each other no matter how straight their legs.

If you have your four-year-old stand as straight as he can and squeeze his knees together as tightly as he can, not more than 6 centimeters should separate the inner ankles. If your physician finds more distance than this, or if any spread suddenly appears in a child whose legs were perfectly straight before, a bone specialist will be consulted.

Severe knock-knees can present a problem when the child runs, so your doctor may consult an orthopedist about the problem, too, The specialist probably won't put wedges in the child's shoes because we've found this time-honored treatment totally ineffective. Wearing leg braces at night has more potential for correcting knock-knees, but it seems a bit drastic for a condition that gets better with every passing year. (See p. 338, **Ref. 53**; see p. 338, **Ref. 58**.)

FLAT FEET *(Pes Planus)*

Nearly all toddlers have beautifully arched feet as long as they aren't standing on them. When the child stands, her weight flattens her feet, and the arches are gone. When she stands on her toes, the arch returns. Her feet can be twisted and turned easily. Such feet are called relaxed or flexible, and resemble a tripod that sinks into the ground when too much weight is put on the top. The reason a toddler's feet flatten when she stands is that the ligaments supporting the arch just aren't strong enough for the job.

In some mysterious way, this most innocent of conditions, flat feet, crept into the closet of "medical monsters and dragons." For those who like to worry needlessly, this is as good an area as any, since flat feet are usually completely harmless and don't interfere with activity. Some of the world's fastest runners also have the world's flattest feet.

Shoe treatments, such as wedges, special heels, and inserts, may protect shoes from uneven wear, but they do nothing for the child. These special devices don't make much sense and may even worsen the problem. Since the basic problem is looseness of the ligaments, the solution should be tightness. The opposite is achieved when you provide the foot with external support. By taking away the need for the foot to develop its own strength, you make it so relaxed that it's practically comatose.

At toddler age, ligaments everywhere in the body tend to be loose. No doubt, if our ancient ancestors had chosen to walk on their hands instead of their feet, we would today be discussing the topic of flat hands. (See p. 338, **Ref. 53.**)

KNEES SWINGING TOWARD EACH OTHER
(Femoral Neck Anteversion)

Legs swing from the hip socket like a pendulum. The swing is straight ahead when the upper end of the thighbone fits squarely in the hip's socket. The swing deviates if the upper end of the thighbone is rotated slightly one way or the other and doesn't fit squarely in the socket.

Since most newborns normally have outwardly rotated hips, their legs tend to swing outward when they start to walk. There's a gradual correction with time, and by age three, most children's thighs are swinging straight ahead.

But many children have inwardly rotated hips, either from birth or from an overcorrection of the outward rotation at birth. When these children lie on their backs, their knees point toward each other instead of straight up. When they walk, the fronts of the kneecaps seem to be kissing.

Children with inwardly rotated hips have a special way of sitting on the floor. Holding their thighs together and turning their lower legs out and back, their legs form a perfect W. For them, it's the most comfortable position imaginable, but since it keeps the hips inwardly rotated, it tends to delay the normal spontaneous improvement that comes with age. For this reason, we suggest that children with inwardly rotated hips be encouraged to sit with their legs crossed in front of them, Indian style. Older children can be made aware of their leg swing by teaching them to skate or ski.

In the past, children with kissing knees were treated with twister cables that were attached to the shoes and ran up the outside of the leg to a belt around the waist. When a child wearing this device tried to walk, the cable pulled and twisted against the ligaments and joints of his legs. Sometimes, they created permanent deformities. The discomfort that they caused was equaled only by their worthlessness. (Twister cables, I suppose, aren't completely without value. They can always be used to pry secrets out of hostile prisoners of war.)

With time, the inturning at your child's hips will correct itself. I've been told that surgery has been performed in the rare cases that don't spontaneously improve, but in my 20 years as a pediatrician, I've never seen a child who needed the operation, so it's clear that time does a very good job with this one. (See p. 338, **Ref. 53.**)

WALKING ON TOES *(Habitual Metatarsal Standing)*

Most babies stand on their toes when they're first held erect. As they get more experience and grow more confident, they gradually begin to plant their whole feet including their heels on the floor. At times, especially when they're excited, some toddlers revert to toe walking. If yours spends part of his time on his toes and part of his time on his planted feet, nothing is wrong. It's only when he spends all of his time on his toes, or when he's no longer a baby, that a problem may exist. For the child under seven years who spends part of his time on his toes, and whose feet can be flexed upward 20 degrees while the knees are straight, this toe walking is nothing more than a habit.

If a child is *always* on his toes, he's referred to as an obligate toe walker, in which case he should be seen by an orthopedist. His problem may be orthopedic if the only tight tendon is the Achilles tendon, or neurologic if other tendons are involved. If the child is older than seven and still walking on his toes and nothing is wrong with his

Achilles tendon, your physician may suggest a search for an emotional cause. (See p. 338, **Ref. 53**; see p. 343, **Ref. 150.**)

SWAYBACK *(Lumbar Lordosis)*

A number of challenges confront your toddler's lower back when he decides to get up off his duff and face the world on his feet. In the first place, his hips are still flexed. This creates an angle between the trunk and the legs, and if the baby tries to put his legs straight to the ground his trunk is forced forward. This would be fine if he always moved forward, but when he has to stop and stand awhile, or lean to the side or back, he's unable to keep his balance.

Now the toddler's only recourse is to compensate for the forward tilt of the pelvis by arching his lower back backward. The hollow, or lordosis, this creates also pushes the already protuberant belly forward, completing the picture of the normal swaybacked toddler.

The extent of the sway is limited only by the ligaments of the spine, and at this age the ligaments aren't any tighter there than they are elsewhere. So, it's no surprise that swaybacks are more exaggerated in loose-jointed children and tend to improve with age as the ligaments tighten up.

The swayback is also helped as the hip flexion gradually lessens and the pelvis gets better support from the developing abdominal, lower back, and buttock muscles. Eventually, only a small hollow persists in the lower back, balanced by a rounding of the upper back called kyphosis, and another hollow or lordosis of the neck.

Thus, the side view of the childhood spine should show three smooth curves, two inward and one outward. Without these curves, the spine wouldn't have its shock absorber capacity, and the child's balancing and flexibility would be impaired. If the spine didn't have these built-in springs, a jump from a few feet up might transmit enough force upward to fracture the skull. (See p. 338, **Ref. 53.**)

VERY SORE CALVES AFTER VIRUS INFECTION *(Transient Acute Viral Myositis)*

Most viral infections produce aches and pains during the period of the fever. But sometimes, when the fever has passed and your child is clearly on the mend, she may wake up with intense pain in her thighs and calves. This infrequent condition follows influenza most often, but sometimes other viruses as well, including herpes, mononucleosis, and hepatitis.

Typically, the child wakes up with excruciating pain and absolutely refuses to walk. The muscles of her legs, especially the calves, are tender and slightly swollen. The event is often so dramatic that children who experience this symptom are frequently rushed to the hospital and subjected to intensive investigation, including muscle biopsy.

But with this condition, unlike more serious conditions that resemble it, there's only minor weakness in the painful muscle. Aside from the severe pain, there are no other signs or symptoms of illness, and the only blood-test abnormality is an elevated muscle-enzyme level, indicating recent muscle injury.

Within a week of this episode, called transient acute viral myositis (muscle inflammation), the child is entirely well. If your physician is aware of this syndrome, he'll have no trouble recognizing it, and will offer his reassurances. If he wasn't aware of it before, you can bet that he'll be waiting for it the next time influenza comes to town. (See p. 343, **Ref.** 151; see p. 343, **Ref.** 152.)

Functional Conditions

1. Respiratory System

TOO MANY COLDS

Little children have lots of colds and some of them appear to be afflicted with an eternal cold. Often, it's hard to tell whether the current cold symptoms represent the cold that's going away or the one that's just starting. This plethora of symptoms is enough to make an otherwise confident parent very nervous, and she usually begins to look for someone or something to blame. Is there something wrong with the child who seems to pluck out of the air every virus that floats his way? Is his diet lacking some essential cold retardant? Is there something wrong with the parents who can't manage to keep their child healthy for more than 20 minutes a month? And why doesn't the neighbor's child ever get sick, even though he's always half undressed and never eats the right foods, and his mother never takes him to the doctor, and so on?

Don't wear yourself out looking for the answers to these questions. The common cold is a common event. Fancy explanations aren't needed for everyday happenings. Still, you might rest easier if you knew just how common the common cold is. Studies done in Cleveland during a ten-year period showed that children under one year of age catch cold at the rate of 7 per year. At one year of age, children catch 8.3 colds per year, and the rate stays above 7 per year until they reach five years old. From age six years until adolescence, there's a gradual decline in the number of colds, until they reach the adult rate of 4 to 5 per year. That's a lot of colds, and goes a long way toward explaining why they're called common.

The above cold rates apply to age groups only and don't take into account other factors that are known to influence infection rates. For example, boys get more colds than girls, children in school or with a sibling in school get more colds, and children in large families have more colds. Colds occur two to three times more often in September through May than they do in the summer months. Children in day care or Head Start or the countless other toddler enrichment programs also have a higher incidence of colds.

The rhinovirus, which is the common cold virus, produces symptoms lasting 7 to 10 days for young adults. Children's colds tend to last 3 days longer than adults', so when you multiply 10 to 13 days of cold symptoms by 6 to 7 colds per year, you get 60 to 90 days per year of cold symptoms. At this rate, is it any wonder that you spend a lot of time wiping your perfectly normal, healthy child's nose?

If frequent respiratory infections are par for the course during early childhood, how can you tell if your child has something more than a common cold? How can you tell if your child's resistance is low, i.e., his immune system is weak? When children who have weak immune systems get sick, the illness is no small matter. True, these children, like any other, catch their share of common colds, but when they do, the cold is only the beginning of their illness. An immune-deficient child's cold invariably becomes complicated by ear infections, lymph node infections, chest infections, and the like. And even the complications become complicated: ear infections progress to ruptured eardrums, lymph nodes need to be surgically drained, and pneumonias don't respond to the customary treatment. In short, simple common infections in children with immune defects tend to spread, often into the bloodstream. These children also have many problems with germs that ordinarily pose no threat to the normal child. As soon as a doctor finds that a nonvirulent germ is behaving in a virulent way, he'll suspect that something is lacking in the child's defense against infection. Furthermore, children with immune defects tend to be small and frail, often have chronic diarrhea and skin infections, and don't look well. A normal child with frequent colds, on the other hand, continues to thrive and, aside from his constantly wet, sticky nose, he manages to look pretty well.

Immune-deficiency states are very rare. Allergies, however, are common, and your doctor may suspect that your child is allergic on the following grounds:

The allergic nose is swollen, oozes lots of clear watery fluid, itches, and does a lot of sneezing, often one sneeze after another. These symptoms may be accompanied by itchy, teary eyes and wheezing. When the doctor looks inside the child's nose, she'll see a pale, boggy, wet, bluish-tinged lining. If other members of the family are similarly afflicted, and if these symptoms are greatly relieved by the use of antihistamines, she'll probably conclude that the child has an allergy.

One feature of allergic problems is called seasonality, referring to the fact that the same set of symptoms always appear at the same time of the year. If the time of the year is one that ordinarily produces a peak rate of colds—such as winter—it's easy to mistake the seasonal, viral common cold for the seasonal allergic sniffle. On the other hand, if the nose blossoms at the same time as the cottonwood, year in and year out, smart money should be put on allergy.

A second feature of allergies is duration. The longer the symptoms last, the more likely they are to be allergic in nature. Sometimes, however, it's hard to tell if the symptoms are caused by one long allergic illness or by a long string of relatively brief viral illnesses. Because it isn't easy to tell the allergic sniffle from the viral cold, what seems like one long illness may be actually a series of colds and allergies, merging with each other. The infection-allergy cycle can get started in either of two directions. The virus-infected nose can become much more sensitive to an inhaled allergen (allergy inciter) than one that isn't infected, and what began as a straightforward infection can end up with typical allergic features. On the other side of the coin, an allergically swollen nasal lining is a less effective barrier to the infecting virus, making it more susceptible to infection. So you see, what starts out in the allergic camp may end up in the infection camp, and vice versa. This can make things very confusing if you're trying to figure out how long the cold has lasted.

The presence of wheezing was once considered a strong indication of allergy, but we've since discovered a large class of wheezers without allergies. The term that doctors use for nonallergic wheezing is *reactive airway disease.* Those with reactive airways look and sound just like allergic wheezers, but they don't benefit from regular injections of the desensitizing treatments used to treat allergies.

Lastly, a child with frequent ear and sinus infections as well as recurrent bouts of bronchitis might be suffering from an allergy. Allergies have been found to be involved in these nagging problems, and all doctors will recall the rare child who had one chest infection after the other and whose problems suddenly disappeared the moment the suspected offending allergen was removed from her environment. Allergies are certainly worth thinking about if your child seems to have endless sniffles, but more often than not, you'll find that removing her favorite toy or taking away her milk bottle won't make the toddler any better or happier.

Allergies aren't the only underlying causes for persistent respiratory symptoms that your doctor will be thinking about. There are a number of categories of causes that she'll consider, ranging from a foreign substance stuck up a nostril to a complicated problem like cystic fibrosis. Most of the time, the child suffering from frequent colds is perfectly normal and the only direction in which the accusing finger can be pointed is toward the nursery school or the day-care center. This isn't to say that children with frequent colds should be taken out of their surroundings. Contact with other children in supervised, socially educational settings does more good for their heads than the colds do harm. In my opinion, common colds are the dues we pay for membership in an active society. Some children pay their dues during the first few years of life, and others pay them later. The reality is that if we want to play, we have to pay, and sooner or later we all pay up. (See p. 343, **Ref. 154**; see p. 343, **Ref. 155**; see p. 343, **Ref. 156**.)

2. Digestive System

NOT EATING ENOUGH

Roughly one third of mothers believe that their children don't eat enough. When the children of these mothers are weighed, we find that as many are overweight as underweight. Notwithstanding parental concerns, nutritional surveys consistently show that children in North America get too many calories, not too few, with the protein intake being particularly excessive.

The only real danger that nutritionists find is that of obesity and protein overload.

How can so many parents be so off base? Why do so many parents see a problem where none exists? I believe that the answer comes from the parents' basic misunderstanding of the child's nutritional needs, and while trying to "correct" what's falsely perceived as a problem, such parents create a genuine eating problem. Here's how this can happen:

Children consume calories only to satisfy their need for growth and energy. During periods of rapid growth, high intakes are required; during periods of slower growth, less is required. From birth until three months of age, the average child gains 210 grams per week. For the next three months, he gains at the rate of 160 grams each week. For the third quarter of his first year, 100 grams per week. During the last quarter of the first year, the baby's growth rate is down to 75 grams per week. The growth rate continues to fall off even more during the second year, and, as the growth rate declines, fewer calories are needed. Can you imagine what it would be like to feed a 2,000-

kilogram six-year-old? That is what the average six-year-old would weigh if his rate of growth remained at the pace set during the first three months.

As the declining growth rate reduces the child's caloric intake, the parents may start to worry that their child isn't eating enough. This usually happens at the same time as the baby's shape is changing from a sphere to more of an ellipse. The baby is still growing and gaining weight; it's just that he appears to be slimmer because his overall configuration is changing. This is the only time in one's life when one can look slimmer while gaining weight, and parents who assume that their child's slimmer lines mean weight loss add this fuel to their worries about their baby's eating. Thus, what starts out as a normal event in the child's life becomes a crisis for the parents and, in response, two major mistakes are commonly made. Either one would be sufficient to wreck the child's eating habits for a very long time.

The first is the use of force. When the baby is very young, his stomach is entirely at the mercy of whoever is wielding the spoon, and no baby is a match for an accomplished practitioner of the art of spoonmanship. As fast as the baby pushes the unwanted food out of his mouth, it reappears on the next inbound spoon. Sometimes the satiated baby is distracted and entertained, and the minute his attention is diverted a spoon finds its way into his mouth. Later on, when this overt use of force fails, covert operations are begun. The baby is offered bribes (usually sweets), threatened with punishments, or held captive at the table until he has eaten a sufficient amount to satisfy his parents.

Now, how are these parents rewarded for all their good efforts? They wind up with a child who refuses to eat. Mealtime becomes the worst time of the day. Tensions mount as the hour for dining approaches. The table becomes an arena where parent and child do battle. (At one point in a child's development—the period of the normal negativism—the child's food resistance is only a part of his general resistance to pressure of any type.) Eventually, the unpleasantness at mealtime conditions the child against food, and a genuine food aversion develops.

The alternate route to nutritional mayhem takes the road of surrender. Battle-weary parents give up the struggle and allow their child to eat and drink whatever, wherever, and whenever they want. Between-meal snacks become the *haute cuisine*. With all the eating going on between meals, there's never a need for meals. For these children, mealtime is often the only time they break from eating. Of the "non-eating" children, these snackers are generally the most overweight.

The mother of a 40-kilogram four-year-old once told me that her child didn't "eat for her" (a not uncommon expression). During the time that it took this mother to complete that sentence, her four-year-old opened her purse, located a package of hard candy, unwrapped it, and in a single mouthful ate the entire package. I was very impressed, and when I pointed out this accomplishment to the mother, she wearily said, "Sure, he eats all right for you, but for me, it's a different story."

The truth is that when it comes to a child's eating, ask not for whom the child eats. He doesn't eat more than he wants to because he wants to compliment the chef. He eats only for himself, and with typically childlike self-interest. Most children like only a handful of foods and have little interest in diversity. In one large study, the average child ate only 3 cooked and 3 uncooked vegetables, though 29 different varieties were available. The same group ate only 4 out of 17 varieties of fruits, and 6 meats out of 20 choices. To no one's great surprise, children's tastes were more varied when it came to candies, choosing 14 out of the 16 offered. With candy being the one exception, children tend to be wary of new foods.

Here's what the preschool diner likes on his plate. He likes his food soft. He prefers it mushed, mashed, and minced. He likes the soft centers of the bread, not the hard crusts. He likes his soup cooled and his ice cream melted. The best temperature is room temperature. He prefers bland flavors and reacts negatively to the slightest deviation from the desired taste. He loves colors. The more contrasting colors on the plate, the better. He likes small portions on his plate.

Children eat first with their eyes, and if they see a plate heaped with an impossible amount of food, they're likely to choke up before they take their first bite. Play it smart and offer very small servings. An uncrowded plate is also easier for the toddler to handle. Small servings are more likely to be finished, and everybody is happier when the child comes back for a second helping.

The last and perhaps most important part of the meal is the "ambience," in the parlance of restaurant critics. Children eat better in a calm, unpressured atmosphere. Mealtime isn't the best hour to solve the most pressing military, economic, and political world crises. You can do that after the children have gone to bed. Table talk should be calm and pleasant with one person talking at a time. Children are easily distracted, and a lot of peripheral noise may ruin the atmosphere for them.

The bottom line is this. Children's eating needs are different from their parents' and, furthermore, they change their eating habits as often as their rate of growth changes. If you're aware of their special needs and can keep an even keel during the periods of change, there's a good chance that you'll avoid the common mistakes, and the needless emotional turmoil and eating problems they produce.

But don't strain yourself trying to make each and every meal perfectly balanced in all the food families. Not only is that quest totally unnecessary, but to succeed at it you would have to serve your child pizza (which happens to be a well-balanced meal) every night. Be assured that your child will, over the course of weeks to months, select a diet that's perfectly balanced, especially if he's allowed to do the choosing. (See p. 343, **Ref. 157.**)

DIARRHEA *(Chronic Nonspecific Diarrhea of Childhood)*

If your child has frequent loose stools for longer than three weeks, she's said to have chronic diarrhea. If she's growing and developing normally, and if your doctor hasn't been able to identify the cause of the problem, the odds are that her problem will be labeled chronic nonspecific diarrhea of childhood (CNDC). About 30 years ago, we would have called this condition mild celiac disease. About 20 years ago, it was described as mild starch intolerance, because many of the children's stool specimens contained starch granules in appreciable amounts. In England, the condition is called toddler's diarrhea, and sometimes peas and carrots syndrome, owing to the frequently seen, recognizable, undigested food in the baby's stool. I don't know what the next label will be, but I feel in my bones that CNDC doesn't have much of a future.

Regardless of what you call it, a lot of children on both sides of the Atlantic Ocean between 6 and 30 months, who have three to six loose stools with mucus daily, are perfectly well nourished and are growing and developing normally. This condition accounts for almost 35 percent of all outpatient referrals to pediatric gastroenterologists, and it accounts for most cases of chronic diarrhea in the thriving child.

Typically, a child with this condition starts the day with a large, formed or partly formed stool. Later in the day, the subsequent stools become smaller and looser, containing mucus and recognizable food particles. Only one such child in ten has more than six stools per day; most have three or four. Most of these children are troubled with constipation before this pattern begins, and to everybody's amazement, the constipation can reappear briefly while the typical diarrhea pattern is still present. Not surprisingly, children with CNDC often have sore, irritated bottoms.

Despite its single clinical picture, CNDC is probably not a single disorder, but a mixed bag of intestinal disorders having two essential features in common. First, there's an initial "insult" to the intestine that originally caused the acute diarrhea, and then there's a secondary insult that leads to the persistence of the diarrhea. We know a lot more about the initial than the secondary insult.

Most of the time, the initial intestinal insult is nothing more than a bout of intestinal flu that occurs in a healthy child of 6 to 20 months of age. Other trigger events in decreasing frequency are: dietary manipulations such as switching from formula to formula, introducing solid foods too early, and the use of certain medicines such as antibiotics or even decongestants. Whatever the insult, the intestine responds with diarrhea that, for most children, subsides when the intestine recovers. For others, there's a secondary insult and the diarrhea hangs on to produce the syndrome of CNDC.

Several medical theories have been offered to explain how the secondary insult comes about. One popular explanation holds that damage done to the intestine's lining by the original insult leads to a transient enzyme deficiency. This contributes to a buildup of highly irritating, partially digested and unabsorbed food particles that add to the intestinal injury, delay the repair process, and prolong the diarrhea.

Another explanation is that children with CNDC are predisposed to it from birth and that the trigger event only brings the problem to the surface. Supporters of this theory point to the high incidence of bowel problems in parents and siblings of children with CNDC, and to the high frequency of colic and constipation in the children before they started having CNDC. The common threat, they say, is a disturbance in the regulation of the intestine's rhythmic, coordinated, wavelike activity. Indeed, when children with CNDC have the rate of their intestinal activity measured, many are found to have an abnormally rapid "mouth-to-anus transit time." According to this theory,

CNDC is simply the child's version of the "irritable colon," an extremely common functional bowel disorder of adults.

The latest theory on CNDC puts the blame on the way we feed the child after the initial insult. The standard and altogether proper diet for a child with acute diarrhea is one limited to "clear fluids," consisting of dilute carbohydrates such as weak fruit juices and flat sodas, which provide the child with water to avoid dehydration, plus calories. This diet ordinarily works and the diarrhea soon improves. When it does, the diet is gradually advanced back to the prediarrhea level.

Sometimes the diarrhea returns, in which case the child is put back on the clear fluid diet and advanced again as soon as improvement is seen. If the diarrhea returns, the cycle is renewed. Soon, the period that the child remains on the low-calorie, high-carbohydrate, no-protein, no-fat diet becomes longer than originally planned. The carbohydrate overload slightly irritates the intestines, stimulating the mucus-secreting cells to produce mucus. Now you have diarrhea with mucus, and the start of CNDC.

If this theory is correct, as most experts now believe, it explains why treating CNDC with dietary restrictions doesn't stop the mucous diarrhea. Furthermore, if there's enough caloric restriction, the child doesn't gain weight during this period. What these children need is more calories, not fewer, especially if they include proteins and fats in well-balanced proportions. But be forewarned that forging ahead with this diet may temporarily worsen the diarrhea. Eventually the stools firm up and rapid catch-up weight gain occurs.

Tests on children with CNCD show that many of them have two dietary abnormalities, both of which result from keeping them on the acute diarrhea diet (a high carbohydrate intake) for long periods of time. The first is a deficiency of fat (less than 30 percent of calories consumed). If the proportion of fat is increased to 40 percent of calories, the diarrhea usually stops. Furthermore, half of the children with CNDC whose fat intake is normal improve when more unsaturated fats are added to their diets. We don't know exactly how or why adding small amounts of margarine or peanut butter to the child's diet works, but we've seen that it does.

The other dietary factor is excessive water intake. If your doctor determines that your child has a fluid intake that's more than two and a half times the required amount, you can help him greatly by restricting his fluid intake to a level that's only 50 percent above his required amount. Restricting fluid intakes of children with CNDC that aren't excessive to begin with won't help. Only about 20 percent of cases of CNDC are caused by excessive fluid intake. We don't know how many are caused by a deficiency of dietary fat, but it may be as high as 50 percent.

For those not in either category, there are still a number of dietary maneuvers to be tried. Since the acute intestinal insult can produce a transient deficiency of certain enzymes, a temporary wheat, milk, or sugar intolerance can follow the acute diarrheal episode. For this reason, it's worthwhile to try avoiding these foods for a few days to see if it helps. If there's a significant improvement, don't assume that your child will have a lifelong problem with that food. With time, the enzyme level will be restored and the food will be fully tolerated.

If none of these experiments work, and your child continues to have mucous diarrhea, what should you do?

Wait for the child to outgrow the condition. While you're waiting, your child will have good days and bad. Some of the bad days will coincide with colds or emotional upsets. Eventually, the diarrhea will stop. Ninety percent of children with CNDC are free of diarrhea by 36 to 39 months of age. (See p. 343, **Ref. 158;** see p. 343, **Ref. 159;** see p. 343, **Ref. 160;** see p. 343, **Ref. 161;** see p. 343, **Ref. 162.**)

CONSTIPATION DURING TOILET TRAINING *(Stool Withholding)*

Many toddlers are so enthralled with their newfound mastery over their muscles of defecation that they make their potty chair the center stage for acting out major acts of compliance and defiance. During the period of early toilet training, the sensation of rectal fullness and pressure isn't always reason enough for them to have a bowel movement; they have to be in the mood for it. And if you are and they aren't, there's no way that you'll prevail. The ensuing tug-of-war will only tear at your nerves. The more coercive pressure you put to bear, the less abdominal pressure you'll get from the child. What begins as a small show of power from headquarters becomes a major insurrection from the rear brigade. As the stool remains in the baby's rectum longer and longer, it gets larger and dryer, and before long it becomes a real problem for the baby to expel. Now we have a truly constipated child, and if the hard dry stool is expelled with pain or bleeding, we also get a frightened child who has just discovered another reason to withhold stool.

The scenario doesn't have to go this far. If you don't make a big deal of the toilet training, it tends to stay in perspective. If you do, it becomes a rallying point of defiance or compliance. If you have reason to anticipate a bit of withholding as your child learns to control her rectal muscles, give her some natural laxatives such as prune juice and raisins in her diet to keep her stool from becoming dry and hard to expel. If the toddler starts to squeeze her cheeks, turn yours. You can't win this one. Let her win the little skirmish or else she'll surely win when the conflict has escalated to a full-blown war. If there's resistance, put her back in diapers until she decides that she's ready. You'll be sparing yourself and your baby a lot of needless grief.

BRIGHT RED BOWEL MOVEMENTS: RED FOOD COLOR

There's nothing scarier than seeing a bright red bowel movement. When you see red, it's natural to think that the reason is blood and, if that turns out to be the case, the cause can be quite serious. But if your child is otherwise healthy, not suddenly pale, and not in pain, stop and consider some of these common mimics of intestinal bleeding.

Red food coloring can turn the stool a bright red color. Red Kool-Aid, Hawaiian Punch, and the all-time monster of the breakfast cereals, Frankenberry, are the best examples in this category. Any medicine, food, or drink that's dyed red can produce a stool that's dyed red. Some foods, such as beets and tomatoes, are naturally red, and if they're only partly digested, the stool may look red.

The sophisticated stool watcher knows that high intestinal bleeding tends to turn the stool black, not red. But even all that's black isn't blood. For example, the pigment of licorice, grapes, raisins, and cranberries can produce black stools. If enough charcoal is eaten, the stool will be black. Medicines such as Pepto-Bismol and iron capsules also blacken the stool. Remember, what goes in red, purple, or black may come out looking like blood. If there's any doubt about the cause of the stool's color, your doctor can do a very simple chemical test to determine if blood is the reason for the stool's worrisome color.

Incidentally, all of the above causes of "bloodlike" stools are equally good at mimicking blood in vomit, so if your baby has a red throw-up after downing a bottle of Hawaiian Punch, don't take off for the nearest emergency room.

3. Nervous System

BREATH-HOLDING SPELLS *(Anoxic Convulsions)*

About 1 child in 20 has at least one breath-holding spell that produces unconsciousness and/or convulsive movements. All in all, the episode resembles an epileptic convulsion. But it's not. Further, it doesn't come from or lead to brain damage. In fact, this particular childhood mimic of real disease is a specialty of the very normal child and can easily be differentiated from the serious epileptic attack.

Medically, the episode is either called cyanotic (blue) or pallid (pale) infantile syncope (fainting spell), depending on the child's color before passing out. The difference in colors results from a subtle physiologic difference in the way the two groups respond to breath holding, but, for all practical purposes, it doesn't matter what color the child turns.

The spells usually start between 6 and 18 months of age, affecting boys and girls equally. They happen only occasionally at first, say once every week, and gradually become more frequent, often occurring several times a day during the second and third years of age. They then gradually decrease in frequency, and by the time the child is six years old, 90 percent of all breath holding stops. Breath holding can be a family tradition. Twice as many parents of breath holders were breath holders themselves as compared to parents of non–breath holders.

The typical breath-holding spell starts when the infant receives a sudden, unpleasant surprise, either a fright, a frustration, a minor injury, or a scolding. Whatever the unpleasant stimulus, it comes as a big surprise and the baby is startled. More angered than hurt, he cries vigorously for a few breaths, or takes a few gasps, and then starts to turn colors. Most turn a lovely shade of lavender around the lips, deepening to an oceanic blue. About one child in five turns white instead. Regardless of the color, the baby loses consciousness. At this point, most children grow limp, but some stiffen out. As a finale, some give a few convulsive jerks of their arms and legs. The whole thing is done in less than a minute, and when it's all over the baby appears sound, but a bit tired.

What makes the outraged nonbreathing infant pass out when he holds his breath, while an underwater swimmer just swims along breathlessly? It can't be the lack of oxygen, because we know that these babies lose consciousness when their blood oxygen saturation is still between 75 and 90 percent, which aren't levels that would produce unconsciousness. We also can dismiss low blood pressure as the cause.

All the information obtained from monitoring breath holders during attacks leads to the conclusion that the breath-holding spell (and, probably, fainting after violent coughing [see p. 311] and forceful urinating [see p. 311] as well) results from the same chain of events that produces the old "mess trick." In this famous old game, the performer, usually a fun-loving undergraduate, breathes deeply as fast as he can and, at the end of a deep breath, suddenly forces all the air out of his chest and keeps forcing until he passes out. The trick always amazes and mystifies his friends and does wonders for the undergraduate's status on campus. When the two-year-old performs it, the only gain is in the number of gray hairs on his parent's head.

After you've sat through a few of these performances, and are wise to what's going on, you aren't so likely to be taken aback. But the grand opening can be terribly anxiety-provoking, especially if you don't recognize the "trick." It may be, for example, that, in your judgment the precipitating event was too trivial to justify such an emotional response, or the period of breathlessness didn't seem long enough to lead to unconsciousness, or the jerking movements lasted too long for your comfort. It's especially confusing if you don't even see, recognize, or remember the precipitating event. When the period of breath holding is very brief, or you didn't see it at all, you might mistakenly connect the unconsciousness or the convulsive movements directly to the stimulus for the breath holding, especially if it was a fall or a blow to the head. Children who quickly lose consciousness with a minimum of crying also tend to turn white instead of the more understandable blue, and this also increases their chances of being confused with children who have a true convulsive disorder.

Your doctor will distinguish the breath holder from one who has a seizure disorder by several methods. In the first place, the onset of these episodes in early infancy is typical for breath holding but distinctly uncommon in the basic epileptic disorder (idiopathic epilepsy). The epileptic attack occurs without warning, often during sleep, and usually lasts several minutes. The breath-holding spell is provoked by a specific incident, never happens during sleep, and rarely lasts as long as a minute. During an epileptic attack the child is hot and sweaty, and has a racing pulse. During a breath-holding episode, the child is cool and clammy, and has a very slow pulse. After an epileptic attack, the child is confused, disoriented, and very sleepy. After a breath-holding spell, the child is clearheaded and maybe a bit sleepy. Although these distinctions make it quite easy to know which situation you're dealing with, your doctor may want to have an electroencephalogram done to be certain.

When breath holding is promptly recognized, the child is, or course, spared the medication given for convulsive disorders as well as the unfortunate stigma that, in the minds of many people, is still attached to the diagnosis of a seizure disorder. The treatment of breath holding requires no medication. This is another of the conditions to which the motto "Don't just do something; stand there" applies. Don't blow into your baby's mouth or splash cold water on him. If he comes out of his spell and finds someone carrying on like this, it might make him angry, and you know what happens when a little breath holder gets angry. Try instead to count to 60 slowly. Remember while you're counting that breath-holding spells have a built-in fail-safe system. As soon as your baby blacks out, his automatic breathing controls take over, bringing him out of the spell.

Many breath holders also have temper tantrums and bang their heads to demonstrate their displeasure and stubbornness. Sometimes these behavioral disturbances occur during the breath-holding years, but sometimes they're saved for later. A sixth of all breath holders grow up to become fainters when frightened, angered, or subjected to pain.

The only dangers breath-holding spells pose result from misinterpretations and overreactions by the child's parents or, of course, a misdiagnosis of epilepsy, in which case the child will be wrongly medicated. Because of the terrifying nature of the attacks, the parent, scared out of his wits, may be inclined to do just about anything to avoid frustrating, disappointing, punishing, or scolding the child. Hoping to avoid even the mildest provocation, the parent may establish a padded-cell atmosphere in an attempt to protect the child from anything that might provoke a breath-holding episode. As you can imagine, this sort of undisciplined, overprotected climate is an intensely unfavorable one in which to raise a normal, healthy child.

If the parents remain calm during the attack, and don't relinquish the responsibility for discipline, the overall outlook for the breath holder is good. The need for discipline of these children is increased, not lessened, by their breath holding.

It might help if you try to keep the image of a velvet hammer in your head when you're pounding out the discipline. To be effective, it must have clout; but it doesn't have to be delivered with anger or harshness. Try to discipline your breath holder while thinking about the "three Fs": firmness, fairness, and fondness; and use the "three Cs": controlling, caring, and consistency. The last thing you want to produce is a "three Ts" child: terrible, terrified, and tyrannical. (See p. 343, **Ref. 163**; see p. 343, **Ref. 164**; see p. 343, **Ref. 165**.)

EPISODES OF DIZZINESS *(Benign Paroxysmal Vertigo)*

Benign paroxysmal vertigo (BPV) is so remarkably consistent in its age of onset, and the nature of each episode, that it seldom needs laboratory confirmation. If you or your doctor want laboratory confirmation, it's available, but most doctors are familiar with BPV and will be able to make the diagnosis after hearing the child's story.

BPV attacks occur suddenly, without warning. The child, between one and three years of age, looks frightened and pale, and begins to cry. He lunges for his mother's skirt or a table leg; if he can't find either, he staggers drunkenly until he falls or maneuvers himself into a sitting position on the floor. He may say "round and round" during the attack. If he's more verbal, he'll describe the house, room, or ceiling as "going around." Some children say they're falling or spinning, others that they're dizzy. They all remain fully alert and may be talkative during the episode.

The attacks last a few seconds to a few minutes. They leave as suddenly as they come, at which point some children announce: "All gone." Vomiting, darting eye movements (nystagmus), and head tilt (torticollis) are all common during the attacks. The child looks entirely well after the attack and stays that way till the next one.

The frequency of these episodes varies from several weekly to several yearly. Most children with BPV have 8 to 12 attacks per year. Sometimes they occur in clusters and don't appear again for a long time. After several months to several years, the attacks stop.

As with most of the benign conditions of childhood, your physician's main task in correctly labeling BPV is to distinguish it from similar disorders that are more significant. Like breath holding (see p. 213), BPV is sometimes mistaken for epilepsy. The complete alertness of the child during and after the attack will tip off your doctor and, if needed, a normal electroencephalogram will keep the distinction between these two entities quite clear. Parents often worry about a brain tumor in this situation, but a tumor seldom causes such dramatic episodic symptoms without also causing some difficulty in between the episodes. If this worry persists, it can easily be resolved with a brain scan. Nor does the BPV represent an emotional problem in this age group, or in any children who show no other signs of having psychological problems. Your doctor might suspect a disorder of the balancing center, the vestibular apparatus, in the inner ear, though this seldom leads to episodic dizziness in BPV's age group. If any doubt exists, a diagnosis of BPV can be readily established by specific tests of vestibular function performed by a specialist.

Treatment of BPV is ordinarily unnecessary, but if the attacks occur more than once each week, your doctor may suggest putting the child on Dramamine, or any other motion-sickness remedy. Either way, BPV is just another indication of an immature nervous system. With time and patience all will be well. (See p. 343, **Ref. 166**; see p. 344, **Ref. 167**.)

BODY ROCKING AND HEAD BANGING
(Rhythmic Habits)

The percentage of infants who rock their bodies to and fro and roll from side to side varies from 35 to 91, though only 19 to 21 percent of normal children are heavy rock-and-rollers. On the average, children begin this habit pattern between six and ten months of age, usually just after they've given up the foot-kicking habit. Both boys and girls do it, and most children stop by two and one half to three years of age. Body rocking occurs most often when the child is listening to music and seldom lasts longer than 15 minutes. The majority of head bangers started out as body rockers.

Three to six months after body rocking, about 6 to 10 percent of both boys and girls begin rolling their heads. Head rolling is most often seen when the baby is left alone in the crib or playpen, but heads also roll when the children are listening to music.

Another 5 to 15 percent of babies are head bangers. They strike their heads rhythmically, monotonously, and continuously against their crib's headboard, side rail, or whatever else they can find. Head banging starts at about the same time as head rolling. In study after study, boys are found to be head bangers three to four times more often than girls, and in one study 22.3 percent of the boys were head bangers. They bang their heads when they're tired, bored, or mad. They also do it when they're in pain, most often from a tooth or an infected ear. I've seen children develop calluses on their foreheads from banging, but I've never seen or heard of anything more serious happening to their heads. Plaster on walls that the crib is touching can be loosened by the repetitive banging, and I've seen hospital walls destroyed in this way. Roughly two thirds of head bangers are, or were, body rockers.

There are countless theories explaining rhythmic body habits, ranging from self-directed pleasure giving to self-directed pleasure taking. Whatever the reason for them, they seem to be closely tied in to the normal maturation and development of infants, and until more is learned about them, I'll continue to view them as an expression of pleasure, tension, or pain in an infant lacking a great variety of ways to express himself. (See p. 340, **Ref. 99**; see p. 344, **Ref. 168**; see p. 344, **Ref. 169**.)

SLEEP DISTURBANCES
Screaming in Deep Sleep (Pavor Nocturnus)

Beginning on page 133, we described how the newborn's sleep is different from the adult's and how, by three months of age, most newborns develop sleep patterns that begin to assume the adult's characteristics. By age two years, though some differences still remain, the child's sleep has, by and large, assumed the adult form; that is, his sleep consists of a series of alternating states of rapid eye movement (REM) with a slow brain wave (non-REM) state, and the latter is clearly divided into four stages. Instead of entering REM sleep directly as he did when he was a few months old, he now must enter REM by ascending through the various stages of non-REM. This sleep-lightening process, called arousal, doesn't always proceed smoothly for the child, and as a result several common disorders of sleep can develop.

The most common disorders of arousal from sleep are nighttime bed-wetting (nocturnal enuresis), sleepwalking (somnambulism), sleeptalking (somniloquy), and night terrors (pavor nocturnus). The first three are described on pages 226 and 315, but since all are disturbances in arousal, they share many of the following common traits.

They are familial; that is, they occur in certain families more than others. They are all episodic, automatic, robotlike acts of which the child has no memory. Ninety percent of these acts take place during the emergence from non-REM stage 3 and 4 to stage 2. All of them occur most often during the first three hours of sleep. They all result from an immature nervous system and, if allowed to proceed normally, all disappear in time as maturation goes on.

Night terrors occur during intense and sudden arousal from non-REM stage 3 or 4. In the typical scene, the sleeping child suddenly bolts up and screams. He's sweaty and his heart rate is speeding. He appears to be staring at some imaginary object, but for about ten minutes there's no way to get through to him. Eventually he relaxes and goes back to sleep. In the morning he has no recollection of the event, and isn't sleepy during the day. The next night he happily trots off to bed having no memory of the incident and, therefore, no dread of night terrors. Although they may appear to be similar in many ways, night terrors are very much different from the nightmares and anxiety dreams that are described next. (See p. 340, **Ref. 92**.)

Nightmares

During his second year, the average child gets into enough conflict with his family and trouble with his environment to generate a measurable amount of tension and anxiety. Furthermore, he now views going to bed and nighttime awakenings as representing separations from his loved ones, and this adds to his anxiety at bedtime. If his day is capped off with wild and vigorous horseplay, the overexcitement adds to the bedtime tension, and the ultimate product is the nightmare (*mare* means evil spirit or goblin that frightens people).

The contents of most nightmares in this age group are limited to reenactments of the frightening experiences of the day, i.e., a replay of the daymares, with the cast of characters switched to animals, ghosts, or monsters. They occur during REM sleep, and can be remembered. The memory aspect distinguishes nightmares from night terrors, and also makes the child reluctant to return to bed, that night or any other.

As the child matures, he gradually learns to separate dreams from reality and, with the development of ego strength, he comes to fear bedtime less and less. Until this happens, most childhood bedtime anxiety is relieved by the bedtime ritual. For some children, the ritual involves placing all the toys in the room in the same position; for some, it's reading the same boring story night after night; for some, it's a highly evolved complex of activities such as going to the bathroom, then taking a sip of water, then saying good night to the stuffed animals, and on and on. More tension needs more ritual. Remember this fact as you go into the bedroom to kiss your baby good night for the final, absolutely, this is it, now I really mean it, last time. (See p. 340, **Ref. 92**.)

Giving Up the Nap *(Maturing Sleep Patterns)*

During infancy, the baby spends more time asleep than awake, but after the age of two years, the total daily sleep requirement decreases. The reduction in the total is entirely at the expense of the daytime napping; night sleep remains relatively constant until age five, averaging 11 hours each night.

The morning nap becomes a cherished memory of the past by age two years, and from two to four years an increasing number of children will relinquish their afternoon naps as well. Four percent of two-year-olds, 10 percent of three-year-olds, and 30 percent of four-year-olds don't take afternoon naps. Those who do take naps take them for as many hours as the younger child. In other words, the length of the afternoon nap remains at slightly over an hour for two-, three-, and four-year-olds who nap. Children under three who take an extra-long afternoon nap have no difficulty falling asleep that night, but there's evidence that the older children who take a long afternoon nap frequently have a hard time falling asleep, and may sleep less at night. Other factors that reduce the amount of the child's sleep are: (1) getting overtired, (2) sleeping in a room with adults, and (3) going to bed later than usual. Children sleep better and longer when they have another child in the room, and when they're put to bed at a consistent time in a consistent way. It also helps to give your child some warning that bedtime is approaching; that way he has some time to get himself ready. It's also useful to make him actively participate in his bedtime routines by getting him to put his toys away, select the book you'll read from, and choose his nightclothes. Lastly, keep in mind that good habits need to be started early and constantly reinforced. Bad habits can be started anytime, and seem to become firmly entrenched after the first experience. (See p. 340, **Ref. 91.**)

RAG DOLL INFANT—FLABBY MUSCLES, LOOSE JOINTS *(Benign Congenital Hypotonia)*

Whenever doctors try to determine the level of young infants' development, we're unavoidably overinfluenced by their gross motor skills, like sitting, crawling, and walking. It isn't that this particular area is more important than language, social, adaptive, and fine motor skills; it's just that the gross motor skills are more conspicuous and easily assessed. For this reason, children who are late in reaching their gross motor milestones tend to get spotted early and may be suspected of being slow. But if such infants happen to be floppy, it's possible that their entire problem is limited to their muscle tone.

It's fairly easy to detect the floppy child. She's one whose muscles feel flabby, whose joints are so loose that almost any position can be assumed, no matter how bizarre, and whose limbs can be passively bent to a greater extent than you might expect. In short, a rag doll.

The medical profession has been burdened with a lot of confusing terminology in this area; many terms are used for the same condition, and several different conditions have been grouped together under the same name. Nevertheless, if your infant is floppy but not weak, is up to date in her other areas of development, and has no disorders in any other body system (such as the thyroid, for example), it's highly probable that your doctor will make a diagnosis of benign congenital hypotonia. It occurs most often in children who have a family history of loose-jointedness and/or very late onset of walking. Incidentally, it's always nice to get a multiple-word diagnosis beginning with the word *benign*.

Children with benign congenital hypotonia may not be able to sit unsupported until 16 months of age, or walk until 36 months, yet they'll be entirely normal by the time they're 4 years old. (See p. 344, **Ref.** 170; see p. 344, **Ref.** 171; see p. 344, **Ref.** 172.)

4. Urinary System

DOESN'T URINATE DURING TOILET TRAINING *(Urinary Retention)*

Chanting resolutely to himself, "Hell, no, I won't go," a child of two to three years, who is making his last stand against the toilet-training establishment, is able to distend his bladder to the size of a uterus in the fifth month of pregnancy. When it dawns on the rest of the family that the child hasn't urinated all day, and that his belly is sticking out, the scene usually shifts to the doctor's office. Where the final curtain falls depends a lot on what kind of office the child was taken to.

Urinary retention is a fairly common problem of older men. If the doctor who has been selected to solve the baby's problem happens to be one who specializes in older people's problems, and if nobody has told this doctor that toilet training is in progress, the chances are good that his approach to the child's acute urine retention will be more applicable to the child's grandfather than to the child.

Here are a few things that you can try even before you rush off to the doctor's office. First, think back to how things were before you started potty-training your child. If there was no problem with his stream then, the odds are good that there's no problem now. Next, take off his "big boy" pants and put him back in his diapers. Most little tykes will feel immediate relief of the toilet-training pressure and will go with their flow. For some, their muscles are in such tight spasm that they still just can't seem to let go. In this case, here are a few, very safe tricks that you can try.

First, even if you see absolutely no humor in the situation, you can tickle the child. The giggling will often lead to a loss of urinary control, especially if the child is a girl. Or you can give the child a nice, warm bath. The relaxation that a bath provides will usually allow the child to let his urine go, but if not, try a rectal enema. There are two reasons for this. In the first place, urine withholding is often accompanied by stool withholding, and by the time the bladder distension is noticed, there may already be a sizable accumulation of stool filling the rectum. Second, the muscles that have to be relaxed to let the enema fluid out are the same ones that let the urine out, so while the child is ridding himself of the enema fluid, he inadvertently empties his bladder. Some doctors believe that the constipated mass of stool usually constitutes an obstruction to the bladder, but in my opinion, both the constipation and the urinary retention are the results of the same cause, namely withholding. If these measures fail to empty the bladder, your doctor should be informed and other measures can be considered.

There's one other possible factor involved in a child's withholding of urine. At times, the reason for withholding is more than willful. Sometimes, there's a sore in the vicinity of the urinary opening, and as soon as urine flows over it the child experiences pain and reflexively clamps down on the muscles that allow the escape of urine. In the case of a boy, the sore may be an erosion at the very tip of the penis, which can fill in with a scab that may actually sit over the opening itself. If the boy is still in diapers, his sore may be anywhere on his bottom, from the shaft of his penis to the tender skin around his anus. If constipation has been a feature of withholding, the odds are pretty good that there will be some soreness around the anus. No matter where the sensitive skin is, if it gets wet, it can sting and the child will turn off the flow.

Since little girls, even out of diapers, tend to dampen a broad area of their bottoms while urinating, they can have the same sort of problem. So, in addition to the above tricks, it's a good idea to look for the sore on the child who is withholding urine.

SEEMS TO URINATE TOO OFTEN OR TOO
SELDOM *(Normal Frequency of Voiding)*

Once your child passes her first birthday, she'll start to cut down on the frequency of urination from 16 to 24 times each day to 8 to 18. During her third year, the average number of daily voidings is 10, and the fourth year, 9. From then until she's 12 years old, the number gradually drops to 4 to 6 each day, where it remains through adulthood.

The amount of urine in each voiding varies greatly from child to child and from day to day, but a rough rule of thumb states that the average amount of urine per voiding is 5 milliliters for every kilogram of the child's weight. In other words, a 20-kilogram child will have an average voiding volume of 100 milliliters. (See p. 344, **Ref. 173**; see p. 344, **Ref. 174**.)

DAMP PANTIES IN GIRLS *(Vaginal Reflux)*

When girls of any age urinate, some urine is invariably detoured through the vagina. For some girls, the amount of urine is considerable enough to distend the vagina, but for most, there's only partial filling. This distension happens regardless of the girl's age, voiding position, or shape and extent of hymen. Radiologists in the process of doing X-ray examinations of bladders first noticed this vaginal reflux, and they came to view it as a normal part of the female voiding process.

Because of vaginal reflux, urine can slowly escape after the little girl has wiped herself. Depending on the amount of reflux, she can either soak her panties or merely dampen a small area. Don't accuse her of wiping herself too carelessly or of not making it to the bathroom on time. Both are "bum" raps. All you have to do to satisfy yourself that her wetness is simply the trickling out of refluxed vaginal urine is to look and see if she's dry before she goes to the bathroom and wet only after she's finished urinating.

The amount of urine that trickles out is usually quite small, and seldom causes more than a little dampness. If this is causing a problem, teach your little girl to stand up and jiggle around a little before applying her final wipe, and that should take care of the refluxed vaginal urine. (See p. 344, **Ref. 175**; see p. 344, **Ref. 176**.)

BED-WETTING *(Enuresis)*

Human beings first grappled with bed-wetting 3,000 to 4,000 years ago, but we didn't get our heads above water until we learned that bed-wetting is a sleep, not a urine, problem. The ancient Egyptians treated enuretic children with a mixture of juniper berries, cyprus, and wine. The Greeks, who gave bed-wetting its name (*enuresis,* meaning to urinate in), modernized the treatment using white chrysanthemums in tepid water. Two thousand years later, the healing arts had progressed from the garden to the barnyard, and the drug of choice became pulverized stomach of hen taken twice daily. Treatment remained somewhat folksy until very recently, when modern technology gave us the information that led us to reclassify the disorder as a problem of sleep.

Depending on what age is used to define when wetting the bed becomes abnormal (the range is three to five years), as well as its frequency, the prevalence of enuresis varies from 2.2 to 26 percent. Factors other than age and frequency, such as whether the children were selected from the general population or from a special group, like an institution, or whether social, economic, or cultural differences were taken into account, also make the true incidence hard to come by. We do know that enuresis occurs frequently during the school-age years, that it gradually decreases, and that 2.5 percent of all World War II recruits were discharged because of bed-wetting.

We also know that there's a psychological aspect to bed-wetting. For example, it's more common in children who are high strung, developmentally delayed, or learning disabled, and in any child whose behavior tends to be infantile. Illnesses, family conflicts, and academic stresses all contribute to bed-wetting, particularly if there's a family history of enuresis, which is true for up to 80 percent of all bed-wetters. We also know that many, if not most, of the psychological problems are the result of the wetting, rather than its cause.

It's no coincidence that all of the above traits are also found in children subject to sleepwalking, sleeptalking, and night terrors, since they all stem from the same basic problem, a faulty process of arousal from deep sleep. Here are a few other characteristics of enuresis that are shared with the other parasomnias, as they're collectively called (see pp. 219 and 315): (1) The event, in this case wetting, tends to occur during arousal from the first sleep cycle of the night. (2) While it's going on, the child is out of contact with his surroundings. (3) Many more boys are affected than girls. (4) There's no memory of its happening the next morning. (5) The child isn't overly sleepy the next morning.

The problem isn't entirely a matter of sleep control. The nonenuretic's bladder has occasional low-pressure contractions during stage 3 and 4 non-REM sleep. These contractions are ignored by the nonenuretic's sleeping brain. In contrast, the enuretic's bladder has spontaneous contractions during deep sleep that are stronger and more frequent than the nonenuretic's, and closely resemble those of the young infant's. All in all, it seems proper to place the blame squarely on the immaturity of the nervous system, since no urine is released unless an immature bladder contraction signals an immature sleeping brain to stop holding back. This is why maturity puts an end to most enuresis.

The question is what to do while you're waiting for maturity. The first thing to do is find out if your child has the kind of enuresis described above, that is, functional enuresis. Not all bed-wetting is simple, functional enuresis. Some wetting results from organic diseases such as urinary infections, bladder malformations, overproduction of urine, or problems within the spinal cord. Since all of these disorders cause daytime wetting as well as enuresis, your doctor will carefully look for signs of poor urine control during the day before she tells you that no organic illness exists, and that the enuresis is functional.

Functional enuresis is called primary if your child has been wetting the bed since infancy, and secondary if your child was once dry at night and is now wetting. In the case of secondary enuresis, your doctor will carefully look for a recent reason for your child to be feeling less secure and more anxious. She'll probably find one, such as the birth of a new baby, a move to a new home, or a bully in school. The management of this problem is straightforward. After identifying the problem, you change the situation. If the problem happens to involve a blessed event, and if you don't plan on returning the baby to the hospital, you'll have to think of some other way to make your older child feel more secure. On the other hand, unless a leaking water bed is found, the management of the child with primary functional enuresis, by far the most common type of enuresis, will be more complex. If obvious psychopathology isn't present, there's no need to get psychotherapy for your child. The emotional problems that accompany primary enuresis are the result, not the cause, and they tend to stop once the child becomes dry at night. If psychotherapy isn't needed, what should you do?

First of all, you should accept the idea that primary functional enuresis is a result of neurologic immaturity, is usually hereditary, and isn't a sign of stubborn laziness, babyishness, or rebelliousness. It's very easy to get furious at the child who defies your best efforts at keeping the sheets dry and who seems to be totally unaware of his own role in the problem. In this regard, fathers are usually much more tolerant of the problem than mothers. Perhaps they see a certain similarity between what's going on with their baby sons and what went on when they were somebody's baby sons. Or maybe it's just the fact that they aren't the ones changing the sheets in the middle of the night and washing the bedding day in and day out.

Next, remember that chances are excellent that the enuresis will stop once the child gets older. Now that you've heard all this wonderful news about enuresis, you may feel consoled and comforted. This does little for your enuretic child, who still wakes up in the morning doing the backstroke. What can we do for him?

Our methods of helping him fall into two groups: (1) things that doctors and parents do *to* him (passive therapy) and (2) things that we do *with* him (active therapy). Included in the first group of passive therapy aids are certain minor surgical procedures, drugs that alter sleep patterns, drugs that alter bladder function, and electrical devices that condition the child to wake up when the bladder feels full. The success rates for these treatments vary from 30 to 100 percent. Thirty percent success is probably what Thomas Phaer, the father of pediatrics, got with his treatment, hedgehog stones, and probably a bit higher than its predecessor, urine from spayed swine. But even when these methods make the child dry, there's still the danger of fostering an impression that the child is somehow defective, sick, or incompletely developed, and in need of other people or things to make him normal. I prefer to use active therapy instead. Active participation makes the child responsible for his wetting and his control. I turn my back to the parent and speak directly to the child. I start out by saying that even though his mother has been the one to deal with his wetting the bed, the problem is really his and not his mother's. I tell him that I know that he would like to stop wetting his bed, and that I know a number of good ways to help him with his problem.

I tell him that it would be helpful if he kept track of his dry nights and his wet nights. I suggest that this can be done by putting a special mark on the calendar for dry and another one for wet. Perhaps, I add, he'll be able to see if there's any pattern to his being wet.

I then explain that he should do a bladder exercise every day to "stretch" his bladder. When he feels the urge to urinate, he should count to 10 and then void. The next day, he should count to 20, and so on, until he reaches 100. (Actually, I suspect that what this does is increase his awareness of his bladder when it's full.)

If his wetting happens to occur at the same general time each night, I tell him to set an alarm clock for one half hour before his usual wetting time. I further instruct him to put the alarm clock a bit beyond the midpoint between his bed and the bathroom. He's the only one allowed to set the clock or turn it off.

He's to take care of laundering his wet bedding. If Mother feels that he can't handle the washing machine, he should do whatever he's deemed capable of doing to relieve her of this extra chore. I tell him that "this is only fair." I assure him that if he forgets any of these suggestions or needs to have any of them explained further, he can call me on the phone. He's also asked to call me after a week to tell me about his results. If he doesn't know how to use the phone, his mother calls me; but he does the talking.

I then turn back to Mother and tell her in a loud, clear tone that I've had wonderful success with these suggestions but only when the child was willing to make a strong effort.

Mother's only responsibility in my scheme is to be attentive to her child's efforts and to heap praise, gifts, real estate, or whatever it takes to make her child feel rewarded for his efforts. If your pediatrician doesn't choose to go through all this, or some other scenario of his own, whichever parent isn't involved daily in the child's toilet training and such might play my role here.

This approach requires a motivated child and patient understanding parents, but when it works the success is twofold. Not only is the child dry, but he also has the sense that he's intact and in control of his functions without the need for drugs or devices.

If this approach still doesn't work, and if the enuretic child is developing feelings of humiliation, embarrassment, and shame about his problem, your doctor will probably prescribe the drug imipramine.

This is a highly effective medication that increases the percentage of time spent in stage 2, non-REM sleep and decreases the number of shifts between stages of sleep. Both of these effects reduce the likelihood that conditions favoring bed-wetting will materialize. Opponents of the use of imipramine argue that chemicals shouldn't be used to treat a condition that will eventually correct itself and that imipramine does nothing to alter the basic problem, immaturity of the nervous pathways. While it's true that the chances of spontaneous cure during the next six months is very high for the child under five years old, the chances for rapid self-cure fall off abruptly for the child who is still wetting after the fifth birthday. In fact, there's a 50-50 chance that the 5-year-old enuretic child will still be enuretic at age 12. So, if using imipramine will make the difference between your child's having self-confidence or no confidence, having fun or not having fun, going to slumber parties or staying home, its benefits can't be ignored. Imipramine certainly isn't as effective as maturity, but it may have to do until we learn how to speed up the maturation of the nervous system. (See p. 340, **Ref. 92**; see p. 344, **Ref. 177**; see p. 344, **Ref. 178**; see p. 344, **Ref. 179**; see p. 344, **Ref. 180**.)

RED URINE *(Beeturia)*

Once again, when you see red, it doesn't necessarily mean that you're seeing blood. As you may have read in the section beginning on page 140, urate salts excreted in the infant's urine give it an orange-red color. In addition, certain medicines, when excreted in the urine, give a red-brown discoloration. But by far the most common and most dramatically red color seen in toddlers' urine comes from eating beets, which is probably something that didn't even enter your mind.

The term that we use for urine that turns a deep pink to red color after eating beets is beeturia. Strictly speaking, it should be called betaninuria, since it's the beet's pigment, betanin, that's in the urine, not the beet, but no matter.

Not every child gets beeturia after eating beets; in fact, only 14 percent of normal individuals are excreters of betanin. This fact was pondered for a number of years, but our understanding finally dawned quite unintentionally when researchers investigating specific food allergies learned that 80 percent of iron-deficient people show beeturia.

The connection between iron deficiency and beeturia is now well established, and its explanation isn't as farfetched as you might imagine. Actually, it's rather elegant.

During periods of iron deficiency, the body becomes iron hungry and increases its efforts at absorption of iron from the intestines. The intestines' carrier system isn't able to distinguish iron from betanin. Consequently, iron-deficient people unintentionally absorb the beet's pigment, and once the betanin is absorbed into the circulation, it's quickly excreted by the kidneys.

So, if your child, or you yourself for that matter, should happen to have pink to red urine after eating beets, think first of beeturia. If the red color can be eliminated by sprinkling a bit of baking soda into the urine, and returns when you add some vinegar, the diagnosis of beeturia is certain. Be comforted by the knowledge that the red is not blood, but be aware of the possibility of iron deficiency. (See p. 344, **Ref. 181**; see p. 344, **Ref. 182**.)

5. Growth

CHANGING RATE OF GROWTH *(Crossing Percentiles)*

For a few months after birth, boys grow at a faster rate than girls, but from six months until adolescence, both sexes grow at the same rate. Following birth, the major factor that determines the rate of growth changes is the child's very own set of genes (instead of the previously predominant maternal or placental factors). In essence, babies are now on their own and, not surprisingly, the majority move to a different growth track, one that's more reflective of their own genetic coding.

During the first 12 to 18 months, the growth rate of a third of all infants shifts upward, that of another third shifts downward to a new channel of growth, and that of the final third remains about the same as it was *in utero*. Babies who start out smaller at birth than their genes are coded for are in a hurry to catch up and start their upward shifting as soon as they're born. The smaller-than-destined babies arrive on their new growth track by 4 to 18 months. Those who are larger at birth than their genetic potential enjoy their view from the top of the growth chart for several months before starting their descent to their intended growth track. These larger babies usually reach their final, lower channel by 8 to 19 months, but I've seen the downward drift last longer.

By 24 to 30 months, the major shifts are over, and the child stays put in whatever growth track he settles on. Shorter children grow at a fairly constant 5 centimeters yearly, taller children at 7.5 centimeters yearly. (See p. 340, **Ref. 100.**)

PART THREE

The Older Child—

From 6 to 16 Years

1. Skin, Hair, Nails

STRETCH MARKS *(Striae Distensae)*

Your adolescent child may show stretch marks because her skin, like the rest of her, is "semimature." The way skin responds to stretch depends a lot on the person's age. Young, elastic skin goes with the stretch, gets longer briefly, and, as soon as the stretch is released, springs back to its original length. If you apply the same force to old skin, it tears. In-between skin does an in-between thing and what results is the stretch mark, a series of parallel, shallow, linear depressions in the skin starting out purple and ending up silver. To understand how the maturing process has such an influence on skin elasticity, it helps to have an understanding of collagen and how it changes with maturation.

Collagen, meaning glue-producing substance, is the complex protein whose physical and chemical properties give skin its elasticity. Specifically, elasticity is determined by two factors: the amount of long, distensible collagen fiber in the skin (the more the better) and the number of short, rigid, cross-linkages of protein molecules between the individual fibers of the same substance (again, the more the better).

Some elasticity is lost with maturation because each passing year of life reduces the quantity of long-fiber collagen in our skin by 1 percent. Partially offsetting this loss is the gain in strength that comes from the increase in the number of cross-linkages that occurs with age. During the intermediate stage of life, adolescence and young adulthood, these changes produce a skin that still has abundant long fibers of collagen, with some rigid cross-linkages, as well. The net result is a semimature skin that gives slowly when stretched, causing tearing of some but not all of the fibers. The outcome is the striae, from the Latin word for furrows or fluting. If the skin has enough elasticity to meet the requirements of the growing teenager, it will simply stretch. If there isn't enough stretch in the skin to accommodate its enlarging contents, some of the fibers within the skin will rupture to allow the whole of the skin to be stretched without tearing.

If I was to say that the adolescent can grow too fast for his skin, I wouldn't be stretching the point. (See p. 344, **Ref. 183.**)

TAN SPOTS *(Café au Lait Spots)*

The café au lait spot (CAL) looks just the way it translates from the French, like a light coffee stain. It's a tan, flat spot. Its discrete but irregular borders are either smooth (referred to as coast of California) or jagged (coast of Maine). CALs are often mistaken for giant freckles, but, unlike freckles, CALs don't darken with sun exposure and are much more common on the trunk and buttocks, which are seldom exposed to the sun.

CALs belong to the group of pigmented birthmarks, which includes the Mongolian spot (see p. 39); CALs, however, are different in one important way. Nobody counts Mongolian spots, but if your doctor finds a CAL on your child, don't be surprised if she examines him from head to toe looking for more. When it comes to adults, we know that it's perfectly OK to have a few CALs, but finding six or more of at least 1.5 centimeters is sufficient to make the diagnosis of neurofibromatosis. This condition, known as Von Recklinghausen's disease, can produce multiple tumors of the tissue surrounding the nerves in the skin and brain, as well as a wide range of neurologic and skeletal abnormalities. There are at least seven subtypes of this disease and each subtype has a different clinical picture. The severity of neurofibromatosis can range from one extreme, the Elephant Man, to the opposite pole, at which the patient's entire "disease" is limited to CALs and is perfectly harmless. For the most part, neurofibromatosis is an inherited disease, and most of the time the symptoms in the affected child are no worse than those in the affected parent, but this maxim doesn't apply to every case.

Since the only way to recognize a mild case is by counting the CALs, doctors who notice one CAL will be inclined to look all over the body searching for more. We know that the adult shouldn't have more than five sizable CALs. What is the growing child's CAL quota? Since CALs tend to increase in number, size, and intensity as the child gets older, children of different ages have different CAL quotas.

Ninety-nine percent of all white children under five years old have no more than two CALs measuring 0.5 centimeters each. Seven out of eight white children don't have any CALs, about one in ten has one, and about one in five has two. Black children, because they have more pigment to begin with, are about twice as likely to have them as whites (22 percent have one and 5 percent have two), though follow-up studies show that some of these supposed CALs turn out to be Mongolian spots, which, unlike CALs, eventually fade away.

When we count CALs in children older than five years, we use 1 centimeter as the minimum size to be included. Less than 1 percent of children 5 to 14 years old have five or more CALs, and those who do are presumed to have neurofibromatosis. Like the younger children, virtually all (98 percent) have two or less.

I generally categorize children with CALs into two groups; those who are normal and have no more than two CALs, and those who have five or more (often too many to count). The second group has neurofibromatosis. Once in a great while, a child comes along with three or four CALs. Whether or not this child has any problem of significance will have to be decided by methods other than CAL counting. (See p. 344, **Ref. 184**; see p. 344, **Ref. 185**; see p. 345, **Ref. 187**.)

MOLES *(Pigmented Nevi)*

Strictly speaking, a nevus (from the Latin word for new) is present at birth and a mole (a pigmented nevus) doesn't appear until late childhood or adolescence. Not every nevus is pigmented, whereas moles are always pigmented. Most doctors use the terms interchangeably, and if the truth be known, nobody really cares what you call a growth as long as you call it benign—which, for the most part, moles are. There are many different names given to these marks, some based on where they are in the skin and some paying homage to the first person to give the particular mole a clear description. Here's a brief rundown on the ten most common moles seen during childhood:

1. Junctional nevus: It's so named because the pigment cells are located at the junction of the two layers of skin, the dermis and the epidermis. The normal furrows of the surrounding skin are preserved as they pass over this nevus. Most are flat, hairless, smooth, and brownish-black, and most eventually develop into the next type of nevus, the compound nevus.

2. Compound nevus: Bumpier than the junctional nevus, the compound nevus's surface may have a warty texture with dark, coarse hairs growing out of it, especially if it's on the face. These nevi tend to appear in older children.

3. Intradermal nevus: This mole occurs more often in adults, but is sometimes seen in children. It's usually dome-shaped, a bit elevated, and warty, and may have hairs. It's especially common on the head and neck.

None of the three preceding moles are particularly menacing; and if they're removed at all, it's for reasons of convenience or appearance.

4. Congenital pigmented nevus: This nevus comes in two sizes, regular and king. For a while, physicians believed that only the king-sized variety, which we call the giant congenital pigmented nevus, was potentially malignant. But there's an emerging sentiment that the risk of a small congenital nevus's becoming malignant is as high as 5 percent. This high estimate is by no means accepted by all physicians; there are some who feel that the risk of malignant degeneration in the small congenital nevus is far less than 1 percent. When it comes to the giant congenital nevus's malignant potential, there's no controversy. Its risk matches its king size: it's a whopping 6 to 20 percent. This is the mole that gave moles their bad name.

There's usually no problem in identifying either small or giant congenital pigmented nevi. Most of the small ones are no larger than 1.5 centimeters in diameter and have a distinctive look. At birth, they appear as flat tan areas containing mottled freckling. Later on, they become raised and may grow a few dark-brown hairs. Giant congenital pigmented nevi are a different matter. They cover vast expanses of the body, often like a garment. For this reason, they're also known as bathing-trunk, coat-sleeve, capelike, or stocking-type nevi. They're unevenly colored a dark brown-black, and their surface is bumpy and leathery. Most are hairy, and almost all have satellite nevi around them. As the child grows, these nevi become darker and the folds become deeper. Because of the risk of malignancy, your doctor will probably photograph a congenital nevus periodically, and if that doesn't get rid of it (which it seldom does), she'll remove it under local anesthesia at some convenient time before puberty. The large congenital nevus must be removed as totally and as quickly as possible.

5. Spindle cell nevus: This mole, named by its dominant cell type, comes with a very rich blood supply that accounts for its pink tint. It's usually a solitary, dome-shaped bump on the face, of 0.6 to 1.0 centimeters in diameter. Sometimes when spindle cell nevi aren't so pink the diagnosis may not be terribly obvious, and when that happens they're best removed.

6. Halo nevus: This mole is surrounded by a 1- to 5-millimeter rim of white skin. It usually appears on the child's torso and goes away on its own. If the nevus needs to be removed, your doctor will be sure to remove the halo as well.

7. Nevus spilus: This one sounds like a Roman general, but it's nothing more than a spot (*spilus* means spot) consisting of a flat patch of tan skin speckled with dark brown-black freckles. It's a hairless, harmless, fairly common nevus that can appear at any time during childhood. It can be as large as 20 centimeters in diameter.

8. Becker's nevus: This mole resembles the nevus spilus in color, size, and shape, but tends to occur on the shoulders and upper torsos of adolescent boys. A few years after it appears, it grows a crop of long, coarse hairs. This nevus may be removed, but the decision is based on cosmetic considerations only. The surgery may leave a scar, and the mole may reappear.

9. Freckles: Everybody loves freckles except those who have them. They are reddish-tan flat spots, usually less than 5 millimeters in diameter, that begin to sprout after two years of age and gradually fade away during adulthood. They tend to be inherited with fair skin and red hair. Freckles are most common in the sun-exposed parts of the body, and they darken and grow during the summer months. Children who have them get teased, but somehow these children turn out to be the most beautiful of adults. I never had freckles.

10. Lentigines: A lentigo is the same size as a freckle but is much darker, increases in number into adulthood, isn't influenced by sunlight, and can appear anywhere on the body, including the lips and

mouth. The earlier in life they appear, the more likely they are to fade away. As with the café au lait spot (see p. 236), lentigines may be associated with more than meets the eye, so don't be surprised if your doctor does a bit more inquiring than you expected. (See p. 325, **Ref. 5**; see p. 345, **Ref. 186**.)

WRITING ON SKIN *(Dermatographism)*

If you run a pointed but not penetrating object firmly over your skin, a predictable series of events occurs. Within 15 seconds, a red line appears over the exact site of the stroking. During the next 15 to 45 seconds, a red flare gradually diffuses outward from the red line. One to three minutes later, a raised white line appears in the original stroke line and it lasts a few minutes before gradually fading away. If you're fast, you can get in a full game of tic-tac-toe.

In some children, the reaction is exaggerated. When the final white line comes, it swells considerably, lasts for hours, and itches all the while. Children who are susceptible to this "skin writing" often scratch where they itch, and this makes more swelling, more itch, more scratch, more swelling, i.e., hives. It becomes hard to tell cause from effect. If your child has a problem with hives and if you can ascertain that severe dermatographism is the cause, you'll be spared a lot of fruitless effort searching for the responsible food, drug, or whatever might be causing the hives. In reality, these children are usually creating their hives by scribbling on their skin with their scratching fingernails. An unusually severe case of dermatographism can be suppressed with antihistamines. (See p. 345, **Ref. 188**.)

ITCHY, CRACKED FEET *(Juvenile Plantar Dermatosis)*

This rash can be blamed on the popularity of jogging and the plastics industry. When everybody began to jog, the shoe industry responded by making a running shoe stylishly designed, lightweight, and colorful. That meant using plastic and other synthetic materials that have less capacity to absorb sweat and more resistance to the passage of water vapor. Shoe manufacturers did such a great job in designing them that, before long, teenagers and others made these shoes, designed for running, their everyday shoes.

"Sneaker foot" is confined to the areas of the foot that have the most contact with the inner surface of the shoe. This usually includes the balls of the feet, the heel, and the ball of the big toe. The affected skin gets thick, shiny, pink, and scaly, and eventually cracks. It looks exactly like the cracked glaze on old porcelain. It also itches, and if the cracks are deep enough it's very painful.

This rash is the direct result of retained sweat trapped for long periods of time in the thickest layer of skin in our bodies. The immediate distress can be relieved by medication, but the long-term solution is to wear other kinds of shoes. Most parents are relieved to know that the rash isn't caused by a hard-to-treat fungus, but when they try to separate their child from their beloved sneakers, they may find themselves wishing for a fungus.

A less common but scarier reaction of feet to sneakers is the "black heel." It is seen almost only in active teenagers, especially basketball players. The black heel is really a painless, horizontal band of dark purple speckling occurring just above each heel. It is the result of repeated pounding of an uncushioned heel against a hard surface and disappears within three to six weeks after stopping the activity. Weight lifters get the same thing on their hands. (See p. 345, **Ref. 189.**)

LITTLE YELLOW BUMPS IN SCARS *(Traumatic Epithelial Implant Cysts)*

If you think that the little yellow-white bump(s) that you see in your child's healed scar looks just like the bumps that he had on his nose when he was just born (which we call milia—see p. 43), you're entirely right. In both cases, the tiny cysts result from the accumulation within the layers of the skin of a cheesy material called sebum. Sebum can accumulate whenever surface skin finds itself living inside the deeper layers of skin. This happens when bits of the outermost layers of skin are torn off by the trauma that produced the scar, and subsequently become stuck in the deeper layers by the healing scar, or if the surface skin got left behind in the deeper layers when the fetal skin was forming.

These tiny epithelial implant cysts need no special treatment and will disappear spontaneously. (See p. 345, **Ref. 190.**)

BODY HAIR *(Hypertrichosis and Hirsutism)*

Just to give you an idea of how common "hairiness" is among young women, a study of 400 girls attending the University of Wales showed that 26 percent had terminal facial hair; 17 percent had chest hair, usually around their areolae; 35 percent had abdominal hair, usually along a line running up the middle of their lower bellies; 15 percent had hair over their lower backs; 84 percent had hair on their lower arms and legs; and 70 percent had some on their upper arms and legs. That's a lot of hair for a bunch of normal girls, even for the Age of Aquarius.

There are two forms of hair (see p. 56): short, light, downy fuzz, called vellus hair; and long, coarse, and often pigmented hair, called terminal. Most of our hair concerns are with the terminal type, since vellus hair is rarely unsightly. On the other hand, terminal hair, especially in girls, can be so unsightly that it's almost a cosmetic emergency, and further, it can herald an important endocrine malfunction, as explained further on in this section.

In addition to the two forms of hair, we also have two categories of hair based on where it's growing. Hair is called sexual if it's found in the pubic, facial, underarm, abdominal, or chest area, and nonsexual if it's growing elsewhere. If the sexual hair is excessive, we say the person has hirsutism, and if the nonsexual hair is excessive, we call the condition hypertrichosis. Often the terms are used interchangeably. Now that the terms are defined, the next question is: At what point is hairiness excessive?

That's easy. It's excessive when it's longer, coarser, and more luxuriant than normally expected in that particular location, considering the person's age, sex, and race. For example, we expect males to have more hair than females, but that the difference won't be striking until puberty. We also expect that some races will be hairier than others. For example, some Negroes, Chinese, and American Indians need very little hair before it's viewed as being excessive for them. On the other hand, we expect to see a considerable amount of hairiness in certain ethnic groups, particularly those with Spanish, Near Eastern, or Semitic blood. Not that children of hairy families are exempted from having endocrine disturbances. It's just that we more or less expect them to be somewhat hairy. For this reason, we might not feel compelled to investigate the cause of increased body hair in a 15-year-old girl with Turkish parents, but we might take a different view of it if her hairiness developed all at once, or if she were 7 and not 15.

Since the difference between normal and abnormal is really one of degree, there are times when the doctor will be uncertain. For this reason, as well as the fact that hairiness can be the first outward sign of a hormonal imbalance, we rarely dismiss a question of hypertrichosis without considering some of the important causes.

There are a few situations where the cause of the hypertrichosis is obvious from the outset. For example, doctors often see a lot of hair growing on an extremity, such as a leg that was fractured and casted for a long period. This hair sheds when the cast is shed. Also, some medicines produce hypertrichosis as an untoward side effect. If the doctor who is evaluating your child's hairiness is unaware of what medicine she is taking, be sure to fill him in. Some severely brain-damaged children develop excessive hair for reasons that aren't well understood. If your doctor has decided that your child is excessively hairy, and if none of these situations apply to her, the physician will have to turn his attention to the endocrine system.

Since it's the male hormones, or androgens as they're called, that are responsible for stimulation of the hair apparatus, your doctor will want to know if other signs of excess androgen activity are present. If he finds no other signs of virilization, and if the androgen level in the blood and urine is normal, he'll assume that the child's hair apparatus is simply particularly responsive to normal levels of androgen. We call this idiopathic hirsutism.

If excessive hair isn't the only feature of virilization, and if the doctor finds deepening of the voice, acne, increased muscularity, enlargement of the phallus (clitoris or penis), hairline recession, and top-of-the-head baldness in any girl or boy under ten years old, he'll worry about an abnormal source of androgen and will refer you to an endocrinologist.

Don't get the idea that virilization per se is such a bad thing. For boys older than ten, nothing could be dandier. But anyone else with hair who is becoming virilized, such as a hairy adolescent girl whose breasts are getting smaller and whose menstrual periods are becoming scantier, should be examined by an endocrinologist.

By far, most children suspected by their parents of being excessively hairy are normal.

The younger children thought to be hirsute usually have nothing more than downy fuzz. The older children usually are truly hairy, but the cause is "ethnic" in the great majority of cases. (See p. 345, **Ref.** 191; see p. 345, **Ref.** 192.)

GROWTHS OF BLOOD VESSELS *(Vascular Growths)*
Reddish Nodule That Bleeds Easily *(Pyogenic Granuloma)*

This growth results from the same causes that gave us the oozing navel (see p. 87). Basically, it starts with a small sore, most often in an area like the face or hands that's especially likely to get injured. Instead of healing, the sore turns into a raised, bright red bump, about 0.5 to 2 centimeters in diameter. It bleeds at the drop of a hat, and therefore it generates much more anxiety than it deserves. It won't go away unless treated, but once treated, it doesn't come back.

Spider Spot *(Nevus Araneus)*

Up to 15 percent of normal children have one or more red spots from which symmetrically wavy, pink, delicate lines radiate. They're little more than permanently dilated little arteries that can occasionally be seen to pulse. Spider angiomas, as they're usually called, are most often found on the face, but can occur anywhere. Although some result from liver disease, most have no known cause. They last indefinitely, unless treated by a skin specialist. (See p. 335, **Ref.** 5.)

2. Head

LUMP ON FOREHEAD *(Organized Frontal Hematoma)*

This type of lump can occur anywhere, but it shows up most often on the child's forehead. You may notice it first during the child's bath time, or after the child has fallen and you check him over for injury.

If it's a firm, irregular, completely painless, dime- to quarter-sized swelling deep beneath the skin, and seems to be attached to the bone, it's an old lump that we call an organized hematoma (*hemato* refers to blood; *oma* is growth). Sometimes there's a dimple in the skin directly over the lump.

An organized hematoma may feel ominously hard, but it's really nothing more than an old bruise that was too large to get completely absorbed. After a while, the body deals with the unabsorbed blood by replacing it with fibrous tissue. The end result is a temporary scar that can be easily felt under the skin.

The process of replacing a blood clot with fibrous scar tissue is called organization, and because the forehead is such a likely place for getting a substantial hematoma, most of them are found here. They can be left alone. Eventually, the scar tissue softens and the lump slowly fades into the background.

3. Face

MUMPS LOOK-ALIKE *(Hypertrophy of Masseter and/or Temporalis)*

Sometimes a muscle enlarges to such an unexpected size that you think that it's something else. If it's in an unexplainable location, you'll undoubtedly take the child to the doctor. If the muscle enlargement is just below the child's ear, it could easily appear to be a swelling of the parotid gland (see p. 174), and the mistaken diagnosis is usually the illness mumps.

Mumps is an infection of the parotid gland, a salivary gland that sits in front of the ear at the angle of the jawbone. The masseter and temporalis muscles, being chewing muscles, happen to be in the same vicinity. You can find your masseter without much trouble simply by clenching your jaw tightly and feeling the muscle just above the back of your jaw. The temporalis muscle isn't as easy to find unless it's enlarged. It fills the normal hollow of the temples and is much higher up on the face than the masseter. (Both of these muscles work to keep the jaws closed.)

A child who chews gum daily or who grinds his teeth when nervous, or any child with a severely abnormal bite, might easily have an enlarged set of masseters and/or temporalis muscles, and there are times when the swelling is so massive that it becomes unsightly. If your child has a swelling of this sort, it's important to tell the doctor about the child's chewing habits. If this connection isn't made, the diagnosis can remain uncertain and the doctor might feel the need to do a number of tests, some of which fall into the category of invasive testing—among them, biopsy of the presumed parotid swelling. In short, if you know of your child's closed jaw habits, open yours and speak up; there's nothing as helpful to a doctor, in this case, as being told about the child's chewing habits.

It's always a good idea, in fact, to speak up when you know something that might bear upon your child's problem. I once saw a teenage boy from Delhi, India, whose father was taking him all over the world in hopes of uncovering the reason for the boy's severe jaw pain. He'd managed to stump the experts in most of the world's capitals, and I was no exception. As is my custom in conundrums of this sort, I briefly excused myself and left the consultation room to scratch my head for a while. When I returned to the room, the boy "told" me what his problem was. I found him hunched forward, sitting at the edge of his chair, with his right elbow resting on my desk and his chin cupped in his upturned palm. When I asked his father if his son sat like that often, he said, "All the time." I told him to stop. He did, and so did his jaw pain.

The same sort of thing happens over and over again. A young wood carver is dragged from physician to physician by worried parents who have noticed a peculiar muscular swelling at the root of their child's thumb. I've seen a number of older children with frightening-looking abdominal swellings that appeared when the children tensed their abdominal muscles. These swellings, as it turned out, didn't debut until the children started a program of maybe 500 sit-ups a day. I've seen little girls with blood in their urine that began to appear when someone gave them rocking chairs for their birthdays. They'd subsequently been spending hours bruising their kidneys against the backs of hard rocking chairs. There are lots of stories like these. The common thread that unites them all is the special thing that the child does that you know about and the doctor doesn't. Do yourself and your child a favor and tell the doctor about these activities, even if you don't think that there's any connection with your child's problem. (See p. 345, **Ref. 193.**)

4. Nose

NOSEBLEEDS *(Epistaxis)*

The bloody nose is an especially common problem for the four-to ten-year-old. In this age group it's mainly a problem for boys, but after the onset of puberty it occurs more often in girls. When a nose bleeds following a punch to it the cause is no great mystery, but most of the time nosebleeds happen without warning, usually in the middle of the night. This is particularly true if the child is sleeping in a dry, overheated bedroom. Nosebleeds also follow very minor trauma such as blowing the nose or attempting to scratch the inside of it, itchy or otherwise, with a sharp fingernail. Further, whatever increases the amount of blood flowing through the nose, such as a common cold or allergy, increases the likelihood of a bloody nose. Doctors, following Hippocrates, refer to the bloody nose as epistaxis, from the Greek word meaning to drop or trickle.

The blood from the nose usually comes from one of the tiny vessels in Little's area, the very front part of the nasal septum (the wall between the two nasal chambers). These blood vessels, because they're so close to the nostrils, are easily subjected to the drying influence of inhaled hot, dry air.

Older noses bleed for other reasons. For example, adolescent girls occasionally have nosebleeds during menstruation for reasons that aren't understood but don't appear to be hormonal. A type of benign tumor that grows in the area of the adenoids also causes nosebleeds. This tumor, the juvenile nasopharyngeal angiofibroma, isn't at all common, but when it does occur it's in adolescent boys almost exclusively. Occasionally, a clotting or bleeding disorder will limit its signs to the nose, but far more often, there's evidence of bleeding in other areas of the body.

Most nosebleeds can be stopped by putting a wad of cotton, wet with decongestant nose drops, into the bleeding side and then squeezing the nostrils shut for five minutes. It's not a good idea to take frequent breaks during the five minutes to check on how well it's doing. Take it from me, it's doing great. Only in the rare situation where the bleeding won't quit will the child need medical attention. If the doctor can find the source of the blood, he'll use a silver nitrate applicator stick or an electric spark to coagulate the bleeding vessel.

Bleeding from the back of the nose, which is uncommon in children, may need to be controlled by the use of a pack. Properly inserting this packing can be a complicated procedure and should be left to the ear, nose, and throat specialist. Plugging up the back of the nose also blocks the normal pathways to the ears and sinuses, and infections in these areas often result, so you certainly shouldn't try this yourself. Furthermore, any form of tight compressive packing anywhere in the body can lead to the development of toxic shock syndrome. Fortunately, nasal packs are seldom needed for children. (See p. 345, **Ref. 194**; see p. 345, **Ref. 195**.)

5. Ears

EAR PAIN WITHOUT EAR DISEASE *(Otalgia)*

Ordinarily, you assume that if your child is holding her ear in pain, she has something wrong with her ear. But you might be wrong. A mother whose memory of her child's early years is filled with nighttime awakenings, screaming earaches, and one ear infection after the other is particularly apt to jump at her teenager's complaint of an earache. Hold on. There are several times when an earache doesn't necessarily mean an ear problem.

Erupting molars are the major nonear cause of ear pain in younger children, but later the most common nonear reason for the earache is a painful temporomandibular joint (TMJ). This is the hinge between the lower jawbone and the skull, and it's located directly in front of the ear. When it hurts, the pain seems to come straight from the ear. The TMJ hurts when it's abused, and all the things that are responsible for masseter and/or temporalis muscle hypertrophy (see p. 246), such as excessive gum chewing, nervous teeth grinding, and bad biting, can irritate the TMJ. Even spending a long time in the dentist's chair with the mouth held open can produce TMJ pain masquerading as ear pain.

Minor trauma to the ear is another cause of brief and usually mild ear pain. In teenagers, the pain can result from phonic booms: telephonic and stereophonic. Telephonic trauma to the outer ear comes from holding a phone tightly against the ear for prolonged stretches of time, and stereophonic trauma comes from wearing improperly fitting headsets.

If any of these scenarios seems familiar, and if you can produce the pain by moving the child's jaw around or pushing on her outer ear, you have nothing to lose if you try to eliminate the pain by correcting the situation. You can keep trying as long as your child has no fever or hearing loss, but if the pain is severe or persistent, you should have her ears examined by a doctor to see if they're truly infected.

6. Mouth

WHITE-RIMMED RED AREAS ON TONGUE
(Geographic Tongue)

Between 1 and 16 percent of all children have tongues that will, at various times, look like a map of the world. The "continents" consist of red, flattened areas from 0.5 to 5 centimeters in diameter. These areas are outlined by 1 or 2 millimeters of a raised white margin that appears on the tongue prior to the debut of the red flat areas. The number of such areas varies from one to as many as eight. They're located for the most part on the top of the tongue, but they can appear on the tip and sides as well. They've even been known to occur on the hard palate and gums.

Like some parts of the world, the boundaries and contours of these areas shift, coalesce, and enlarge, creating an ever changing pattern of geographic shapes. You may have noticed these shapes on your child's tongue and decided, quite rightly, that they weren't ominous enough to lead to an office visit. Unfortunately, however, the situation is ripe for adults who are involved in the subject of adult nutrition to volunteer the opinion that the child is suffering from a vitamin deficiency. That usually brings the child into the office.

The geographic tongue does appear to have some relationship to a number of other skin disorders, including psoriasis and seborrhea, and children who have such tongues are more likely to have allergic tendencies. However, geographic tongues should not be mistaken for tongues that are infected, for example with herpes or yeast, because these agents cause blisters and heavy white curds on the tongue. Deficiencies in the B-complex vitamins can lead to a diffusely sore and red-all-over tongue, but the soreness of a geographic tongue is seldom more than a mild sensitivity to hot foods. In essence, the geographic tongue is nothing more than one way that the tongue responds to a number of different underlying conditions, only a few of which we can identify at this time.

The other variety of tongue that deserves comment is the one with deep furrows along its length. This type is called plicated, scrotal, or fissured, and it's found in 2 to 5 percent of children with otherwise normal tongues and in 40 percent of those with geographic tongues. Like the geographic tongue, it's harmless.

While we're on the subject of tongues, I might mention that some tongues can bend, curl, and roll, while others can't. If your child has one that can't, don't spend a lot of time in training. It's a genetically determined trait and the potential for tongue rolling is determined from the moment of conception. All the practice and coaching in the world won't change things; if your teenager wants to sharpen his lingual skills, he'll have to learn a foreign language. (See p. 336, **Ref. 21**; see p. 345, **Ref. 196**; see p. 345, **Ref. 197**; see p. 345, **Ref. 198**.)

YELLOW-WHITE PLUGS STICKING OUT OF TONSILS *(Tonsillar Debris)*

Each tonsil has from 15 to 20 deep crypts that burrow from its surface to its core. During bouts of tonsillitis, these crypts usually fill up with pus, which studs the exposed tonsillar surface like pieces of cold butter over a cold waffle. Sometimes tonsillar crypts fill up with matter even when they're not infected. The matter can be food particles, but most often it's a soft, yellow-white, cheesy substance similar to dental tartar and about the size of a grain of rice.

Tonsillar debris is especially common in older children whose tonsils have been scarred by battle and are pockmarked. Some of these children report a sensation of something caught in their throats, something that they try to pick or rinse out, but more often the debris sits around quietly, waiting to be discovered. Sometimes a child spots it and, regarding it as "icky," spends a lot of time tidying up her tonsils.

Most of the time, Mother makes the initial sighting, and most of the time, she thinks it's pus. This is an understandable error since, thankfully, most mothers don't routinely inspect their children's throats, complaints or no, and therefore don't get the chance to see tonsillar debris in its innocence.

If you do happen to go on a tonsil hunt, there are some easy ways of knowing what you're seeing: Pus on the tonsils is a sign of infection, and if the tonsils are truly infected your child will show other signs of infection such as pain, fever, redness, and swelling. Tonsillar debris, on the other hand, accumulates on the uninfected tonsil. Tonsillitis usually involves both tonsils in a fairly homogeneous way. Tonsillar debris, in contrast, appears in randomly selected crypts. Of course, having tonsillar debris doesn't protect your child against tonsillitis, and she may actually have both at times. The main thing is not to confuse the two, or to think that your child has a chronic infection in her tonsils simply because each time you look in there you see a yellowish kernel of debris staring you in the face. If it offends your child's throat, or your eye, vigorous gargling will ordinarily rinse it away. If the debris is particularly stubborn, a Water Pik can be used to blast it off. (See p. 336, **Ref. 22.**)

7. Neck

APPARENT SWELLING OF THYROID
(Pseudogoiter and Modigliani's Syndrome)

A goiter (*guttur* means throat in Latin) is a swelling of the throat that comes from an enlargement of the thyroid gland. Until fairly recently, medical students were taught that the thyroid gland naturally swelled during adolescence as a response to the increased endocrine demands of puberty. In the past, whenever doctors saw a healthy teenager, especially a female, with a smooth, nontender enlargement of the thyroid, they would confidently assure the mother that this was a natural process and indeed a healthy sign that puberty was progressing. They were wrong. We now know that 90 percent of these healthy teenagers with diffusely enlarged thyroids actually have a chronic inflammation of their glands and should be treated for it. Medical students now learn that the only time that the thyroid gland is expected to enlarge is during pregnancy.

On the other hand, children are often brought to the doctor's office because there's a suspicion of a swollen thyroid gland, or goiter, when in reality no swelling exists. What, then, is creating the illusion?

Most often, the pseudogoiter is created by the forward curving or lordosis of a long and slender neck, giving the normal-sized thyroid greater prominence. The illusion can be immediately erased by having the child, usually a girl, sit up with straight posture and relinquish her adolescent slouch. This phenomenon has been dubbed Modigliani's syndrome after the painter whose subjects were so often young women with long, curved necks. You can think of it as a sign of grace and beauty, but it has no medical significance.

The other common misinterpretation in this area applies to children whose necks are short and chubby. In this situation, a roll of skin can develop around the lower neck, and this chubby roll can look much like a swollen thyroid gland. Since short, plump children are often suspected of having thyroid disease, they're especially vulnerable to this error. To be completely sure that the thyroid isn't a part of the "swelling," a thorough feel of the neck by a specialist may be necessary. While you're waiting for your appointment, put your child on a diet. If the swelling vanishes, you can always cancel. (See p. 245, **Ref. 202.**)

8. Chest

BREAST ENLARGEMENT IN ADOLESCENT BOYS *(Gynecomastia)*

With the growth in total body size that occurs during adolescence, individual body parts grow as well. To some extent, the overall growth accounts for the increase in the size of the breasts' areolae that we see in boys (as well as girls) during their rapid-growth phase of puberty. There's also a direct stimulation of the areolar tissue during puberty due to the secretion of hormones. This growth is normal and permanent. But for many boys, there's also a temporary growth in the breast tissue itself that can be confusing, disturbing, and embarrassing. This growth is called gynecomastia (*gyneco* means femalelike; *mastia* equals breast), and occurs in up to 60 to 70 percent of normal boys during puberty.

Occasionally, an eight-year-old boy may develop gynecomastia precociously (see p. 178). In this case, it appears as a firm, mildly tender, discrete plate of breast tissue directly beneath the nipple. It's usually one-sided, causes great havoc until it's identified as normal breast tissue, and goes away in 6 to 12 months. Its departure is appreciated but not understood.

Gynecomastia in teenage boys may reveal itself as a disklike, silver-dollar-sized plate of firm tissue under the nipple, or it may be a more spread-out mass of tissue that feels firmer than the surrounding fat. It can be tender, and the affected boy often holds his shirt away from his chest to avoid painful contact. Since boys of this age group invariably roughhouse, they usually assume that the soreness and swelling are the results of bangs on their chests. They're often embarrassed by the situation, though, and frequently try to avoid undressing in front of their friends. Thus, enthusiastic swimmers may ask for an excuse to avoid swimming or the group shower after the physical education class. You can suspect normal gynecomastia if you have a faintly moustached 14-year-old boy whose rapid growth makes the tops of his socks show when he walks, who holds his shirt away from his chest, and who smells like his high-school locker room.

Gynecomastia is less frequent in black than white males. It involves only one breast in about 25 percent of the boys affected. When it's one-sided, it's on the right side twice as often as the left. The enlargement may not go away immediately. It lasts for up to two years in 27 percent of the boys, and for three years in 7 percent.

Typically, the age for gynecomastia is 12 to 15 years, particularly 14 to 14½ years. Not that there's any magic to these numbers. It's just that, at that particular age, most boys have reached the part of their puberty called Tanner stages 3 to 4. At that point, boys are in the midst of their height spurt, their voices are starting to deepen, hair is growing in the pubic and underarm regions and on the upper lip and chin, and the genitals are growing. At this particular stage of development, gynecomastia is completely normal. (If the teenage boy has reached full sexual maturation, i.e., Tanner stage 5, any breast enlargement isn't normal gynecomastia.)

After World War II, we found that many starved prisoners of war acquired gynecomastia when they were fed. Since then, we've seen it occur in many young men who were recovering from prolonged illness, especially if the recovery involved regaining a considerable amount of weight that had been lost during the illness. This syndrome is called refeeding gynecomastia, and, like normal gynecomastia, it regresses after a few months or years. We believe that, as these young men recovered, their endocrine status became analogous to a "second puberty."

About 20 illicit drugs can cause gynecomastia, some of them in the group of "best-sellers." Among the illicit drugs, marijuana is the best-known cause of the condition. The bad news here is that, when gynecomastia is caused by drugs, the breasts may not fully return to normal size after the drug is discontinued.

If the gynecomastia occurs at some time other than puberty, or isn't drug related or refeeding related, your doctor may refer you to an endocrinologist for a thorough investigation of the less common but more serious causes. Otherwise, it's normal and will pass. (See p. 345, **Ref. 203**; see p. 346, **Ref. 204**; see p. 346, **Ref. 205**; see p. 346, **Ref. 206**.)

LUMPY BREASTS IN GIRLS *(Fibrocystic Disease)*

Although breast masses in females under 20 years of age are rarely malignant, they're always suspected of being so, and rarely fail to generate a great deal of anxiety and excitement when they're found. As already described (see p. 178), some turn out to be nothing more than normally enlarging breast buds, and, as can't be said often enough, these should be left alone.

When the swelling turns out to be a lump *in* the breast, not a lump that *is* the breast, the answer is usually found within a tiny group of common conditions. One of these conditions is called fibrocystic disease of the breast, and it has recently been welcomed to the ranks of the nondiseases. This condition affects most women. It usually starts after a few years of menstruating and lasts throughout the reproductive years. It consists of painful, tender lumps that are, in fact, cysts in the breasts, fluctuating in size with the menstrual cycle, and getting progressively larger and more tender until the menopause. These lumps are firm, very mobile, and smooth. There may be many in each breast, or only one dominant one. Some women—and even some young girls— are so accustomed to them that they view them as belonging where they are.

Today, fibrocystic "disease" isn't considered a disease at all, but the normal response of the breast's different components, i.e., glands, fat, and supporting fibrous tissue, to hormonal cycling. A certain number of lumps in the breasts, with varying degrees of pain and tenderness, are the physiologic rule rather than the exception. Some breasts are lumpier than others, and where to draw the line between normal and abnormal depends on the doctor's judgment. If the breast swelling is judged to be too large, too tender, or too persistent it should be seen by a surgeon. He may simply decide to see if it persists. The majority of girls with breast masses diagnosed as cysts referred to the gynecology clinic of the Boston Children's Hospital no longer had them after two to three months of observation.

If a breast mass thought to be a cyst doesn't oblige us and get lost, it can be carefully punctured by a skilled specialist armed with a needle and syringe; if the mass collapses, it can be assumed to be a cyst. Just to play it safe, we always send the fluid obtained to the laboratory to see what kind of cells can be found floating in it.

If your adolescent daughter has a breast lump that isn't diagnosed as a cyst, can't be needled, and must be surgically removed, find a surgeon who will take great care not to disturb the rest of the breast. Four fifths of such masses in adolescent girls will turn out to be fibroadenomas, entirely benign tumors, and the rest will, in great likelihood, be an assortment of equally benign tumors. Some will even turn out to be breast cysts that somehow managed to escape the needle. (See p. 346, **Ref. 206**; see p. 346, **Ref. 207**; see p. 346, **Ref. 208**.)

9. Abdomen

ABDOMINAL MASS *(Abdominal Aorta, Fecaloma, or Pregnancy)*

The aorta, a garden-hose-sized blood vessel, after exiting the heart, follows a course just in front of the spine. This vessel can be felt as a pulsing cylindrical mass in many children's abdomens, especially if they have a fair amount of lordosis (see p. 199) pushing the lower spine forward, or a thin, flat tummy, bringing the aorta's pulsations within close range of the belly wall and the doctor's hand or your own. In some cases, you can actually see the heart beat in the abdomen when the child is lying on her back. So if your completely healthy child tells you that her belly surface beats rhythmically in tune with her heartbeat, you can believe her.

Sometimes, during a routine physical examination of the child's abdomen, a doctor may come across another mass. This one is about the size of a lemon, smooth, round, firm, nontender, and movable. The child appears to be entirely healthy and about the worst the parent can report about the owner of this citrus-sized swelling is that she tends toward constipation. If this child is examined later, particularly if she had a bowel movement during the interval between examinations, the mass will be found somewhere else. Eventually, the mass disappears when it finds its way to the child's plumbing system, because it's nothing more than an accumulation of hard stool within a loop of large intestine. Such masses are called fecalomas (*fecal* refers to stool; *oma* is growth). If there's any doubt about the identity of this swelling, a series of enemas will provide the diagnosis and cure.

The last of the abdominal masses that don't require removal is the pregnant uterus. It's an unfortunate fact, but a fact nonetheless, that a growing number of today's teenagers are getting pregnant. Their bellies grow just like adult women's, but unlike most adults, they may not share the information about their pregnancy with you or anyone else. Either embarrassment or ignorance may keep the child, the parent, and the doctors in the dark about the reason for the youngster's enlarging abdomen. As a result, all too often, the diagnosis of pregnancy is made in the darkness of an X-ray room when, during the evaluation of the "abdominal mass," the radiologist finds a picture of the fetus's bones.

There are easier ways to make the diagnosis of pregnancy. There are also safer ways that don't involve exposing the fetus to X rays. So if your doctor orders a urine or serum pregnancy test on your teenage daughter who has a growing tummy, he's only being thorough and considering the well-being of everybody, including the unsuspected fetus.

FIRM SWELLING ON SURFACE OF
ABDOMEN *(Hypertrophy of Asymmetric Rectus Muscle)*

If you look at the belly muscles of young people devoted to physical fitness, you'll see that the upper half of the muscle covering the middle of the abdominal wall, the rectus abdominis, has several horizontal grooves dividing it into three or four segments. These grooves are created by narrow bands of fibrous tissue that inscribe a line from the outer surface of the muscle through most but not all of its depth. These lines are only found above the navel, and usually number three or four. They differ in length and shape; some reach from side to side and others run upward or downward for varying distances. About one fifth of us have more of them on one side than the other and, as a result, one fifth of us have upper recti whose sides don't match.

Under ordinary conditions, this unevenness isn't noticed, but when a youngster develops his belly wall by performing hundreds or thousands of sit-ups daily, each segment becomes clearly defined and the "extra" segment of rectus stands out like a sore lump. In the same way that enlargement of the masseter and temporalis muscles simulate mumps (see p. 246), this muscle impersonates a tumor.

You may notice this phenomenon as a well-defined swelling beneath the lower rib cage on one side of the midline, if your teenage boy has recently thrown himself into physical fitness in a big way. (I've never seen it in girls, but anything is possible.) Often, the boy himself finds the swelling, usually when he's "pumped up" after his exercises. The key to recognizing this tumor imposter lies in appreciating that its size, prominence, and firmness are all enhanced when the boy tenses his abdominal muscles. At that time, the "mass" feels exactly like the other segments of the upper rectus muscle. If your doctor isn't absolutely sure that this mass represents an enlarged muscle, she can refer your child to a specialist who will insert a fine needle into it and record its electrical activity, thus determining whether or not the mass is muscle. Unusually developed muscles can masquerade as tumors in other areas of the body, such as the back and the extremities, as well. Most often, the mystery is over as soon as the child tells us about the physical activity he engages in that produced the enlargement. (See p. 346, **Ref. 209.**)

10. Genitalia

SOFT SWELLING IN LEFT SIDE OF TEENAGER'S SCROTUM *(Varicocele)*

Varicoceles (*varix* means dilated vein; *cele* is a hollow cavity) have become more common nowadays than they used to be—why, I can't fully explain. Once considered rare, these swellings are now found in 10 to 20 percent of adolescent boys. Maybe physicians are finding more because we've been looking harder for them ever since fertility clinics began reporting lower sperm counts in men with varicoceles. Or perhaps we're finding more because we've learned that there's a right way and a wrong way to examine for a varicocele.

Only 20 percent of all varicoceles cause symptoms, usually a dull scrotal aching after exercise. And after hearing that complaint, the doctor usually discovers the varicocele. If the teenage boy himself discovers the swelling, he seldom shares the news with anyone. The remaining 80 percent of affected boys have no symptoms, regardless of the size of the swelling, and unless the varicocele happens to be found by the doctor during a routine checkup, it remains undetected (and the doctor has to make a special effort to find it, at that).

A varicocele results from the dilation of the coiled section of the spermatic vein as it winds around the cord that suspends the testicle in the scrotum. Just like its varicose relative in the leg, it must be engorged with blood to be detected. Since the only time these veins distend is when the patient is standing, the doctor won't notice the varicocele if the boy's scrotum is examined when the boy isn't standing up. If the boy is on his feet, the veins will fill more and more the longer he stands, and eventually the varicocele will start to look and feel like a "bag of worms."

The varicocele is almost always found on the left side of the scrotum, probably because our anatomy provides unequal routing for the two sets of veins that drain the testicles. The vein that drains the right testicle is favored with a direct access to the main abdominal vein. The vein draining the left testicle has to make a difficult connection en route. Varicoceles range in size from the barely detectable to the massive, but even a massive one can escape detection if the boy is examined when he's lying down. The great majority of them don't appear until full sexual maturation (Tanner stage 5) is reached.

Interest in varicoceles has skyrocketed since their association with adult infertility was publicized. Once known as harmless "bags of worms," they're now considered to be a cause of male infertility, correctable by surgery. By operating on infertile males with varicoceles, urologists have been able to improve the semen characteristics of about 65 percent, and about half of the surgically corrected adults became fertile. Some of these urologists now suggest that it would be advisable to surgically remove an adolescent's varicocele before it does irreparable damage to the growing young testicle. Others advise that surgical correction be undertaken if the testicle on the side of the varicocele is significantly smaller than its mate on the other side. If their advice is heeded, seeing that at least 10 percent of teenagers have varicoceles and 77 percent of these have one shrunken testicle, then 1 teenage boy in 12 will be subject to varicocele surgery.

Needless to say, a great deal more information is called for before any conclusions such as this should be drawn. For now, the only facts you should rely on are: (1) Varicoceles are commonly found in the left sides of many healthy teenagers' scrota. (2) Varicoceles are much more common in men who are attending infertility clinics than in those who are not. (3) The reason for the varicocele's presence should be investigated if it appears in a child before puberty, persists when he lies in the supine position, or is on the right side of the scrotum. These factors mark a varicocele as unusual. (4) Varicoceles should be operated upon if they cause considerable aching or bulging. Until some very carefully designed studies are done on the long-term effects of teenage varicoceles on fertility, don't jump into surgery. (See p. 346, **Ref. 210**; see p. 346, **Ref. 211**; see p. 346, **Ref. 212**.)

URINARY OPENING ON PENIS SEEMS TOO SMALL *(Apparent Meatal Stenosis)*

Too small for what? Definitely too small to drive a recreational vehicle through. But how about being too small to allow the urine to pass through unimpeded? How can you tell? Some doctors do it simply by looking at the opening and judging if it's adequate or not. By this method, a lot of little boys who think they're all right can be diagnosed as having meatal (opening) stenosis (narrowing). When a group of 1,800 healthy third-grade boys in Ohio were inspected by a pair of urologists, 32 percent were judged to have significant meatal stenosis. Now that's a lot of abnormal findings from a normal group of kids. Furthermore, these urologists felt that they'd actually underestimated the frequency of meatal stenosis, since their method wasn't terribly sensitive. They were, nevertheless, amazed by the large number of boys with meatal stenosis and wondered what happened to them as adults. A third of all adult men certainly don't have meatal stenosis. Another, more realistic conclusion that they might have drawn is that visual inspection isn't a good way to screen for meatal stenosis.

Which it isn't. That fact has been demonstrated by the studies that involve making actual measurements of the urinary opening. By inserting a succession of rods of increasing size into the opening until significant resistance is met, an examiner can determine the size of the opening. Using this method, we frequently find no correlation between how small the meatus looks and how small it actually measures. Does that mean that every little boy should have his urinary meatus measured and compared to the statistical norm for his age? Not at all.

The body's blueprint doesn't come with a size specification for the meatus. The meatus's only requirement is that it be large enough to allow a decent stream of urine to flow out. To determine this, all you have to do is watch your boy's stream while he urinates. If the stream's caliber, force, and rate are normal, nothing is wrong with the meatus, no matter how small it looks or measures. If doubt still exists, your friendly urologist can have your son urinate into a special urinal called a flowmeter. This will accurately measure the rate and tell him if it's normal or impaired. (See p. 342, **Ref. 146**; see p. 342, **Ref. 147**.)

LONG INTERVALS BETWEEN MENSTRUAL PERIODS *(Adolescent Menstrual Irregularity)*

Most young girls' periods are far from regular. The question is: How irregular can they be and still be normal? To avoid needless worry and scurry, what needs to be known is how many months you can comfortably wait for the second period to come, and then the third one, and so on. It's also helpful to know how many days the earliest periods normally last and, while you're at it, how many years you can wait before you're entitled to worry about your daughter's menstrual irregularity.

Much of our understanding of early menstrual cycles has come from records kept by a group of teenage girls attending a boarding school. We learned that to complete their first five menstrual cycles, a range of 127 to 519 days was required, the average being 276 days. That's quite a range. The average number of days between each of the first five periods was 69 days. More than half of the girls recorded gaps between periods of three months or more. Many had gaps of six months.

Cycles 6 through 10 were a bit more regular. They were completed in 106 to 293 days, a narrower range, with an average of 181 days. The average number of days between periods was down to 45. Only 10 percent of the gaps were longer than two months, and none was greater than five months. Clearly, after only five cycles there's an obvious lessening in the individual variations as well as a reduction in the really long intervals.

By the time these girls reached their 11th to 15th cycles, none had gaps greater than four months between periods, and less than 10 percent had gaps longer than two months. In essence, the really long gaps disappeared by the time 15 cycles had been completed, and most of the girls began to approach regular periods.

Often, adult-type consistency isn't achieved until cycles 25 to 39. By then, two thirds of the cycles are within ten days of each other. But until then, some degree of menstrual irregularity is the rule rather than the exception.

Young girls who have a great deal of menstrual irregularity at the onset of menstruation are especially likely to join the 11 percent of college girls whose cycles are 35 to 90 days long. The likelihood of this happening is increased if the girl loses 20 or more pounds or engages in intensive physical exercise. So far, research doesn't support the view that "stresses" of college life are factors causing any increased rate of menstrual irregularity in the college girl.

The variability seen in the length of the cycles of adolescents isn't seen in the length of the periods themselves. Eighty-eight percent of all the periods reported by adolescents run from three to seven days in length, with an average of five days. From all this, it's pretty evident that worrying about irregular periods during the first two years of menstruating is a waste of worry. When, then, is worry appropriate? Only if the periods are extra-frequent or extra-heavy. Then an evaluation by a specialist is definitely in order. (See p. 346, **Ref. 213**; see p. 346, **Ref. 217**.)

VAGINAL DISCHARGE STAINING ADOLESCENT'S UNDERWEAR *(Physiologic Vaginal Discharge)*

Prior to a girl's adolescence, the only time when a vaginal discharge is considered normal is during her first few weeks of life (see p. 90). At that time, the discharge is merely the normal outpouring of mucus from the baby's estrogen-stimulated cervix. The estrogen was made by the mother and placenta, the mucus by the baby. Baby girls eventually mature, and when they reach puberty and start to make their own estrogen, their cervical mucus-secreting glands start production once again. That's the basis for physiologic vaginal discharge.

In Budapest, Hungary, this secretion is called the natural puberty discharge. When 1,000 normal 13- to 14-year-old girls were examined there, 447 were found to have such a discharge. Perhaps if the other 553 girls had been examined at another time of the month, they, too, would have been found to have a discharge.

You may notice the discharge as a dried yellowish stain on your 11- to 12-year-old daughter's panties, especially if the panties are tight-fitting nylon, since these garments don't allow the discharge to escape or evaporate. The girl may be just about to have her first period, or she may have been having periods for about a year. If she happens to be examined by a doctor, he finds no sign of inflammation on her genitalia, only a gray-white, thick, mucous, odorless discharge. The discharge is usually scant, but it's not uncommon for some girls with more active secretion to have a copious, thinner discharge that requires their wearing a pad. An analysis of the discharge would show normal cervical mucus, desquamated vaginal cells, and the usual bacteria that harmlessly inhabit the area.

Not every vaginal discharge is benign. If, in addition to the discharge, there's itch, redness, and pain, the condition is called vulvovaginitis (the vulvar area is the external genitalia of the female). This, too, is extremely common. Of the 1,000 "normal" girls examined in the survey to determine the normal incidence of physiologic discharge, 183 had some degree of vulvovaginitis.

Vulvovaginitis is the common cold of the external genitalia. Although its treatment is ordinarily left to the pediatrician or family doctor, it still accounts for 87 percent of visits to gynecologists by prepubertal girls over ten years old, and for 54 percent of visits by postpubertal adolescent girls. It's an infection, so it isn't "normal," but it's so common that it deserves some discussion here.

Most of the time, vulvovaginitis is caused by vulvar contamination by bacteria that normally and harmlessly inhabit the rectum. While it's common in adolescents, it's even more common in prepubertal girls. We hold several factors responsible for vulvovaginitis, including the closeness of the anus to the vagina, the lack of an acid vaginal secretion to inhibit bacterial growth, improper wiping after bowel movements, and the use of harsh soaps, particularly bubble baths. Pinworms, germs that are normally present in the respiratory tract, foreign bodies of any kind, even shredded toilet paper inadvertently trapped within the vagina are all common causes of vulvovaginitis, and each needs its own specific treatment. And of course if the teenager is sexually active, she's subject to all the specific causes of vaginitis that produce it in the adult. Vulvovaginitis, unlike normal physiologic vaginal discharge, needs some form of treatment, and a doctor should be consulted. The condition usually does lessen after a few years, and is usually helped by the substitution of loose-fitting, frequently changed cotton panties for the tight-fitting nylon ones. (See p. 346, **Ref. 214**; see p. 346, **Ref. 215**; see p. 346, **Ref. 216**.)

PAINFUL MENSTRUAL PERIODS *(Dysmenorrhea)*

Half of all teenage girls have painful periods, called dysmenorrhea (*dys* means difficult; *men* equals month; *rhea* refers to a flow) by doctors, and known to the girls as "the curse." Dysmenorrhea is the number one cause of school absenteeism in teenage girls, and it brings one fifth to one half of all teenage girls to a doctor's office seeking relief. For the rest, it tends to be underdiagnosed, since many doctors don't ask about it; and if they did, many teenagers wouldn't tell them. Until very recently, this problem was treated primarily by self-medication, but we now believe that we know the cause of dysmenorrhea, and we have effective treatment for it. This is a breakthrough.

Since ovulation is required to produce dysmenorrhea, and since most girls don't ovulate during the first year or two of menstruating, nearly all cases of dysmenorrhea start within two years of the first period. If you're the kind of person who believes that every cloud has its silver lining, you could say that the onset of painful periods after a year or two of painless periods is the silver-lining reassurance that ovulation has started. Unfortunately, being reassured of normal ovarian function doesn't compensate for the painful periods. But understanding the pivotal importance of ovulation has led doctors to the successful use of birth control pills to suppress ovulation and thus prevent dysmenorrhea. For sexually active teenagers with dysmenorrhea, that's exactly what most physicians, myself included, recommend. For teenagers who aren't sexually active, a pill that isn't a contraceptive, but instead inhibits a certain group of chemicals called prostaglandins, is effective for the following reasons:

During menstruation, the uterus normally contracts. The uterus of the menstruating, dysmenorrheic girl has contractions that are particularly strong and particularly frequent. These contractions can generate pressures that are 1.5 times the level of the average labor contraction peak. No wonder they hurt. These powerful contractions we now believe are caused by one or several prostaglandins. Prostaglandins affect many different organs in many ways. In this situation, they stimulate the uterus to contract and the arteries within the uterus to narrow. They also increase the sensitivity of the uterus's pain receptors. It's easy to see that anyone having too much of this stuff would be subject

267 Bones and Joints

to painful periods, which is exactly what current research has revealed. Adult women with dysmenorrhea have two to ten times more prostaglandin in the muscles of their uteri than those without dysmenorrhea, and dysmenorrheic women have a higher than normal amount of prostaglandins in their menstrual blood.

We don't know why dysmenorrheic women have more prostaglandins than others, which prostaglandins are most important, or even if the studies done on adult women are relevant to the adolescent population. What we do know is this: When we give a drug that turns down the production of prostaglandins, we can almost completely eliminate the pain of dysmenorrhea.

A normal pelvic examination should suffice to reassure you and your daughter that there's no abnormality that accounts for the dysmenorrhea. Once that's established, your doctor can prescribe either birth control pills or prostaglandin inhibitors as suits the situation. (See p. 346, **Ref. 218.**)

11. Bones and Joints

PAINLESS SWELLING BEHIND KNEE
(Popliteal or Baker's Cyst)

A painless, balloonlike swelling in the inner side of the space behind a child's knee is usually caused by a popliteal (in Latin, *poples* means back of the knee) cyst. These swellings are also commonly known as Baker's cysts, although the swelling that William Morant Baker described in 1877 was painful, not painless.

Popliteal cysts appear twice as often in boys as they do in girls. They occur in children from 2 to 14 years old, with a mean of 6 years, and can be found on either leg, but rarely on both of them. They range from the size of a Ping-Pong ball to that of a grapefruit. Regardless of the size, you'll probably worry—unnecessarily—when you find it.

In the past, doctors used to excise these cysts in the operating room. The results were disappointing. If cyst fluid was inadvertently released during surgery, often it would interfere with the healing of the wound. If the fluid worked its way down to the calves, it was so irritating to the calf muscle that it looked as if a deep vein within the muscle was inflamed. To make matters worse, about half of the cysts returned. Many children had to undergo a second operation. By the time some children were having their third operation, most of the popliteal cysts that had been left alone had already disappeared. These cysts were trying to tell us something.

The next approach we doctors took was to put our hands in our pockets and wait and see what happened. When we simply stood back and admired the natural courses of 70 of these popliteal cysts in children, we noted that 51 had spontaneously disappeared during a mean period of 20 months.

Nowadays, we first satisfy ourselves that the swelling is truly a popliteal cyst. Other things can inhabit the space behind the knee, and at times the swelling may be a sign of an enlarged lymph node (see p. 171), a collection of fatty tissue, a swollen nerve, a weakened dilated artery, or that great lump imposter, the unexpected localized muscular enlargement (see p. 258). If the swelling is none of those, and if the doctor can illuminate the swelling by holding a bright light against it, he'll feel confident that it's nothing more than a popliteal cyst.

After this has been established, your doctor will do a very thorough examination of all the child's joints, and if he's satisfied that the cyst isn't the result of a joint disease (a true Baker's cyst) that hadn't been noted before, he'll advise that nothing be done. If the cyst is, in fact, the result of a joint disease, it will disappear when the joint disease gets proper treatment. In the very rare event that the cyst is the first sign of a rheumatoid disease, only time will make that fact known, and there's still no reason to remove the cyst.

Your doctor will only remove the cyst if it gets so massive that it interferes with the movements of the knee. Fortunately this, too, is extremely rare. (See p. 343, **Ref. 151**; see p. 346, **Ref. 219**; see p. 346, **Ref. 220**; see p. 346, **Ref. 221**.)

ROUND, SMOOTH SWELLING OVER TOP OF WRIST *(Ganglion)*

Hippocrates used to refer to any lump under the skin as a ganglion (meaning knot in Greek). His physician descendants now use the word to refer to the firm, rarely tender, cystic swelling that's most often found on the tops of the hands or feet. A ganglion can be as small as a pea or as large as a plum. If it's filled with a firm, jellylike fluid, it can feel quite hard. Like the popliteal cyst (see p. 267), it will "light up" if a bright light is held tightly to it. Ganglions often appear over joints, and unless the skin over the joint is pulled taut by the swelling, many small ones go unnoticed. They're so common that if you happen to have one, you mightn't react to seeing one on your child. We don't really know for sure if ganglions are outpouchings from the joint cavities, outpouchings of the sheaths that surround the tendons, or simply accumulations of degenerated collagen from injured tendons, ligaments, or joint capsules. They probably result from local irritation, either from a blow or from overuse of the tendon. Like their close relative, the popliteal cyst, ganglions are often found in children with rheumatoid arthritis, but in that context they're usually very soft and multiple.

In the recent past, ganglions, like popliteal cysts, were treated surgically. The results were no better than those obtained with popliteal cysts. Much earlier, ganglions were subjected to the force of religion, being smashed repeatedly by a heavy family Bible. Some doctors, apparently believing that "scientific" treatment would be more effective than faith, used their *Gray's Anatomy* textbook in place of the Old Testament. Neither approach had striking success; the ganglions withstood both forces and tended to recur. At the present time, unless the ganglion is very large and interferes with the joint's movements, doctors suggest benign neglect.

Again, like popliteal cysts, they go away. (See p. 343, **Ref. 151.**)

BONY, HARD BUMP ABOVE HEEL *(Pump Bump)*

If the back of a shoe presses hard against the back of your child's heel month after month, the skin there will thicken and form a callus. The swelling will make the shoe's fit even tighter, and unless something is done to take the pressure off the growing heel bone, an extra lump of bone will form directly under the skin lump. It's usually at the top of the back of the shoe, and can be alarming by virtue of its hard, bony feel.

Since this whole problem came about from an ill-fitting shoe, this extra bone is called a pump bump. Change the shoes. If the doctor advises surgery, change doctors. (See p. 338, **Ref. 53.**)

POOR TEENAGE POSTURE *(Adolescent Slouch)*

I've never seen a teenager come to the office believing that he had poor posture. It's always the parent who does the worrying about the child's posture. At times, a parent will bring her adolescent to the office on some pretense, and before I enter the examining room, she will, in hushed tones so no one else will hear, ask me to tell her slumping child to stand up straight before it's too late. Sometimes, parents even plead with me to threaten the child with the necessity of wearing a brace. I do neither.

Rapidly growing adolescents slouch because they're trying to avoid attention. They don't feel comfortable yet with their new height, or breasts, and their frequent physical and social awkwardness makes them especially self-conscious. Without being aware of precisely what they're doing, they slump, shrug, sag, and slouch. Parents, being what they are, become concerned and exhort the child to sit up or stand up or straighten up. Adolescents, being what they are, react with resistance, denial, and, often, frank hostility. Before too long, the situation becomes tense, and the parents, in desperation, turn to the old pediatrician to straighten their child out. This isn't too good a position for us pediatricians to be in.

If a pediatrician assumes the parent's point of view, she's now in league with the Establishment. If she takes the child's position, she's part of the Resistance. The pediatrician therefore has to approach this problem with caution. In talking to your child, she must avoid lecturing him. If the physician becomes too directive, the adolescent will be apt to choose the opposite course. The doctor must calmly and carefully present the facts and let the adolescent make the choice. With a little skill and a little luck, she can show the teenager what constitutes good posture, what he's doing that isn't so good, and what can be done to make it better. Having a full-length mirror helps. It also helps if the child will part with most of his clothes for this examination. For some teenage girls, putting on a bathing suit works very well.

When your doctor does this examination, what is she looking for?

As viewed from the rear, the middle of the youngster's head should line up perfectly with the midpoint between the shoulder blades, the buttock crease, and the point between the ankles. Your doctor may use a plumb line from the local hardware store to line up these points. As viewed from the side, a plumb line held behind the ear should pass over the tip of the shoulder and across the hip, pass just in front of the middle of the side of the knee, and end up just in front of the outside ankle.

If the plumb line doesn't go that way in your teenager, your doctor can show the child where it deviates. She can then show him what changes he can make to correct the deviation. She can explain that poor posture, although completely painless at his age, may cause problems later on.

If your child's posture is significantly abnormal, and doesn't improve as his self-confidence and body awareness improve, your doctor can refer you to a physical therapist for postural exercises that are often very useful.

Most teenagers will cooperate as long as they understand what they're doing wrong, how they can correct it, and why they should bother at all. (See p. 346, **Ref. 222.**)

MILD CURVATURE OF THE SPINE *(Scoliosis of Less Than 20 Degrees Found During School Screening)*

A few years ago, most cases of curvature of the spine (scoliosis) weren't identified unless the deformity was extreme. A recent study in Ontario, Canada, showed the following breakdown: About one third of children in whom scoliosis was diagnosed had such advanced curves that surgery was recommended immediately. Another 40 percent needed a brace, and of these, 10 percent eventually required surgery. It's no wonder that the public equated the diagnosis of scoliosis with years of wearing a brace or with a major operation, and sometimes both. While that assumption may have been true for the severest cases, no one, including doctors, had anything to say about the mildest cases, since they never came to anyone's attention.

The advent of routine, compulsory screening of preadolescent schoolchildren for scoliosis changed all that. Mass screening has turned up such an enormous number of children with very slight curves that we're seeing the complete scoliosis spectrum for the first time. As you might imagine, most of the curves found are extremely mild, representing very early, previously undetected scoliosis. Once these mild cases are detected, some will need treatment, either at the time of initial discovery or later. While there are differences of opinion, most spine specialists begin bracing if the child's curve is 20 degrees or more, especially if the child is young and the curve has been increasing with time.

But not every child's spinal curve does increase. Some children's curves stay mild, and some disappear. Here's the rub: At the present time, we have no way of knowing which way the very mild curve will go when it's first found, but our experience has become so vast that we can quote the odds.

When over 25,000 boys and girls in their first year of high school were examined for scoliosis by trained school nurses, 7 percent were found to have a curvature. All of these children then had X rays of their backs to confirm the nurse's impression. Some (about 27 percent) were found to have no curve at all. (These children obviously weren't standing straight for the nurse's screening test, and therefore looked curved when they actually weren't.) The overwhelming majority of X-ray-confirmed cases were mild: slightly more than one half had curves measuring 6 to 10 degrees, another 40 percent had curves of 11 to 20 degrees, and 6 percent had curves in the range that specialists begin bracing—21 degrees or more.

What happened to the mild curves?

A very small proportion (3 percent) disappeared entirely. This was most apt to occur in boys, especially if the curve was less than 15 degrees when it was first found. More than 90 percent of the children's curves remained more or less unchanged, and nothing had to be done. A total of 7 percent of the curves progressed, and those children eventually needed some form of treatment (93 percent had to wear a brace and the rest required surgery). The larger the curve at the initial measurement, the more likely it was to progress, especially in girls. (Of the curves that initially measured 6 to 10 degrees, only 2 percent progressed to need treatment, but among those of 11 degrees or more, 10 percent were progressive.)

So where does this leave you if your child is one of the 7 percent of screened children who bring home the note from the school nurse stating that the scoliosis screening test was "flunked" and advising the parents to get in contact with a doctor? The odds are about 3 to 1 that the X ray will confirm the nurse's impression. Once it's been confirmed, the odds are 15 to 1 that the curve won't need immediate treatment. If your child does need treatment, the odds are only 1 to 13 that the treatment will be surgical. In fact, if the curve wasn't treatable when first found, the odds are 13 to 1 that it never will be. The odds are even better if your child is a boy.

Even if your child's curve does worsen and does need to be treated, don't panic. It has been diagnosed at a very early stage, and the doctor won't allow it to progress too far before he starts treatment. (See p. 347, **Ref. 223**; see p. 347, **Ref. 224**.)

GROWING PAINS IN LEGS *(Idiopathic Leg Pains)*

No group of complaints epitomizes the harmless childhood condition that mimics disease better than "growing pains." Practically everybody knows just what you mean when you say that your child suffers from growing pains. Many people also have their own ideas of what causes them, and how to make them go away. The problem is, most of their explanations are either wrong or unproven, and the recommended treatments, if children have them, are either worthless or harmful. Furthermore, some doctors aren't overly convinced that growing pains even exist, and even those who believe in their reality aren't sure of their cause or significance. The latter dilemma doesn't arise because doctors know less about the subject than laypeople do, but because they know how little is really understood about it.

Despite their widespread mentions in popular jargon, growing pains are seldom discussed in medical literature or medical schools. Of the three more-or-less-standard pediatric orthopedic textbooks in use today, two have nothing to say about growing pains, and one devotes a single paragraph to them. As a result, your physician's answers to many of your questions will probably be derived from a source similar to yours, namely, the pediatrician's mother.

Depending on the definition used, growing pains occur in 4 to 50 percent of children. It's hard to know the true incidence of the condition because every survey uses different criteria for the diagnosis. In one, 2,178 schoolchildren were asked if they had growing pains; 12.5 percent of the boys and 18.4 percent of the girls said yes.

Regardless of the true frequency of growing pains, however, we all know that intermittent and sometimes severe leg pains do occur all through childhood, most often during the years 3 to 12. Despite the name of the condition, it doesn't increase during the period of the great growth spurt—12 to 14 years of age.

Growing pains tend to occur after a youngster has had a particularly active day. He usually feels them in both legs, deep within the thighs, in the calves, or behind the knees. On rare occasions, a child may complain of pain in his back, shoulder, arm, instep, or groin. Most of the time, children locate the pain in a muscle, but sometimes they point to a vague area around a joint. If your child does point directly to a joint, the joint itself will appear entirely normal to you, with no redness, warmth, swelling, or limitation of motion.

Typically, a child's leg pains wait for him to fall into a deep sleep and then hit, causing him to wake with a cry. His pain can be brief or it can last for half an hour, or even longer. You can relieve it by massage, heat, and hugs and kisses. When the pain subsides, the child will fall asleep again and wake up the next morning absolutely pain free. By the time he reaches maturity, the attacks always subside.

Your doctor will ask a number of questions before he decides that your child's problem is actually nothing more than growing pains. He'll want to know if the pain is definitely localized in one spot, especially if the spot is over a bone or joint. (If so, the diagnosis will probably be something other than growing pains.) If your child's joints are painful, your doctor will check to see if they're swollen as well, since 90 percent of children with juvenile rheumatoid arthritis have joints that are not only painful but also swollen. Your doctor will also want to know if your child limps or has enough pain during the daytime to require aspirin to control it, and if there's a family history of arthritis. A yes answer to any of these questions lessens the chance of a yes for the diagnosis of growing pains.

Your physician may also try to distinguish between growing pains and something more significant by finding out how your child responds to being handled when he's in pain. This is a very helpful method. Children whose joints are inflamed or whose bones are tender don't like to be touched, because any movement tends to increase their pain. Children with growing pains respond in quite the opposite manner. As noted earlier, they like to have their legs massaged and feel better when they're held and cuddled.

Of the many identifiable causes of leg pain in children, trauma (that is, a bump of some kind) is the most common. It needn't be a big trauma, and it often doesn't help much to ask the child if any trauma has occurred. For many children, just spending the day out of bed is enough reason for repeated minor injuries to the leg. If the injury is minor, the child won't remember it, which is why it doesn't do much good to ask. If the bump is more than trivial, the youngster may not want to mention it for fear of being punished for being careless or being where he wasn't supposed to be. Of course, he could have some bruises, but since they may not surface for days after the injury, and may not even show at the point of injury, it would take a highly sophisticated computer to ascertain which bruise was connected to which pain. If you're interested in assigning a particular pain to a particular bruise, it might help you to know that the initial color of the bruise, a reddish blue, becomes bluish brown by day 1 to 3, shades to greenish yellow by day 7 to 10, and then turns a yellowish brown that slowly fades over a two- to four-week period. If your child's leg pain is over a bone, and if there's tenderness along with a bruise, trauma is the likely explanation. If the pain doesn't lessen a bit day by day, his leg can be X-rayed to determine if a minor stress fracture of a leg or foot bone (such as occurs after jogging) is present.

Your doctor will make a diagnosis of growing pains only after excluding the other less common, but more serious causes of leg pain. When he's reached that point, he may look to your child's feet for the cause. He'll probably find that they're flatter than pancakes. The explanation may be that, since your child's feet pretty much lack an arch (the most stable base yet designed for supporting weight), the stresses of bearing his weight have been turned over to the muscles and ligaments of his legs. After a busy day that strained these auxiliary supports to their limits, they developed painful muscular spasms and aching ligaments, i.e., growing pains.

Maturation helps the condition greatly. As your child gets older, his loose joints tighten. The ligaments in his feet grow stronger and he doesn't tire as quickly. Furthermore, his habits change. He begins to spend more time sitting and less time running. Instead of going to bed early in the evening immediately after physical activity, he goes to bed later in the evening after a period of quiet. These changes in habits are probably beneficial because they provide the opportunity before sleep for the child's body to dispose of lactic acid, the waste product of the muscular activity that accumulates around the muscles of the legs. Heat and massage, by increasing the local circulation, also remove the excess lactic acid, which may be the reason why children with growing pains find massage so comforting.

Not every ache and pain in the leg of a healthy child is caused by growing pains, but the causes of all the others are usually readily apparent or become so with the passage of a little time. The vast majority, however, are just what your mother—and mine—said they were. Growing pains. (See p. 337, **Ref. 38**; see p. 338, **Ref. 53**; see p. 343, **Ref. 151**; see p. 347, **Ref. 225**; see p. 347, **Ref. 226**; see p. 347, **Ref. 227**.)

1. Cardiovascular System

HEART DISEASE SUSPECTED IN YOUNG, CONDITIONED, HEALTHY ATHLETE *(Athletic Heart Syndrome)*

About the last thought that would enter your head would be that your muscular, highly conditioned, regularly exercising athletic son had something wrong with his heart. Yet, when that same Herculean hulk gets a thorough heart examination, there's a distinct chance that the doctor will discover a loud murmur, a very slow pulse rate, an assortment of rhythm irregularities, some electrocardiographic changes, and, after a chest X ray, an enlarged heart. This constellation of findings is called the athletic heart syndrome (AHS).

Do you take your son with AHS directly to the nearest intensive care unit?

No. Take him back to the Nautilus training center, or wherever he got his superb conditioning. What his examination revealed was nothing more than the physiologic and anatomic changes of the heart in response to regular, intense physical conditioning. What's more, there's nothing bad about these changes. They're actually helpful adaptations to training, should be viewed as beneficial, and will go away when the training is stopped. Everyone involved in physical fitness these days is aware that the slowing of the heart rate is one of the indications of improving fitness. It's called improving vagal tone. When the

277

conditioned athlete gets his resting heart rate down to 40 or 50 beats per minute (some are as slow as 35 beats per minute), the heart compensates by increasing the volume of blood pumped per beat. The heart really has no choice; since there are fewer contractions per minute, each contraction has to squeeze more blood out of the heart. The result of this increase in volume of blood per stroke is an increase in the flow rate, and this is what heart murmurs are made of (see p. 82).

Another result of an increased volume of blood per stroke is an increase in the size of the heart's cavities (they need to hold more blood). Thus, the hearts of athletes conditioned by endurance training, such as marathon runners and skiers, will be dilated to handle the increased volume. Interestingly, athletes engaged in strength training, such as weight lifters and shot-putters, don't need to increase their volume, and therefore their hearts don't dilate. Instead, their hearts, which must pump against an increased pressure, respond by increasing the thickness of the muscular wall.

There are times when your doctor may find electrocardiographic abnormalities that actually resemble those of a blocked coronary artery. Some athletic careers have actually been interrupted by this sort of finding. As a rule, though, any ECG abnormality in the athletic heart syndrome that suggests coronary disease will disappear under the influence of exercise, and doing a stress test should adequately show the health of the athlete's heart.

Several years before the discovery of AHS, doctors discovered a closely related condition called hyperkinetic heart syndrome (HHS), which is a greatly enhanced vigor of heart muscle contractions. Among those who had HHS (a group that included children as young as seven), a third were conditioned athletes and probably had AHS, but the others had no obvious reason for such overly vigorous hearts. At first the physicians assumed that anxiety might be causing the exaggerated activity of the heart, but they found that it continued even when the patients were deep in sleep. Half of the original HHS group had variably high blood pressures and a few went on to develop blood pressures that were permanently high. The great majority, however, were perfectly healthy and remained so. It's probably a benign condition, but the last word on its connection with high blood pressure remains to be written.

As for the athletic heart syndrome, all the observed changes are beneficial responses of the heart to sustained conditioning and they regress when the conditioning is stopped. An athlete should be proud of his AHS. (See p. 347, **Ref. 228**; see p. 347, **Ref. 229**; see p. 347, **Ref. 230.**)

HEART DISEASE SUSPECTED IN CHILD
WITH CHEST WALL DEFORMITY *(Normal Heart in*
Child with Scoliosis, Pectus Excavatum, or Straight Back Syndrome)

Chest wall deformities aren't normal, but most of the time, the heart that beats within them is. This is true despite the fact that many children with these deformities also have heart murmurs, electrocardiographic changes, and strange-looking chest X rays.

The three most common chest-wall deformities are pectus excavatum, scoliosis, and straight back syndrome. If your child has one of these deformities, your pediatrician may find the above irregularities when he tests the child's heart, in which case he'll refer you to a cardiologist. But if your child does end up in a cardiologist's office, the chances are good that you'll leave smiling. Most often, nothing is wrong with the workings of the heart; all of the findings arose in a completely normal heart whose only crime was being in the wrong place at the wrong time. Here's how this happens.

Pectus excavatum is a spooned-out depression of the lower end of the breastbone found in 3.5 percent of first-grade children. Depending on the shape and depth of the depression, it can be described as funnel-, cup-, or saucer-shaped. If the depression is deep enough, it pushes the heart back toward the spine and off to the left. The compression of the heart's chambers and great vessels changes the circulating blood's normal laminar flow pattern (see p. 185), creating turbulence. The turbulence sets up vibrations that end up in the doctor's ears as a murmur, a particularly loud one because the depression in the chest wall allows the stethoscope to get extra-close to the source of the turbulence.

In another finding, a chest X ray may show the heart displaced to the left, a sign that, under other circumstances, can signify enlargement. The electrocardiogram is also influenced by a heart's leftist leanings, and at times has fooled doctors into thinking that a heart attack has occurred.

A generation ago, children whose hearts showed these findings were suspected of having heart disease and suffered a lifetime of prolonged, enforced bed rest and needless restriction of physical activity. They were advised to choose a livelihood that wouldn't "overly tax" their "diseased" hearts. For the vast majority, these restrictions represented another waste of good health.

The past association of pectus excavatum with true cardiac symptoms can be explained, at least in part, by the fact that some children with pectus excavatum do indeed have significant heart defects—in addition to the chest wall deformity. Recently developed techniques for testing lung function also show that some children with severe pectus excavatum have restrictions in their lungs' capacity. It seems reasonable to assume that the child with a pectus excavatum will have a murmur and an "abnormal" X ray and ECG. But he shouldn't have heart disease symptoms such as shortness of breath, chest pain, or fatigue. If he has any, your doctor will give him a complete examination to see if the symptoms come from an associated heart problem, limited lung expansion imposed by the chest wall deformity, or (an extremely remote possibility) a subtle derangement in blood flow. The odds are that the doctor will find that the symptoms are caused by the anxiety that results from the child's belief that he has a heart problem.

Another chest wall deformity that causes the appearance, but not the reality, of heart disease is the straight back syndrome (SBS). This type of deformity doesn't become apparent until adolescence, and affects boys and girls alike. Your doctor may not notice it unless he takes an X ray that shows a side view of the chest. In SBS, the normal backward curving of the upper back is replaced by a straight line and, at times, an inward curve. As a result, there's less room in the upper chest cavity, and once again the heart gets squeezed. This time, the compression comes from behind. The effect is the same: A murmur is heard, a chest X ray shows a displaced heart, and an ECG shows an assortment of strange wiggles. Since this type of chest wall deformity has also been occasionally associated with heart defects, a thorough cardiac evaluation is usually needed to be sure that the murmur, X ray, and ECG are of no significance. Once it's documented that the problem is SBS alone, nothing more needs to be done.

The third chest-wall deformity is scoliosis (see p. 272). Its influence on the heart is the most variable since the spinal curvature varies so much in degree, level, and direction. What's more, a number of children with scoliosis also have pectus excavatum and SBS at the same time. Scoliosis also affects the ECG findings. Like youngsters with other chest wall deformities, a child with scoliosis has an increased chance of having a heart defect (perhaps as high as 5 percent), so it's wise to have complete heart and lung examinations of children found to have "abnormal" ECGs with scoliosis. For the most part, though, their hearts are fine. ECGs on children are being performed more and more these days, not only in children with chest wall deformities. Overinterpretation of heart findings is increasing with the increasing popularity of "diagnostic centers" where unselected screening tests (like ECGs) are performed on young children and interpreted by examiners who aren't familiar with children's ECGs. Errors range from the ridiculous (confusing the effect of a hiccup with that of an extra heart beat) to the sublime (failing to appreciate that certain findings that have grave significance for adults are normal for persons under 20). The bottom line is to be aware that your child's cardiac findings can be overinterpreted, especially if he has a deformity of the chest wall. (See p. 347, **Ref. 230**; see p. 347, **Ref. 231**; see p. 347, **Ref. 232**; see p. 347, **Ref. 233**; see p. 347, **Ref. 234**; see p. 347, **Ref. 235**.)

THIN, NERVOUS FEMALE WITH PALPITATIONS AND MURMUR
(Mitral Valve Prolapse Syndrome)

Some people who have a heart condition known as mitral valve prolapse syndrome are quite ill, but most are entirely symptom free. The condition is diagnosed with increasing frequency and, as of this writing, 6 to 10 percent of healthy young women are reported to have it. Furthermore, doctors are finding increasing numbers of younger people, especially teenage girls, with mitral valve prolapse syndrome. In terms of the number of cases alone, the condition can now be considered statistically normal.

Thin, nervous people who complain of chest pain, palpitations, shortness of breath, and racing pulses have been pacing our planet for a long time. For some reason, the cases seem more frequent during periods of war. An army doctor who had served in the Civil War described it in 1871, and the syndrome surfaced again among English army recruits during World War I. It was called by many names, among them soldier's heart, effort syndrome, and finally neurocirculatory asthenia (*a* means without; *sthenia* refers to strength), or NCA, in 1918. By World War II, psychiatry had become a well-entrenched specialty and most doctors, including some cardiologists, regarded NCA as a psychiatric disorder. They renamed it anxiety neurosis.

While some cardiologists were debating the question of whether or not NCA was a physical or psychological issue, others were busy trying to figure out the significance of certain inexplicable sounds coming from certain patients' hearts. These sounds, called systolic clicks and late systolic murmurs, were ultimately traced to the mitral valve, which regulates the flow of blood from the left atrium into the left ventricle of the heart. (This valve consists of two leaflets, which billow upward when the left ventricle contracts. Together they form a seal that prevents blood being pumped out of the left ventricle from backflowing into the left atrium. Wiry bands, called chordae tendineae, secure each leaflet to the ventricular lining and keep the leaflets from billowing all the way into the left atrium itself. For a description of how the entire heart operates, see p. 82.)

About 60 years after we learned where the sounds came from, we learned how they were actually produced. The systolic click and late systolic murmur turned out to be the results of the protrusion of a floppy mitral-valve leaflet into the left atrium. This became known as mitral valve prolapse (MVP), and when it was connected with palpitations, chronic fatigue, chest pain, high anxiety, and a tendency to panic, the term *mitral valve prolapse syndrome* (MVPS) was born. (It also meant the sad end, for many of us who follow sports, of MVP's standing for most valuable player.)

The term has flourished. Patients with mitral valve prolapse syndrome are turning up everywhere, and many don't even have the click or the murmur that started the investigation in the first place. With the use of an echocardiogram, we can now actually see the prolapsing leaflet poking its head into the left atrium. We've learned that the basic fault is in the collagen structure (see p. 235) of the valve, and we now understand why mitral valve prolapse is such a common finding in patients who are known to have a defect in their collagen production.

MVPS is inherited. If you have it, the chances of your child's having it can be as high as 50 percent, especially if your child is a girl (women outnumber men with this condition three to one). We know that among the vast numbers of patients with MVPS, in only a few will the condition be severe enough to interfere with the normal functioning of the mitral valve. Those who do have severe MVPS may be adding a strain to their hearts that can eventually cause major problems. Many have heart rhythm disturbances, which some doctors suspect is the cause of their dizziness, fainting, palpitations, and possibly all their so-called neurotic symptoms as well. Some people with MVPS may develop serious complications, such as an infection on the floppy valve, or tearing of the chordae tendineae. Fortunately, however, these serious cases are rare. A great deal of research on MVPS is under way now in an attempt to uncover the connection (if there is one) between a ballooning valve inside the heart and a tendency toward neurotic behavior. Most likely, mitral valve floppiness is a matter of degree (perhaps all mitral valves flop, some more than others), with mild prolapse representing an everyday occurrence in so many people that it will have to be considered entirely normal. (See p. 347, **Ref. 236**; see p. 347, **Ref. 237.**)

HIGH BLOOD PRESSURE IN TEENAGER
(Incidental Hypertension)

Hypertension is not benign. Just the opposite is true. Hypertension kills a quarter of a million adults each year and is directly responsible for many more heart attacks, strokes, and other serious problems. Because physicians respect hypertension, we've made measuring blood pressure an important part of the routine physical checkup, and we've worked to make the public aware of the importance of hypertension. As a result of both efforts, we've been finding elevated blood pressures in many people in whom we wouldn't have found them before. What to do about these elevated blood pressures isn't always obvious, and the problems posed are particularly acute when it comes to children.

If your child comes home with a warning slip after having had his blood pressure taken by the school nurse, at the state fair blood-pressure-testing booth, or at the mobile blood pressure truck, don't panic.

Many children who "fail" a blood pressure test on one occasion will pass it with flying colors the very next time. The news of your child's hypertension shouldn't become the basis for your hypertension. Rather than launching a full-scale investigation of the diagnosis, your doctor will first test the child to see if the hypertension is real in the first place. (Hypertension is defined as a blood pressure greater than the 95th percentile for the age of the child; a pressure that's at the 95th percentile is, by definition, high normal and not abnormal.) And if the hypertension is real, is it sustained? And if it's sustained, what's causing it, and what, if anything, should you do about it?

There are countless reasons for the first recording of high blood pressure to be inaccurate. First and foremost is the equipment used. Before the importance of the size of the blood pressure cuff was well known, using too narrow a cuff (a width less than two thirds the length of the upper arm) was the number one cause of findings of "hypertension" in children. Even if the cuff is the right size, it must be at the child's heart level, and the mercury column read by the examiner must be at eye level for the readings to be accurate.

Even if the tests are performed correctly, there are countless reasons for your child's blood pressure to be fleetingly elevated. His blood pressure can be influenced by a recently eaten meal, certain medicines, coffee or tea, or exercise. It can also be elevated if the child is ill, in pain, or frightened, if his bladder is full, and even if the room where the measurement is being made is hot or noisy.

Assuming none of these conditions exists and his pressure is truly elevated, what happens next depends on the magnitude of the elevation, the age of the child, and whether or not the child appears sick. Very elevated pressures in children under ten years old need to be attended to very quickly. They're usually hospitalized promptly, both to lower the pressure and to begin the search for the explanation. On the other hand, if your child is older than ten and has a pressure that's only mildly elevated, your doctor will get more measurements before he makes a further medical judgment.

Doctors have been doing additional blood pressure measurements since we learned that most mildly elevated pressures found incidentally in any group of healthy children don't stay elevated. In one group of 6,622 children 5 to 18 years old, over 13 percent had high pressures on the first reading, but less than 1 percent of these levels stayed up. How often, how many, by whom, and where the follow-up blood pressures are taken varies from doctor to doctor, but if your older child has a mildly elevated pressure, you can expect your doctor to take more measurements. You can also expect her to ask you about high blood pressure, heart attacks, and strokes in your family, to do a very careful examination of your child (especially of the pulses), and to do a urinalysis.

If these measurements still show that your child has elevated blood pressure, and if she weighs at least 20 percent more than she should, she should be put on a diet before anything else is considered. The youngster will probably lose her hypertension as soon as she loses her excess 20 percent. (Overall, obesity accounts for more than 50 percent of children with persistent hypertension.) If the child is lean to start with, her pressure won't drop if she gets leaner. In this case, her hypertension is likely to be the result of an abnormal narrowing of the aorta (the main artery exiting from the left ventricle of the heart), or some kidney or endocrine or other condition known to cause hypertension. This is called secondary hypertension, and it accounts for only about 10 percent of childhood hypertension. We once thought that most hypertension in children was secondary, but we have learned that most is unexplained and therefore primary.

Doctors always try to find a simple reason for sustained hypertension, but unfortunately the rate of discovery is low. Children undergoing orthopedic operations are especially likely to have raised blood pressures, particularly if the procedures involve prolonged bed rest with immobilization, lengthening limbs, and surgically releasing extremities that were held tightly flexed. In these circumstances, the hypertension is usually mild and brief, but there have been isolated incidents where it was extreme. If your child is undergoing an orthopedic procedure requiring immobilization or traction, you may notice that he'll be getting his blood pressure taken more often than his roommate who just had his appendix removed. If you don't notice that this is happening, you might remind the nurse that you would like it to.

Hypertension that results from taking certain medications is also easily corrected (see p. 111). For this reason, you must remember to share what you know about your child's medicines with the person taking the blood pressure. Teenage girls have become hypertensive while taking oral contraceptives, and they've sometimes been known to withhold from their parents the fact that they're on the pill. If you have a teenage daughter, ask for and insist on getting whatever information you need. Even small children can elevate their blood pressure by the use of a chemical. For example, children "hooked" on large amounts of licorice can become hypertensive. Licorice contains a chemical that closely resembles the hormone aldosterone, which in large amounts will raise blood pressure temporarily.

Now what about the hypertensive older child with no identifiable reason to have high blood pressure, and who is, therefore, said to have primary or essential hypertension? If the child is overweight, of course, she should reduce, and that may even put an end to her hypertension. Excessive use of salt should be avoided. It's hard for anyone, especially a teenager, to accept a restricted salt diet, so try to settle for avoidance of high-salt foods (which are, admittedly, most of the foods teenagers like to eat), and keeping the saltshaker off the table. It helps to know which foods are high in salt and, as you might have guessed, the list includes such favorites as A.1. sauce, bacon, catsup, chili sauce, Dorito chips, frankfurters, luncheon meats, peanuts, pickles, pizza, potato chips, pretzels, relish, soy sauce, and Worcestershire sauce. If this list makes your mouth water, just think of what it does to your teenager. You might have more luck with the following additional recommendations:

Mildly hypertensive teenagers should partake in regular exercises, such as running 3 to 5 miles a day, bicycling 10 to 15 miles a day, or swimming 1 to 2 miles a day (all four times per week). Participating in competitive sports should be encouraged, not, as you might assume, discouraged. Aside from helping youngsters lose weight, the improved conditioning also has a direct effect on lowering the blood pressure. Isometric, strength-building exercises such as weight lifting may not be as harmful to hypertensive teenagers as they are to adults, but they shouldn't be encouraged. Smoking increases a teenager's risk of having a heart attack or stroke, so smoking should be avoided.

Doctors have worked out a number of different strategies for dealing with mild hypertension in children, but we still haven't solved three key questions: (1) Is childhood hypertension the beginning of adulthood hypertension? (2) Is the child who was found to have high blood pressure on the first but not the subsequent test at more risk of developing persistent hypertension than the child whose pressure was never elevated? (3) Is the child whose pressure is at the 95th percentile (high normal) any more likely to become hypertensive than the mid-normal or low-normal child? Until we know some of the answers, it doesn't seem fair to make a big fuss about hypertension in otherwise healthy teenagers, and to thereby jeopardize their insurability, employability, and feeling of health and well-being at such a critical time in their lives. (See p. 336, **Ref. 20**; see p. 347, **Ref. 238**; see p. 347, **Ref. 239**; see p. 347, **Ref. 240**; see p. 347, **Ref. 241**; see p. 347, **Ref. 242**; see p. 347, **Ref. 243**; see p. 348, **Ref. 244**; see p. 348, **Ref. 245**.)

2. Respiratory System

CHEST PAIN IN HEALTHY BUT FRIGHTENED TEENAGER
(Adolescent Chest Pain)

Teenagers may be blasé about many of their problems, but not about chest pain. According to one government report, chest pain brings 650,000 patients between the ages of 10 and 21 to their doctors each year. In one survey of black adolescents, chest pain was their seventh most common health complaint. That's a lot of hurting chests for an age group that we don't normally think of in relation to chest problems. If your child has chest pain, and if you're like most parents, the thought of a heart attack (if the child is a boy) or cancer (in the case of a girl) has probably crossed your mind.

If your doctor doesn't respond to the youngster's complaint with the same sort of worry, don't immediately change doctors. If you do, you may be setting the stage for a useless cycle of testing that will probably yield negative results, frustration over the absence of any answers, and more anxiety—which will then provide the impetus for more testing, and so on. As negative data accumulate, the complaint acquires more "mystery," and with this, more importance.

Heart attacks and breast cancer are virtually unheard of in this age group, so you may want to know (1) where such dire thoughts about chest pain originated, and (2) what's really causing the pain. Knowing the answers to these questions will help you avoid the vicious testing cycle and point you in the direction most likely to provide relief.

When doctors looked for the reasons why so many parents curtailed the activities of their children with innocent heart murmurs (see p. 183), they found that most mothers and fathers make no distinction between heart disease in adults and heart disease in children. Most people are under the mistaken impression that children are subject to the same sudden, catastrophic cardiac events that can occur during adulthood. Since this misunderstanding is widespread, it follows that a child's chest pain arouses the same immediate concern as chest pain in an adult.

But chest pain in children is rarely an omen of serious disease, and research has shown that in the extremely unusual event that a major problem is found, it isn't even the source of the child's chest pain! While most adolescents who have chest pain usually say that they don't know "fer sure" what's actually causing their pain, many, if queried further, say that they're afraid that the pain is coming from their hearts. Some children actually believe that they're in the midst of having a heart attack. This adolescent fear may fly in the face of everything that we know about the way adolescents regard themselves as invulnerable to serious disease, but there it is.

Typically, a youngster describes the pain as a sharp stab beneath the breastbone. He usually reports that the pain has been coming and going for several months before he sought attention. Many such children stay home from school and most give up their normal activities. If, when your doctor examines your child, nothing is found, the odds are overwhelming that no useful information will come from laboratory testing, especially chest X rays and electrocardiograms. If your child has an accompanying complaint, such as coughing or nausea, your doctor may suspect that the source of the pain is the lung (potentially bronchitis), or the esophagus (potentially esophagitis), but this rarely turns out to be the case. If, during examination, something is actually found (which is also rare), it's usually tenderness of the chest wall. If so, the precise location of the tenderness will determine which diagnosis your doctor will make.

The most common, most consistent chest-wall complaint is called the precordial (*pre* means in front of; *cor* equals heart) catch syndrome. (In one group of "normal" doctors, one third said that they themselves had experienced it.) In this condition, the pain is sudden, stabbing, and needlelike. It occurs beneath the left nipple, is very brief, and feels as if something is "catching" around the heart when a deep breath is taken. If you were to have this sort of pain, you would breathe very shallowly and be very reluctant to take a deep breath. The precordial catch syndrome occurs when the person is at rest, or only minimally exerting himself, usually when he's in a slightly slouched position. Classrooms and libraries are popular places for this pain to strike. When the pain departs, usually after less than one minute, it may leave a mild, vague aching in the same area.

Precordial catch syndrome is as common in boys as in girls, and it usually scares the wits out of them, because they think they're having a heart attack. If the child also has an innocent murmur (see p. 181), the doctor may refer him to a cardiologist. The cardiologist will quickly recognize this syndrome and explain that it doesn't come from the child's heart. Pain that arises from the heart is typically in the center of the chest, beneath the breastbone, and is crushing in nature. Cardiac pain usually comes during exertion, not rest, and frequently radiates down an arm or up to the tongue. In short, it doesn't behave like the pain of the precordial chest syndrome. Telling the youngster that the pain isn't coming from his heart and that he doesn't need a doctor should go far toward relieving his anxiety.

If the child's point of tenderness is closer to the middle of the chest and directly over the cartilage that connects a rib to the breastbone (rather than the space between two ribs), the condition is called costochondritis (*costo* means rib; *chondro* refers to cartilage; *itis* equals inflamed). Many doctors refer to costochondritis as Tietze's syndrome, but Dr. Tietze himself wouldn't. The patients he described in the medical literature had walnut-sized swellings over their inflamed and tender areas, and most patients with costochondritis don't.

If the child's tenderness is on the chest wall, but somewhere other than beneath the left nipple or over the costochondral area, and if the pain typically occurs when he's resting and worsens when he moves his torso, be prepared for any number of diagnoses, including xiphodynia, slipping ribs, fibrositis, and the chest wall syndrome. These terms are used more or less interchangeably. This mixed bag of complaints has anxiety as its common-denominator cause. The pain probably results from muscle spasm or strain coming from the increased muscle tension that accompanies anxiety.

Hyperventilation is another common, anxiety-based cause of chest pain. The overbreathing is at times obvious huffing and puffing, but it can also be extremely subtle and consist of only sighing. Almost all people who hyperventilate develop complaints of dizziness, light-headedness, and a tingling of the hands or feet, or around the mouth. Several kinds of chest pain can accompany hyperventilation, but the most frequent is similar to precordial-catch-syndrome pain. The pain is probably caused by a distension of the stomach that results from the air swallowed during the hyperventilation.

Anxiety is also involved, though indirectly, when the source of the pain is the breast. Girls with this pain usually imagine that they have cancer (see p. 256), and boys with it think they're developing into carnival side-show freaks (see p. 254). But breast cancer is almost unheard of in children under 16 years old, and your doctor will have little difficulty recognizing your daughter's perfectly normal breast tissue. When your son learns that most adolescent boys develop firm or tender nodules under their nipples during puberty, and that the condition normally goes away, his anxiety over his impending female transformation should vanish.

Most of the time, doctors can find no explanation at all for an adolescent's chest pain. In that case, they usually describe the condition as idiopathic (*idio* means self-originated; *pathic* equals disease). The longer the child has had the pain, the more likely it is to be idiopathic. Two thirds of children who have had chest pain for more than six months are idiopathic, in contrast to only one third whose duration of pain is less than six months. Like the chest wall syndrome and hyperventilation, idiopathic chest pain is probably a result of anxiety.

Besides being *caused* by anxiety, chest pain also *produces* so much of it that you should put considerable effort into reassuring your child. A youngster needs to know how chest pain differs from heart pain, or how the breast tenderness differs from breast cancer. (Both of these distinctions are made earlier in this section.)

He should be helped to understand that the doctor's reassurances don't mean that he considers the child's complaint frivolous or insincere. Try to convince your adolescent that both parent and doctor accept his complaint as genuine and important, even if its cause is not physical. Brief counseling from your pediatrician or therapist in anxiety control and/or coping skills may help here.

Chest pain is a common symptom in adolescence. It may indicate that the child could use some extra help in dealing with the stresses of his age, but it's hardly ever an indication of a physical problem. (See p. 348, **Ref.** 246; see p. 348, **Ref.** 247; see p. 348, **Ref.** 248; see p. 348, **Ref.** 249.)

TROUBLE BREATHING IN ADOLESCENCE
(Dyspnea)

When an adolescent experiences difficult or labored breathing, both she and her parents usually get very frightened. Visions of heart disease and, for the same price, lung disease, abound. Trouble with breathing isn't as common a complaint in this age group as chest pain (see p. 287), and those who have it don't wait long before going to the doctor for help. Just as in the case of chest pain, however, the reason for most adolescents' breathing difficulty is anxiety, not disease. Nevertheless, several identifiable, and treatable, conditions cause difficult breathing in the apparently healthy adolescent.

Don't be surprised if your doctor tells you that your short-of-breath teenager is actually overbreathing or hyperventilating. Her complaint of light-headedness and tingling, hearing herself sigh as she breathes, will be the physician's major clue. If the doctor can get the child to reproduce all her symptoms in his office by coaxing her to overbreathe, his diagnosis of hyperventilation will be solid.

Another common cause of breathing trouble is exertional asthma, or exercise-induced asthma. This form of asthma occurs following exertion, and at no other time. In that regard, it's different from the more common asthma related to pollens and infections that worsens during or after exercising, but isn't limited to exertion. Since children with exertional asthma wheeze at no other time, unless the doctor's office is in a six-story walk-up, the child won't be wheezing when your doctor examines her. If your doctor suspects that your child has exertional asthma, he'll have her exercise right in his office, and bring on an attack. Don't get angry. By correctly diagnosing your child, your doctor is doing her a great service. Before medical science discovered this form of asthma, many children with exertional asthma were considered neurotic or lazy because they shunned exercise. They can now lead very normal lives.

Swimming seems to be the exercise that's best tolerated by such children (unless the water is very cold). If the child has to exert herself in cold, dry air, and if she didn't take her preventive dose of asthma medicine, remind her to wear a face mask or to tie a scarf around her mouth to keep her airway warm and moist. (See p. 345, **Ref. 199**; see p. 347, **Ref. 230**.)

PERSISTENT HOARSENESS *(Functional Voice Disorder)*

During certain times in childhood, hoarseness in an otherwise healthy youngster is not uncommon, and the child may be sent to a specialist. When the specialist inspects the child's voice box (larynx), he may see a bump or sometimes an ulceration that explains the symptom. But often, even in children whose voices are equally hoarse and husky, the specialist will see nothing to explain the symptom. The problem for children in this group is not with the larynx itself, but with the way the child is using it, and such disorders are termed functional.

Persistent hoarseness of this sort often occurs after a bout of laryngitis. During the illness, your child may have a cough, a sore throat, and a hoarse voice. When he gets well, everything but the hoarseness clears up. You'll probably be more distressed by this symptom than your child. He may actually be deriving some benefit from being so hoarse, such as being excused from giving verbal reports in school (such benefits might be regarded as "secondary gain"). After a period of such hoarseness, your doctor may refer your child to an otolaryngologist, who will look at the larynx and tell you that everything looks normal. All you need to do then is to reassure the child that his voice will return to normal, and get him back into the mainstream of activity. If you want more correction, a trip to a vocal coach will do the trick. Vocal therapy helps all forms of functional voice disorders, but particularly the raspy hoarseness that follows an acute episode of laryngitis.

Most often, the children who get hoarse are chronic shouters. Their voice strain may produce sore throats as well as hoarseness. Such a youngster is often a cheerleader, an athlete who exhorts his teammates to reach athletic heights with shouts of encouragement, or the youngest child in a large family, for whom shouting is the only means he has to be heard or noticed. There are two ways to minimize the voice strain of a shouter. You can buy him a megaphone, so he can still make the big sound but not at the expense of his vocal apparatus (only your ears). The second way, and for some reason the more popular, is to encourage the child to rest his vocal instrument for a while and communicate either by writing notes or by whispering.

Shouters sometimes need voice training to prevent the development of swellings (called singer's nodules) on their vocal cords that eventually require excision.

Not every child who develops persistent hoarseness needs to have his larynx examined by an otolaryngologist to be certain that the disorder is functional. If your child's story is similar to one of those above, and if your doctor finds everything else to be in order, he may not feel a need to further confirm the diagnosis. This is one diagnosis that most doctors can make with their eyes closed. (See p. 348, **Ref. 250.**)

3. Digestive System

YELLOW SKIN *(Benign Hyperbilirubinemia)*

There are innocent reasons for children to have yellow skin in every age group (see pp. 46 and 145). The adolescent has three innocent liver conditions, all of them actually present from birth but seldom noticed before the child reaches her teens.

All three conditions stem from the fact that the liver, although a magnificent organ, isn't always perfect. A complex set of enzymes is required for each of the countless functions of the liver, and an otherwise adequate liver can sometimes be found lacking in the performance of one function at one time or another.

If the youngster's liver weakness is in the area of processing the blood constituent bilirubin, as during the first week of life, the yellow-red bilirubin accumulates in the bloodstream, and if the level gets high enough the child's skin turns yellow. The most common resultant condition is called Gilbert's syndrome, after its French discoverer at the start of this century.

Up to 7 percent of the adult population has Gilbert's syndrome. It's usually undetected during most of childhood (the average age of diagnosis is 18 years), because the level of elevation rarely gets high enough to discolor the skin. At times, especially after a prolonged fast, strenuous exercise, or an infection, the level of bilirubin may double or triple, and it will then produce visible jaundice. When this happens, nine times out of ten the doctor will suspect hepatitis, a viral infection of the liver. If the physician then orders a battery of liver function tests to confirm his suspicion, he'll be surprised at the results. The only abnormality that will show up in the tests is an elevation of the unconjugated bilirubin; every other aspect of the liver function will be normal. (To appreciate the benign nature of low levels of unconjugated bilirubin, read the section beginning on p. 46). The doctor could also do a multiphasic chemistry panel of blood tests on the child, which, coincidentally, includes a bilirubin test. Either way, the test results add up to Gilbert's syndrome.

Sometimes a doctor will make a diagnosis of Gilbert's syndrome because he knows that a family member has it. The gene for this condition is dominant, meaning that only one gene is needed for the child to have Gilbert's, and, therefore, only one parent has to have the gene for the condition to be passed down to the children. Fifty-five percent of the siblings in the families of patients with Gilbert's, and 26 percent of the parents have it as well. For some unexplained reason, four times more males have Gilbert's than females.

Once a diagnosis of Gilbert's is made, nothing more has to be done. The condition should be viewed as a laboratory finding only; it has no other significance.

Dubin-Johnson syndrome and Rotor's, the two other syndromes of benign hyperbilirubinemia, aren't as common as Gilbert's but they're equally harmless. Both of these conditions are transmitted by a recessive gene; that is, two genes are needed and, therefore, both parents must contribute a gene for the condition to appear in their offspring. Since these syndromes consist of elevations in the conjugated as well as unconjugated fractions of bilirubin, and since conjugated bilirubin will spill into the urine when its level is high (the unconjugated won't), sometimes the child's urine will appear unusually dark. The livers of children with Dubin-Johnson can enlarge and become briefly tender at times.

Despite the minor differences, all three syndromes have the important major traits in common, namely an excellent prognosis, no need for treatment, and a probability that the doctor may discover it while searching for something else. (See p. 339, **Ref. 83**; see p. 348, **Ref. 251**.)

FREQUENT STOMACH PAIN *(Recurrent Abdominal Pain)*

Somewhere between infantile colic and the adult spastic colon fall countless episodes of unexplained abdominal pain during childhood. There are many causes of chronic abdominal pain in childhood, but the most common, which affects roughly 10 to 15 percent of all schoolchildren, is called recurrent abdominal pain (RAP).

RAP is more common in girls, and they're older than boys when it begins. RAP is over for most boys at eight years of age; half of all girls who will get it don't begin having the episodes until they're eight to ten years old. Because RAP is so common, it has been studied extensively, especially in Great Britain, and the worldwide consensus is that RAP is a stress-related disorder.

The pain of RAP is cramping, dull, and located exactly beneath the navel. It occurs most often during the daytime, especially during the hours spent at school, and almost never shows up if the child is hospitalized for evaluation. Vomiting, paleness, weakness, dizziness, and loss of appetite tend to follow the pain. Headaches and pain in limbs often appear between the episodes. RAP is responsible for a staggering number of days absent from school, but a child with RAP almost always vigorously denies that she dislikes going to school. A few years ago, many children who actually had RAP were diagnosed as having "chronic appendicitis." Even today, in some parts of the world, these children are suspected of having "worms," and if pinworms are, indeed, found, it's assumed, incorrectly, that the source of the pain has been found. The composite picture of the child with RAP is one of a shy, introverted, high-strung perfectionist. She usually has a great dread of failure, whether social, athletic, or academic. She may often ask for a note excusing her from physical education.

Children who have RAP can be at the top, middle, or bottom of the class, but no matter where they are academically, they seem to feel that they could and should be doing a lot better.

When children with RAP are thoroughly tested medically, about

1 in 20 is found to have a physical explanation for the symptoms (half of the answers are found in the child's urinary tract, and the other half are scattered among the remaining million or more causes). The other 19 out of 20 children with RAP are "sick to their stomachs" from the stresses of their lives. More than once, such a child has told me that she has "a headache in my tummy." Some children with RAP will outgrow their complaints and go on to lead normal lives. They're the lucky few. Most children with RAP grow up to become adults with RAP, or with severe, disabling headaches, or both. Long-term studies in the United States and in Europe have made it clear that we shouldn't dismiss children with RAP as "little bellyachers."

On the other hand, intensive reassurance and a little informal, supportive therapy will help the great majority of these children. To make an impact, two conditions must be met. First, everybody (the child, her parents, and her doctor) has to be convinced down to his toes that the child is (1) having genuine pain and (2) physically normal. Any doubts about either point must be thoroughly purged. To do this, your doctor may first put your child on a milk-free diet (see p. 297). He may then call for laboratory tests, consultations, and X rays, but whatever is needed to convince all of you *must* be done. It's often very hard to accept the fact that the child's pain is real; it's tempting to get angry at her when you learn that nothing is physically wrong, and to suspect her of faking the pain. Instead, however, once everyone is convinced that there's no physical cause for the pain, your attention should be directed away from the painful symptom and toward getting your child back into the mainstream of activity.

The next goal is to teach your child how to deal with life's stresses more effectively. This doesn't mean eliminating all forms of stress from her life, although it will help if you can reduce the stress coming from areas outside her control. If, for example, excessive marital discord and violent arguing are factors causing the child's pain, try to avoid exposing the child to the hostility, and assure her that she isn't responsible for any of the marital difficulty.

You can also encourage your child to identify events that are apt to be stressful to her, as well as those that aren't. Some children are thrilled to be invited to a birthday party, while others view the expected turmoil and noise with dread, apprehension, and anxiety. Some children can't wait until the next school play while others hope against hope that they'll be passed over when the roles are given out. (The latter are usually more comfortable in smaller gatherings with one or two close friends, and prefer to have more of a say in choosing activities that make themselves rather than others happy.)

If your child seems to need perfection to maintain her self-esteem and feels disappointed and inadequate with anything less than 100 percent, you should make a special effort to show her that she's accepted and held in high esteem regardless of her performance.

If a child with RAP is aware that a stressful event is on the horizon, she may be able to prepare for it. Physical education classes, for example, are connected with abdominal pain for many children with RAP. If a child is aware that such a class is coming up, and that she usually reacts to it with abdominal pain, she may be able to carefully tune in to herself and become aware of her bodily responses when she begins to accumulate tension. She may also begin to learn what sort of mental or physical tricks can work for her to release the tension. Some children doodle, some roll paper between their fingers, some chat with friends, some go for a stroll, some create mental images of restful scenes, and some tighten and relax different groups of muscles to ease tension. All of these are better than chewing on the lower lip, gouging out skin around the thumb, or nail-biting. When the child learns which techniques will "externalize" and thereby unbottle the tension, she'll have less of it inside and, it's hoped, less abdominal pain. (See p. 348, **Ref. 252.**)

ABDOMINAL PAIN AND BLOATING AFTER DRINKING MILK *(Lactose Intolerance)*

Traditionally, milk, mother, apple pie, and the American flag have always enjoyed a special status. So far, mother, apple pie, and the flag are still safe; milk is in big trouble. Our confidence in milk got a big shake when we found that most of the world's population can't digest lactose, milk's sugar. At that point, the don't-drink-the-milk movement acquired a political flavor. Nestlé's has been branded as racist and accused of attempted genocide for aggressive marketing of milk-based formula in certain parts of Africa. A California action group has asked the state to spend $15 million on a program that will educate the public about milk's hazards, and has demanded that milk producers label their products "CAUTION: If undue gastrointestinal upset develops or increases, discontinue use and consult physician. Persons with a tendency towards heart disease, gastrointestinal disorders, anemia, or food allergies may wish to consult their physician before extended consumption of this product."

If your child experiences gassiness, bloating, or cramping abdominal pain and diarrhea after drinking milk, he may be one of the millions who can't absorb lactose. The fact that he had no difficulty at all as a milk-fed baby won't get milk off the hook, either. But how did the food that was "perfect," when he was a baby, change into his intestinal enemy number one? The answer is quite simple.

Being members in good standing of the mammalian family, we humans feed milk to our young. To handle this diet, young mammals have a high level of lactase, the enzyme needed to digest lactose, in their intestinal lining. Once weaned, most of nature's mammals never consume any more milk and, appropriately, their lactase levels decline (usually to levels less than one tenth of the peak activity). Humans, and sometimes cats, are the exceptions who continue to drink milk after weaning. Unfortunately, however, we aren't exceptions to the disappearance of lactase with maturation, and there's the rub. Lactase levels begin to fall from their newborn heights between three (for black children) and five (for white children) years of age, and from then on, every added year means less and less intestinal lactase. Some ethnic groups have more lactase than others. Ethnic groups descended from societies that domesticated dairy herds seem to have higher levels of lactase than those that didn't. For example, only 3 to 7 percent of Danes and less than 1 percent of Finns have hypolactasia (*hypo* means low levels). In contrast, peoples that existed without dairy herding, such as the Chinese, Koreans, Japanese, American Indians, and Eskimo, have late-onset lactose deficiency in as many as 70 to 100 percent. The most compelling evidence that ancestral dairy herding and the persistence of lactase activity go together comes from the discovery that the Hamitic tribes of central Africa, which depend on dairy herds, have high lactase activity, while the Bantus, who live in the same area but don't domesticate dairy herds, have very low levels.

With millions of children suffering from recurrent abdominal pain or RAP (see p. 295), and millions of children with hypolactasia, it doesn't take much imagination to put the two conditions together. Indeed, there was a time when lactose intolerance was thought to be the cause of RAP. For this reason, if your child suffers from RAP, after your doctor rules out a urinary source for the pain, he'll probably put your child on a milk-free diet for several weeks. He may even feed your child a measured amount of lactose to test her absorption (this is a lactose tolerance test). If your child is indeed lactose intolerant, restricting this substance will unburden her intestines and relieve her of those symptoms that result from her lactose intolerance (unfortunately, lactose intolerance is rarely the cause of the pains of RAP, and the RAP goes on).

If your child is lactose intolerant, don't assume that her lips will never be allowed to touch milk again. In the first place, lactase is rarely totally absent from the intestinal lining. Most of the time, the levels will only be reduced to 5 or 10 percent of normal, and under certain circumstances some milk consumption will be tolerated. Some "milk-intolerant" children can drink milk if they do it slowly, in small amounts added to other foods, like cereals. Others limit their dairy intake to buttermilk, cheese, and yogurt. Many children, especially if their symptoms are mild, prefer to drink the milk and tolerate their mild distress.

Even if your child is unable or unwilling to consume his daily quart of milk, don't despair. Children don't need a quart of milk a day, and there are nondairy sources of calcium that can be substituted for milk if necessary. Cereals, fish, beans, figs, molasses, cabbage, and nuts are all rich in calcium. You can even save the dandelions from your lawn and serve the greens, because they're also very rich in calcium.

Finally, not all the problems caused by milk are the result of lactose intolerance. Milk in the stomach is known to delay stomach emptying, and as a result it tends to suppress hunger for the next meal. If you give your school-age child a milk-and-cookie snack at three-thirty in the afternoon, don't be surprised if he says that he isn't the slightest bit hungry two or three hours later when you offer dinner. His stomach is still full of milk. You should also remember that milk contains more than just lactose. It also contains a protein to which some children are allergic, and they may develop intestinal, respiratory, and skin symptoms, all of which subside when milk is withheld. (See p. 348, **Ref. 253**; see p. 348, **Ref. 254**.)

CHILD WEIGHS TOO MUCH BUT NOT MORE THAN 20 PERCENT OVER IDEAL WEIGHT *(Overweight)*

If your child weighs more than she should, she's overweight. (Nothing else that I have to say on this subject is as certain.) If her weight isn't more than 10 percent over her ideal weight, and if she likes the way she looks, leave her alone. She may not find work as a model, but she's as healthy as she needs to be. If she weighs 20 percent or more over her ideal weight, and if her excess baggage is fat and not muscle or water, she has an illness known as obesity (more about that later). If the child is "only" 10 to 20 percent overweight, she may be called a variety of names from plump (if she's soft and flabby) to stocky (if she's firm and sturdy). Regardless of what she's labeled, she's in limbo; she isn't certifiably obese, but you certainly shouldn't ignore her problem.

It used to be a lot easier. When calling a spade a spade was accepted procedure, children who looked fat were called fat. All this changed when life insurance companies found out that body weight was a health risk factor, and that it cost them more to insure fat people. From their studies, tables of ideal weights were constructed, and nowadays every height comes with an ideal weight. If you weigh more than your ideal weight, like your luggage at the check-in counter at the airport, you're overweight.

Strictly speaking, obesity refers to having too much fat, not too much weight. Ideally, one's fat content should be the main criterion for obesity. Total body fat can, in fact, be measured, but it isn't easy. One method requires a water tank large enough to contain the whole body, and the other, radioisotope techniques. As you might have guessed, neither technique is sweeping the nation. Since half of the total body fat can be found directly under the skin, most fat measurers settle for measuring the thickness of skin folds in specific areas of the body. This requires special instruments that aren't found in every doctor's office. Scales, on the other hand, are standard equipment, so most physicians reply on the scale to decide the question of obesity.

One relatively new method for defining obesity is actually a rediscovery of a method used during the 19th century by a Belgian mathematician named Lambert Quételet. By dividing the weight (in kilograms) by the square of the height (in meters), a number called the body mass index (BMI) is obtained. For those who are resisting the metric movement, pounds and inches can be used, but you have to divide the number by 703.07 to get the same BMI. Normals have BMIs of 19 to 20, overweights are 24 to 25, and obese is defined as 29 to 30. This definition is gaining ground for adults, and something like it will probably be used soon to determine children's ideal weights for their heights.

Regardless of how we try to define the problem, dividing those who have it into mild, moderate, and severe is too artificial to be of much value. Many overweight children are just one meal away from obesity. A ten-year-old boy of average height weighing 62 pounds won't be diagnosed as obese since he's only 15 percent over his ideal weight of 54 pounds. If he gained less than 3 pounds more, he would qualify. Is a parent supposed to relax and "enjoy" the child's 15 percent cushion, and then start worrying as soon as he reaches 65 pounds? It makes more sense to view overweight as a continuum, and the more overweight your child is, the more reason you have to worry. Try a few of these worries on for size:

Childhood obesity doesn't always go away. Predictions vary enormously, but up to 80 percent of obese children two to eight years old become obese adults. The most obese adults and the ones who are most resistant to losing weight are the ones who were obese during childhood. The question of early childhood obesity increasing the number of fat cells, which then persist into adulthood demanding to be filled, remains unanswered and controversial.

In addition, fat children get tormented by their friends. Young tormenters are particularly uninhibited in their attacks and can make a hell of an overweight child's childhood. Many overweight children prefer to stay home from school, just to avoid their taunts. Others who go to school find themselves ostracized. It's worse for the adolescent who lives for only one purpose: to look, act, and dress exactly like his cronies. Finding that he can't, he becomes an oversized outsider and withdraws to become even more sedentary than before, compounding his problem.

If the obesity continues into adulthood, there are at least ten types of medical problems that are known to be connected with it. They are: hardening of the arteries, diabetes, menstrual and reproductive problems, enlargement of the heart, arthritis, gout, high blood pressure, gallbladder disease, cancer of the lining of the uterus, and surgical complications. If an adult is massively obese, variously defined as being 100 pounds overweight or weighing twice his ideal weight, his chances of living to age 50 are slim.

Obese children can have physical problems before they reach adulthood (see p. 284). Obesity is a cause of adolescent high blood pressure. Obese children tend to suffer from injuries to the growing zones of their bones, which are softer than other parts of the bones and are more apt to slip when injured. Massively obese youngsters may have difficulty staying awake, since they quickly tire from such basic acts as breathing. Lastly, they're statistically more likely to be hit by a moving car, probably because they're less agile and move more slowly.

Overweight children are also vulnerable to a few nondiseases as well. Because they tend to be taller as well as heavier, they're often wrongly suspected of having an endocrine disturbance. Overweight boys may have a lot of fat surrounding their penises (see p. 193) and they're often wrongly suspected of having too small a penis. Because the equipment used to measure their blood pressure may not be of the appropriate size, they may also be wrongly suspected of having high blood pressure (see p. 284).

Furthermore, the overweight are discriminated against. If they're competing against a normal-weight person for a job or a place in college or graduate school, they have a fat chance of getting the spot.

To make matters even worse, it used to be taken for granted that overweight children were overeating. Since this implied that their problem was of their own making, they weren't judged to deserve our sympathy. Occasionally, overweight children do overeat, especially when a surrogate feeder, like a grandmother, is involved in the feeding. In which case, the child's weight becomes a measure of the quality of care being given: the fatter the child, these feeders seem to feel, the better the care. But more often than not, even though we assumed that the child was overeating, the source wasn't found.

While the conviction that obesity results when more calories are consumed than spent remains etched in stone, we only recently discovered (to our amazement) that most overweight adolescents actually eat less than their normal-weight friends. Their problem stems from their failure to burn off what they consume. In the slow lanes in which they travel, they're experts in energy conservation. They are, in fact, eating too much for their needs, but the basic fault lies with their needs, not with their eating. This finding has led some of our nutritionists, such as Jean Mayer, to suggest that the best diet for overweight teenagers is exercise.

It may not seem to be much of a task to get your overweight preadolescent to exercise. You might assume that all you have to do is organize family activities, such as long hikes and bicycle riding, and enroll your child in league sports. In this way, of course, your youngster can have fun and lose weight at the same time. This simple plan may work for the preadolescent. But usually, when a parent suggests that her overweight teenager get involved in athletics and exercises, she can expect to be told to "bug off." The only movements to result from such advice will be probably a barely perceptible upward curling of the upper lip, and a deeper slump into the easy chair. Adolescents, being what they are, tend to be rebellious. You'll do better if you suggest to your overweight teenager that she can use more calories by changing the way she carries out her regular daily activities. Instead of adding new activities, she can incorporate more movement and exertion into her regular endeavors, and thus more calories will be spent. The catchword is *animation*.

Here are some guidelines:

First, encourage your overweight teenager to spend one additional hour each day up on her feet and off her derriere. She can do this while talking on the phone, while putting on makeup, or any time when she's "hanging out."

The second skill she should learn is the art of inefficiency. Instead of thinking up ways to save steps, overweight children should be working on ways to waste them. Rather than jockeying around for the closest possible parking spot and then sitting in her car waiting for the spot to become vacant, your plump teenager should look for the one that's in the most remote outreaches, and walk the extra distance. Whenever possible, body power should be substituted for machine power. Describe to her the not so distant past when people used to climb stairs, walk to the stores, get up and answer the front doorbell, and so on.

The third way she can waste energy is to add movements to situations that are ordinarily motionless. She can watch TV in a rocking chair. She can pace instead of stand still, wiggle her toes instead of sit still, and stand up and take frequent breaks for stretches and breathing.

Finally, suggest that she add oomph to her movements. Rather than sluggishly move about, she should walk briskly, and turn sharply with more arm swinging and gusto. She should try to imagine that she's living in one long Pepsi commercial.

For the teenager who's 10 to 20 percent overweight, the role of dieting should be understated. If she's still actively growing, you can direct her to eat just enough to keep the weight where it is. As more inches are added to her height, she'll gradually grow into her weight. You can actually do irreparable harm to the actively growing child if you put her on too strict a diet. This can have a severe impact on her overall metabolism, and permanently interfere with the growth of her bones and muscle.

It's also a good idea to lose weight slowly. If your overweight child can manage to combine a daily reduction of only 150 calories consumed with a daily increase in expenditure of only 100 calories, she'll lose a pound every two weeks. Such sustained effort deserves to be rewarded, and an appropriate way to do this is to buy her some new slim-line clothes every time she sheds enough to drop into a smaller size. Give the old clothes to charity.

If your child starts to slip back into her old habits and weight, one way to secure her weight loss is to suggest that she befriend an overweight child (they aren't too hard to find) and become that child's "therapist." By becoming a teenage weight controller, she becomes a model for her "patient," and her continued success becomes the basis for her role. She won't dare to put her weight back on, since that would mean losing face, and teenagers are particularly sensitive to the need to save face. (See p. 348, **Ref. 255**; see p. 348, **Ref. 256**; see p. 348, **Ref. 257**.)

ADOLESCENT CONTINUOUSLY DIETING AND EXERCISING *(Weight Preoccupation)*

Serious students in the field of eating disorders are aware that centerfolds in *Playboy* have been getting slimmer every year. We've become a nation that yearns to be thin, but in which one third of the adult population is overweight enough to be called obese. In recent years, jogging has become a national obsession. I don't know if there's any connection, but there also appears to be a rising rate of eating disorders, especially anorexia nervosa (AN), beginning in the middle adolescent years. An estimated 1 out of every 100 teenage girls suffers from AN, and the rate is much higher among female models, athletes, and dancers. Given these two trends, it's inevitable that some adolescents will trim down enough to look like someone with AN, and some adolescents who actually suffer from AN will pass as being "really trim." Naturally, slim girls are brought to the doctor's office because their parents are worried that they might have AN. As a result of media attention and public awareness, interest in AN has gone from famine to feast.

Clearly, if your overweight teenager has dieted and is now a bathing beauty, you needn't worry about AN. But if she's now under her ideal weight or heading toward this low weight rapidly, you may have a legitimate cause for concern. The key question is: Does your daughter have AN? There are several strict criteria that must be met before your doctor will make a diagnosis of AN:

1. The person (a female in 90 to 95 percent of the cases) must be young (under 25 years old) and have no known prior or current medical or emotional problem preceding the weight loss.

2. The weight loss must be significant. According to the most strict criteria, at least 25 percent of the original body weight must be lost. (Obviously, anyone meeting all the other criteria who has only lost 24 percent of her weight shouldn't be dismissed as normal.)

3. The person must vigorously defend a highly distorted set of attitudes and practices connected with eating, food, and body image. These attitudes have been dubbed the starving crazies, and include various food rituals, an all-consuming preoccupation with calories and food preparation, hoarding food, excessive use of laxatives, and countless more that your doctor is fully aware of. The starving crazies are the result of starvation from any cause and, though they aren't necessarily related to AN, they're always present in a person who does have it.

4. At least two of the following must be present as well: no menstruation (see p. 329), fuzzy, downy body hair (see p. 56), a resting heart rate below 60 per minute (see p. 277), intense hyperactivity, binge eating, and self-induced vomiting.

As you can see, at least half of these requirements for a diagnosis of AN are standard equipment for many perfectly healthy children.

Most normal teenagers wish to avoid obesity. Some wish harder, and try harder, than others. Still others are obsessed with their weight.

Not surprisingly, teenagers in this group are called weight preoccupied (WP), and if your child is one of these she has a common eating disorder; she doesn't have AN. Several basic differences distinguish the WP teenager from the one who has early AN.

A youngster with AN will deny feeling hungry. She'll also deny feeling tired after exhausting herself in exercise, and will, in fact, deny almost all of the feelings that arise from within her body. In sharp contrast, the WP teenager is hungry and would love to dig in, if only it wouldn't make her (or *him;* there's less female predominance in WP) fat. The child with AN feels that she isn't in control of the changes in her body or around her. To her, the only thing in the world that she can control is her intake. In contrast, the WP child feels directly in control and believes in his effectiveness in his life. Finally, the WP child is eager to receive advice from others. If you bring her to the doctor's office for nutritional advice, she'll be eager to comply. Teenagers with WP don't show the intense distrust of others, especially people trying to help, that's so characteristic of AN. Weight-preoccupied teenagers seldom lose more than 15 percent of their original weight, but if they do, they may develop endocrine changes, such as delayed sexual maturation, similar to those of AN. Sometimes, WP teenagers achieve weight reduction by means of too much exercising. This has been called anorexia athletica, and is a lot like WP in the other regards that have been discussed.

Most thin mid-adolescents concerned about their weight aren't anorectic, or even preanorectic. If they're "into dieting" and exercising, they're doing nothing more than conforming to the prevailing attitudes and values of society at large, and their peer group in particular. As such, their attitudes must be considered normal. WP youngsters may go beyond the precise norm, but they stay within the broad range of the limits of health and need no medical attention. (See p. 348, **Ref. 258.**)

4. Nervous System

TWITCHING *(Tic)*

Watching your child go through a sudden, purposeless jerking movement over and over again can be very scary. (It's scary for the child, too.) If it's a repetitive, senseless motion that worsens under emotional stress, but can be somewhat controlled by a strong exertion of will-power and stops altogether when the child is asleep, your doctor will recognize it simply from your description. This is a tic (*tic* is French for spasm), the most common movement disorder in childhood. Between 4 and 24 percent of children have it, and it usually begins after the age of four years but before the onset of adolescence. The peak age of incidence is six to seven years. It runs in families and boys with tics outnumber girls by three to one. The good news is that the great majority of tics either stop entirely or greatly slow down on their own.

Tics are divided into two groups: simple, if the child has only one tic at a time, and complex, if many different tics are present at the same time. Most children who have them display movements called simple motor tics, which consist of eye blinks, head twists, or shoulder shrugging. If sniffing, throat clearing, or coughing is the only tic the child has, it's still a simple tic, but is called a phonic tic. Many simple tics are never noticed by anyone, especially when the children are able to incorporate them into a series of controlled movements. A child can camouflage the spasm by pretending to have hair in his eyes when he's suffering a head-tossing tic, or a cold when he's having a sniffing tic.

If your child has a simple motor tic that doesn't change its repertory with time, there's a 40 to 50 percent chance that it will stop entirely within the year. All but a few of the others will taper off and come to a full stop before adulthood. Simple motor tics that last less than one year are called transient motor tics, and they're the most common in childhood. Sometimes—though this is rare—simple motor tics continue beyond one year, at which point they're called chronic motor tics, and at times they become more elaborate and evolve into complex tics, such as licking, rubbing, hand washing, squatting, skipping, making animal sounds, and shrieking. These tics can't be concealed or camouflaged, and can be terribly embarrassing for the child and those witnessing the events. As you might imagine, the prognosis for spontaneous cure isn't as good toward this end of the tic spectrum.

At the very far end of the spectrum of complex tic disorders is the one described by Gilles de la Tourette 100 years ago. It consists of bizarre, repetitive behavior, yelping noises, and often obscene and blasphemous utterances. I sometimes wonder if the film *The Exorcist* was inspired by an experience with this condition. Like great floods that begin with a single drop of rain, Gilles de la Tourette's syndrome begins with a single tic. But just as single drops rarely progress to great floods, so single tics rarely progress to the syndrome. Fortunately, its frequency is ⅟₅₀₀ that of transient motor tics, which means that if you spot a simple motor tic in your child, the odds are only 1 in 500 that it will progress to the syndrome.

A note of warning: You should be on the alert for tics if your child has been prescribed a stimulant drug to improve an attention span disorder. Drugs in this class and several others, such as anticonvulsants, have been known to increase the risk of Gilles de la Tourette's syndrome, but not if they're stopped at the first sign of a tic. (See p. 348, **Ref. 259**; see p. 348, **Ref. 260**.)

FAINTING SPELLS *(Syncope)*

There's a long list of possible reasons why your long-legged teenage daughter could keel over and briefly lose consciousness while standing in line at school, sitting in her seat, or just about anyplace. Fortunately, the most common reason, vasomotor syncope (*syncope* means sudden loss of strength), is also the most innocent. It's a result of a very primitive bodily response called fight or flight, and occurs when the body is notified that it's about to be threatened. The purpose of the reaction is to prepare the body for one of two choices: either to stand its ground and engage the enemy, or else to run as fast as it can. In either situation, more blood is needed by the muscles in the arms and legs, and less is needed by the internal organs. (This explains the sinking feeling you get in the pit of your stomach when you're frightened.) If your teenage daughter, confronted by something she finds unpleasant (for instance, "a discussion of bleeding" in health education class), immediately exercises her option to slug it out or run for the hills, she'll be fine physically, though she might have trouble with the teacher. If, however, she merely stands her ground and doesn't exercise her limb muscles, the blood will pool and accumulate in the extremities (the longer and more muscular the extremities, the more blood is pooled). Her heart gets a temporary cutback of blood, and has less to send upstairs. The brain's blood circulation then drops and it has a temporary power failure, which your daughter experiences as a transient loss of consciousness. Because this temporary diversion of the circulation is orchestrated by the vagus nerve, these episodes are sometimes called vasovagal attacks.

Just before this type of faint, your daughter might be nauseated, dizzy, and sweaty. If she were examined at that moment, she would be found to have a very slow pulse and a dropping blood pressure. The episode can last a few seconds to a few minutes. Immediately after waking up, she may be confused, embarrassed, and weak, and have a headache. Don't be upset if a brief anoxic convulsion (see p. 213) occurs while she's unconscious. In one study of fainting blood donors, 53 percent of them had brief convulsions while they were unconscious. This has no connection at all with a seizure disorder.

Fainting spells are regular happenings at blood donation centers and in high schools, particularly among girls who have missed breakfast or are dieting, feeling menstrual pain, standing in a hot crowded room, standing in morning prayer, overhearing a particularly sickening story (in this case, "grossing out" prior to passing out), or in any way frightened or anxious.

If your child is given to fainting, she'll eventually learn to keep herself out of situations that are ripe for fainting. If some can't be avoided, she'll learn to recognize the presyncopal (fainting) symptoms and engage in flight, fight, or a change in posture. As anyone who ever took part in giving injections to military recruits can attest, vasomotor syncope isn't limited to adolescents or females. The bigger they are, the harder they fall.

The next most frequent cause of a momentary loss of consciousness is equally benign, and also a result of blood pooling in the legs. It's called postural hypotension, or sometimes orthostatic (*ortho* means straight; *statos* equals standing) hypotension, since it occurs when the person suddenly sits or stands up. It would never happen if we'd stayed with our original game plan of walking on all fours. When humans took to standing up on their feet, nature had to safeguard the brain's circulation against the effects of gravity. Over the years, a complex set of automatic responses evolved for this purpose. Normally, as soon as you stand up, gravity drains about a pint of blood down to your legs, and your systolic blood pressure drops 10 to 15 millimeters of mercury. Sensitive pressure and volume gauges in the vessels in the chest react to these changes, and they immediately signal the heart to pump faster by 5 to 25 beats per minute in order to maintain its output at a constant level. At the same time, the vessels in the legs are directed to constrict, correcting the drop in blood pressure and returning the blood to the chest. These clever devices usually work, and getting upright usually goes fairly smoothly.

If these compensatory mechanisms fail, for some reason, and the systolic pressure suddenly drops 20 to 30 millimeters, the brain gets shortchanged and you feel dizzy, light-headed, and faint. Postural hypotension tends to occur in the morning, presumably because the pressure and volume gauges in the chest are sluggish after having had the night off. For this reason, it's even worse after periods of prolonged bed rest. It differs from vasomotor syncope in several regards.

First, orthostatic hypotension occurs only when the posture changes to upright; vasomotor syncope occurs after being upright for a while. Second, overly thin people are predisposed to orthostatic hypotension, whereas vasomotor syncope occurs in those who are thin or heavily muscled, too. Lastly, the pulse in orthostatic hypotension is faster than normal; the pulse in vasomotor syncope is extremely slow, even after recovery from the faint. But, as in the case of vasomotor syncope, the treatment for orthostatic hypotension is simple and the prognosis is excellent. Those who get it must learn to get up in slow motion.

Another fairly common situation that can lead to fainting is hyperventilation. It *can* be intentional. Prolonged deep breathing followed by a sudden compression of the chest, a stunt commonly called the mess trick, or fainting lark (see p. 214), will briefly deprive the brain of its needed circulation, leading to a sudden short loss of consciousness and an entertained audience. More often, hyperventilation occurs unintentionally, when the child is under emotional stress. Before the faint, most hyperventilators describe chest tightness or pain (see p. 289), and light-headedness. If these early symptoms are recognized, breathing into a paper bag will prevent the problem from progressing any further.

There are several other precipitating events in which fainting is an understandable response to what's occurring and not an indicator of an unrecognized problem in the nervous or cardiovascular system. In children, the most common such faint occurs after a burst of violent coughing, and it isn't too different from the syncope that follows breath holding. It's called cough syncope, and in the typical scenario the child, most often an asthmatic, has a burst of forceful and emotionally excited coughing, turns purple, and then passes out. We think that the asthmatic chest may be especially vulnerable to the chain of events that overbreathing and breath holding can precipitate. At any rate, the problem is strictly in the chest, and in this context, cough syncope can be prevented by relieving the child's asthma.

Another special event, which occurs frequently in adult men but also occasionally in adolescents, is fainting while urinating. This is called micturition (*micturire* means to urinate) syncope. In this case, like the others, a suddenly lowered blood pressure is at the core of the problem. Bladder distension raises blood pressure (see p. 284) and it's equally true that emptying the bladder lowers blood pressure. In its typical scenario, micturition syncope occurs within one minute of the time the boy assumes the upright posture and while he's emptying a very full bladder. It happens most often to a late-adolescent boy who has spent the better part of an afternoon lying on a sofa watching TV and emptying a six-pack of beer immediately prior to emptying his bladder. Witnesses usually assume that the boy has succumbed to the effects of the beer, not its passage. The blow to the young man's pride is minor compared to the injury that can result from a blow to his head as his unconscious body hits a hard surface in the bathroom. If micturition syncope happens repeatedly, he'll have to suffer the additional indignity of urinating while safely seated.

If your otherwise healthy child has recurrent fainting spells that can't be explained by the event that immediately preceded it, your doctor will suggest laboratory tests to uncover some metabolic (example: low blood sugar), cardiac (example: mitral valve prolapse), or neurologic (example: drop seizures) basis for the fainting. Overall, these diseases account for a very small percentage of fainting spells in children. The explanations for most children's fainting spells will be found in one of the above descriptions. (See p. 336, **Ref. 20**; see p. 337, **Ref. 38**; see p. 348, **Ref. 261**; see p. 348, **Ref. 262**; see p. 349, **Ref. 263**; see p. 349, **Ref. 264**.)

TIRED TEENAGER *(Fatigue)*

When a parent drags a teenager who's "tired all the time" into the pediatrician's office, her major question is likely to be: Does he have infectious mono, weak blood, or a sluggish thyroid? Pediatricians, having heard this complaint so often, have a different key question, to wit: How did the teenager happen to come to the office in the first place? All too often, the teenager's only question is: What am I doing here? On the other hand, if the visit was prompted by the teenager's own concern over his sudden loss of pep, the odds are fair to good that a physical reason for the fatigue will be uncovered. The odds drop if the parent is more interested in the child's fatigue than he is. The odds drop still further if the youngster makes it clear that he's in the office under duress, and the odds approach zero if the tired teenager's only participation in the dialogue between the parent and the doctor is to counter each of the parent's statements with his own version of the truth. I don't mean to imply that no answer will be found, only that the problem isn't likely to be physical. Since the physical is usually the primary concern, let's look at that first.

Because of the widespread awareness of the association of fatigue with infectious mononucleosis, a viral infection enormously popular among adolescents, the answer to the parents' first question about mono must be "possibly." Fatigue can be a feature of every disease known to medicine. But when there are no additional features, such as fever, sore throat, swollen lymph nodes, or enlarged spleen, infectious mononucleosis is very improbable. If there's any doubt about mono, your doctor can clear it up by doing a simple blood test.

For that matter, a handful of very basic tests, including a urinalysis, a complete blood count, a TB skin test, and a sedimentation rate, can rule out most physical reasons for tiredness. If the tired teenager is also overweight, or has any other feature of inactivity of the thyroid gland, it's simple enough to test the level of thyroid hormone in the blood. If there's a reason to suspect iron deficiency, such as heavy menstrual periods or fad dieting, a specific testing of the body's iron stores will be helpful. Your doctor won't rely solely on the absence of anemia to rule out iron deficiency.

The overwhelming majority of tired teenagers, after examination, turn out to have one of two problems, each identifiable and correctable. The first problem is simply too much activity. The adolescent is up at 5 A.M. to begin his newspaper delivery route, attends classes (many of them honor classes), goes to team practice, and doesn't stop running until he crashes in the "early" evening. His "fatigue" is only evident at home, and for that reason, his parents never see him when he isn't fatigued. More often than not, the activities for which he shows the most enthusiasm and energy don't rank high on the parents' favorite activity list. This child will lose his fatigue if he has fewer activities or more hours.

In the other, more common pattern, the teenager spends most of the time that he isn't in school alone in the bedroom. He has lost interest in his friends, old activities, and school. His mood is melancholic and he's quarrelsome, easily irritated, and negative. Nothing is good enough, including himself. Despite being tired, he can't fall asleep until very late, and then he can't get up in the morning. He's most tired in the morning and although, as the day goes on, he gets more energy, it's never quite enough to feel right. This is the typical day in the life of a depressed teenager. If you probe more deeply into the psyche, you'll usually find a considerable amount of stress, with his family or friends, or in school. While it's true that psychosocial stress appears to be a basic component of adolescent life, stressed teenagers who are tired and depressed are carrying it a bit too far. They need to be helped. If your pediatrician succeeds in convincing your adolescent that she's really interested in hearing his story, not yours, and his feelings, not yours, and so on—whose fatigue is it, anyway?—there's a good chance that his problem can be talked out. If not, and if the problem continues, more formal therapy will be recommended. (See p. 349, **Ref. 265**.)

TEMPORARY ABNORMALITIES AFTER HEAD INJURY

Personality Changes (*Posttraumatic Syndrome*)

Some children just don't seem to be the same after receiving a blow to the head. They may have striking personality and behavioral changes, headaches, loss of memory, dizziness, and changes in sleep patterns. The most disturbing personality changes occur in the area of anger control, and some of the rage reactions can be so severe that treatment with drugs may indeed be needed. Collectively, these complaints are known as the posttraumatic syndrome, and up to 30 percent of children develop it after a bona fide head injury. There are three things that you should know about this syndrome: (1) The injury that preceded the Jekyll-and-Hyde personality switch need not be a concussion. Before doctors were aware of this fact, we called the problem postconcussion syndrome. (2) The child's behavior isn't really his fault, so try not to get too angry at him. (3) It goes away, usually after a few months. (See p. 349, **Ref. 266.**)

Temporary Blindness (*Transient Cerebral Blindness*)

Sometimes after a child has a trivial head injury, what follows seems like a total disaster. We don't know how often this happens, but doctors have been aware of the problem since it was first described in 1918. Typically, the child falls on his head, and either immediately or up to four hours later goes totally blind. (If you find this frightening, imagine how your child must feel.) After what seems like a very long time, but rarely longer than 12 hours, the lights get turned on again, and the child and his vision are back to 100 percent. The good news for the child is that he's almost always unable to remember being sightless. You'll have little difficulty forgetting it, but if it happens again, which it might, you'll know that the blackout is temporary. Since fleeting visual disturbances are also a feature of migraine, and since some children who have had transient blindness following a head injury subsequently develop migraine, some doctors suspect that these two conditions are related. (See p. 349, **Ref. 267.**)

SLEEPWALKING AND SLEEPTALKING
(Somnambulism and Somniloquy)

These conditions are the older child's version of night terrors (see p. 219) and bed-wetting (see p. 226), and often occur in the same child. Only 1 to 6 percent of the population repeatedly walk or talk in their sleep, but up to 15 percent of children 5 to 12 years old have done it at least once. It usually happens like this: Sometime between 1 and 3 hours after falling asleep, the child, usually a boy, suddenly sits up in bed. His eyes are open but unseeing. If the child remains in bed, the episode ends in less than a minute. If he leaves his bed, the jaunt may last for half an hour. It usually consists of wandering around opening and closing doors and drawers, or (rarely) walking into furniture or hurting himself. He may mumble a few words, but nothing coherent. The episode ends with the child returning to bed, and since the entire affair happened during non-REM sleep (see p. 134), he has no recollection of the event and feels very well rested in the morning. Like all the other parasomnias, or sleep-arousal disorders (p. 219), sleepwalking isn't an emotional disorder, but like the others it's worsened by psychological stresses.

Sleeptalking may be a part of sleepwalking, or it may occur alone. It also occurs during arousal from deep, non-REM sleep. Rarely do the talkers say anything of consequence, so it really doesn't pay to strain your ears while they're talking. (See p. 340, **Ref. 92.**)

RHYTHMIC TREMBLING OF HEAD AND HANDS *(Benign Essential Tremor)*

There are times when a trembling hand is a sign of an emerging disease of the nervous system. Some neurologic disorders that begin with shaking hands eventually progress to become handicapping illness, but at other times the child's trembling hand is the only sign of a mild nervous-system malfunction. The latter is called an essential tremor because it's an isolated event. It's usually seen in middle life, but trembling hand movements can begin at any age, including childhood.

The tremor is rhythmic, fine, and rapid (about 8 to 10 cycles per second). It usually starts with the hands and sometimes ends there, but more often than not, other parts of the body, like the head and voice box, join in. Sometimes the trembling is confined to the child's chin or head, in which case your doctor may give it its own designation, such as "trembling chin," but these are all variations on the same theme. Regardless of location, the tremors come and go, and are closely influenced by the child's level of anxiety. For this reason, most teenagers with tremors are suspected of having a psychological problem, and if no one makes the correct diagnosis, they might get referred for psychiatric evaluation.

Half of all cases of benign essential tremor are inherited, transmitted by a dominant gene, meaning that only one parent has to have the gene for the condition to be passed down. It will be fairly easy for your doctor to diagnose the condition in your teenager if an older family member has it. If not, and if the diagnosis is uncertain, your doctor may refer you to a neurologist to be certain that the trembling isn't the result of a more serious condition.

The overall outlook for this condition is much better than that of other neurologic disorders involving trembling, but the tremors do tend to get worse with age. Recognizing this condition before the teenager makes a career choice can be very valuable, especially if she aspires to be a concert pianist, miniaturist, or surgeon.

Another, less common involuntary-movement disorder, which includes trembling but is more handicapping than benign essential tremor, is benign familial chorea. This condition can begin at any time from infancy to adulthood. It's an inherited condition that consists of jerking, writhing movements of any part of the body. This condition is only benign in the sense that, though at onset it resembles many other progressive and lethal processes, unlike those illnesses it doesn't progress and the child's intellectual function is spared.

Like benign essential tremor, familial benign chorea is transmitted by a dominant gene, and its diagnosis during childhood is made considerably easier by knowing that the condition exists in the family.

All of these benign tremors are rare and, when severe, can be helped by mild sedatives or muscle-relaxing drugs. For the most part, though, the child with such tremors needs only a clear explanation of the condition, and some reassurance or counseling. (See p. 349, **Ref. 268**; see p. 349, **Ref. 269.**)

5. Urinary System

URINATING VERY OFTEN, BUT ONLY BY DAY *(Pollakiuria)*

If your son keeps running to the bathroom to urinate every few minutes all day long and you suspect the problem to be in the urinary tract, you could be right. However, if this same trigger-happy child has normal urinary frequency during the night (perhaps once, or not at all), don't be surprised if his urinary tract turns out to be entirely normal, and the diagnosis is pollakiuria. What kind of "urinary problem" is this pollakiuria that compels a child to stay within a 30-second dash to the bathroom all day, and then takes the night off?

The answer is the "nervous bladder." Like the nervous stomach (see p. 295) and chest pain (see p. 287), pollakiuria is but one more response of the child's body to its old foe, high anxiety. Nothing is wrong with the child's urine, bladder, or kidneys. Your son's bladder is simply the screen onto which his anxiety is projected. Different children use different screens, and this one is his.

As with other stress-related disorders, you and your doctor must first try to relieve the child of the stress, then work on improving the child's coping skills. (For advice on how to do this, see pp. 296 and 297.) Your doctor may ask for a urine analysis or urine culture, but it is hoped that he will make this diagnosis before your child is subjected to a full-scale urologic investigation, including X rays. (See p. 349, **Ref. 270.**)

BLOOD FOUND IN URINALYSIS THAT'S NORMAL IN EVERY OTHER WAY

After Exercise *(Exercise Hematuria)*

Motorcyclists have it. So do boxers, football players, rowers, swimmers, and, of course, joggers. Physicians used to believe that the blood and protein that appeared in the urine after exercise was the result of repeated jolts to the kidneys, but this idea never satisfactorily explained the presence of blood in a swimmer's urine. We now suspect the kidney's circulation rather than the organ itself is temporarily affected by sustained and vigorous exercise. The bloody urine that bicyclists sometimes get seems to be different since it can be greatly reduced by lowering the nose of the saddle 10 degrees below the horizontal or by riding off the saddle altogether. Regardless of the reason or the activity, the changes don't last more than a day or two. If they do, your doctor will look for some abnormality within the urinary system. Usually, the blood is temporary and harmless. (See p. 349, **Ref 271.**)

Blood Repeatedly Found in Urine *(Benign Recurrent Hematuria)*

About 20 years ago, testing urine required making dilutions, adding chemicals, heating the mixture, then interpreting color changes, all of which took a long time to complete. Today a urinalysis can be performed with the same ease as checking the oil level in your car's engine block. Doctors simply dip a strip of special paper into the urine specimen and within 45 seconds read off the results of no less than eight different tests. Not surprisingly, many more urinalyses are being done these days.

As a result of the dipstick urinalysis, many children who show no outward signs of a urine problem are found to have abnormalities in their urine. Since many serious kidney diseases can remain "silent" for long periods, these abnormal urinalyses might provide the only clue to the diagnosis of these diseases. Therefore, your doctor will probably recommend additional testing for your child if her urinalysis reveals an abnormality. If the only abnormality is the presence of blood, and if there's a chance that the urine specimen was contaminated by menstrual bleeding, the doctor will undoubtedly wait a while and then test the urine again. If the blood persists and a complete kidney evaluation shows no other abnormalities, either the doctor himself or a kidney specialist may diagnose the condition as benign recurrent hematuria (*hemat* refers to blood; *uria* is urine). Your physician might discover benign recurrent hematuria (BRH) in your child in one of two ways. The first is by chance. During a routine screening urinalysis, such as described above, the physician may find a tiny amount of blood, too little to discolor the urine. One recent study showed that 4.1 percent of children 8 to 15 years old had blood in their normal-appearing urine. The doctor will then do further tests to see if anything else is present that might indicate a kidney problem. The diagnosis of BRH is made after all other possibilities are excluded; that is, the doctor has found nothing other than the blood in the urine. Furthermore, every time he tests the child's urine he finds some blood, but at the same time the corroborating tests for kidney disease show normal results.

When most children with BRH reach adulthood their urine ceases to contain blood.

BRH can also show up in a school-aged child who develops painless, bloody urine several days after a respiratory infection. The doctor, suspecting that the child's bloody urine may be caused by a type of kidney inflammation associated with a streptococcal infection, will begin testing. While the tests are under way, the child's urine clears and, once again, the test results show nothing abnormal. This child also has BRH, and from time to time, particularly after viral respiratory infections, he may have grossly bloody urine. BRH is harmless, but the blood may upset the child. If so, tell him to look away from the toilet bowl while he urinates. The bathroom floor may get a bit wet, but the child can be spared needless worry. In between such episodes, the child's urine will appear clear, but if tested will be found to contain small amounts of blood. Most BRH is familial. The kind that appears after viral infections tends not to be, but it does have the same excellent outlook for remission as the first group. (See p. 349, **Ref. 272**; see p. 349, **Ref. 273**.)

PROTEIN FOUND IN URINALYSIS THAT'S NORMAL IN EVERY OTHER WAY

During Fever (Febrile Proteinuria)

Protein can appear in the urine of 1 child in 20 if the child has an illness with fever, especially one over 38.4 degrees Celsius. When the fever leaves, the protein stays, but rarely for more than two weeks. No one knows the cause of this febrile (fever) proteinuria. Doctors differ over the question of whether the protein results from whatever caused the fever or from the fever itself. In any event, febrile proteinuria may or may not come back with the next fever the child has, but it's of no medical importance. (See p. 349, **Ref. 274**.)

Urine Repeatedly Found to Contain Protein (Benign Persistent Proteinuria)

Just as the isolated finding of blood in the urine (see p. 318) can be a red flag indicating serious kidney disease, so can an isolated finding of protein. One tenth of all children 8 to 15 years old show such protein at least once, and 2.5 percent show it repeatedly. If your child's urinalysis shows a significant amount of protein and your doctor is certain that the specimen wasn't contaminated by a vaginal discharge, he'll thoroughly test the child to exclude a serious kidney disease. If all the tests are negative, and the proteinuria lasts, the situation exactly parallels benign recurrent hematuria (BRH; see p. 318), and is called benign persistent proteinuria.

Benign persistent proteinuria is treated the same way as BRH. As long as it persists, your doctor will continue to reassess your child's kidneys periodically, looking for new evidence of malfunctioning. If the protein in the urine remains the only problem, nothing more has to be done. While most doctors feel that the long-term outlook for benign persistent proteinuria is as excellent as that of BRH, there are some who think that longer periods of follow-up are needed before they can be certain of the benign prognosis.

A corollary proteinuria is caused by exercise. Exercise proteinuria disappears within a day of the exertion. Proteinuria is also fairly common for a period following abdominal surgery. (See p. 349, **Ref.** 275; see p. 349, **Ref.** 276.)

Protein Appears in Urine Only When Child Stands Upright (Orthostatic Proteinuria)

If your doctor asks you to collect two samples of urine from your child, one when he's lying down and the other when he's standing up, the physician is testing your child for orthostatic proteinuria. This is the most common reason for proteinuria during adolescence. It accounts for 70 percent of all proteinuria in this age group, and occurs in 10 percent of all teenagers. Why standing up can cause protein to leak into a child's urine is a question that has intrigued doctors for many years and, as of this writing, it's still a mystery. At one time, we thought that it was caused by changes in the kidney's circulation imposed by standing up, but that notion has been thoroughly refuted, and we're now back to being intrigued. Most orthostatic proteinuria is only temporary, but if your child's is constantly present, your doctor will follow him closely to be certain that nothing else develops.

Fourteen- to 16-year-old boys seem to have kidneys that are particularly susceptible to the effects of posture. In fact, proteinuria can be induced in 75 percent of them by having them stand with their backs arched as far backward as possible for a sustained period of time. (Maybe that's why teenage boys slouch.) For whatever reason, orthostatic proteinuria becomes less common after adolescence, as does the ease of producing proteinuria by sustained, forceful arching of the back. Long-term studies of orthostatic proteinuria continue to support the excellent prognosis that doctors have been assuming for many years. (See p. 349, **Ref.** 277; see p. 349, **Ref.** 278; see p. 349, **Ref.** 279.)

SHE LAUGHED SO HARD, SHE ALMOST WET HER PANTS *(Giggle Incontinence or Enuresis Risoria)*

Roughly 25 percent of young women will admit to wetting their pants when they laugh. Many of the rest admit feeling the need, but manage to resist the urge. Those who are too ashamed to bring the subject up will never find out how common their problem really is.

If a youngster has giggle incontinence—enuresis risoria, as it was called by ancient Roman doctors—laughter (or giggling) suddenly produces an extreme and urgent need to urinate. Within a moment, her bladder starts to void and it continues to do so until it's empty. Her giggle incontinence is distinctly different from the other type of involuntary wetting, which occurs without warning and is only a very partial emptying of the bladder.

Giggle incontinence occurs in girls much more often than boys, and is often familial. It tends to be a problem during the school years, and in most cases improves or disappears with adulthood. If your daughter has it, there's no reason to have her urinary tract or nervous system evaluated, because the results are sure to be normal. Laughter seems to be one of many triggers that can activate the voiding reflex, and some youngsters are seemingly better than others at fighting it back. (See p. 349, **Ref. 280.**)

6. Size and Maturation

MUCH SHORTER THAN OTHER CHILDREN OF SAME AGE

During their first three years, the growth rate of most infants either speeds up or slows down as they head for the precise growth-track percentile that their genes coded for them (see p. 231). From then until the onset of puberty, the healthy child grows at a constant rate. Short children grow 4 centimeters a year, and tall children grow 7.5 centimeters a year. This is how, in a certain sense, the short get "shorter" and the tall get "taller," and by the time the child reaches puberty, the range of normal heights is wide.

Every interest group seems to have its own ideas about what constitutes shortness. Doctors consider a child to be short if he has a standing height that's two standard deviations or more below the mean height for the youngster's age. Children know they're short if they go to the front of the line when the teacher calls "size places." Parents deem their child short if it appears that he isn't going to reach the height of the shorter parent. While these are all important considerations, the most practical concern is whether something other than the stretching rack can be employed to make the short child taller. The answer depends on the cause of the child's shortness and this isn't as hard to determine as you might imagine.

To make the diagnosis, your doctor will take the following steps: (1) He'll compile a thorough family history. (2) He'll examine your child—again, nothing unusual. (3) He'll take a good look at your child's growth chart. (4) He'll obtain a skull and a wrist X ray. (5) He'll do a few blood and urine screening tests.

From these few tests, your doctor will be able to tell you if your child belongs to the small handful (less than 5 percent) of short children with an endocrine problem, children who need referral to an endocrinologist; whether your child is one of the 15 percent who have some underlying and unrecognized illness that must be treated before normal growth will occur; or whether your child belongs to the largest group (80 to 85 percent) for whom explanation and reassurances are all that's usually needed. A child who belongs to one of the first two groups may need treatment. Chances are good, though, that your short child belongs to the third group, and that his small stature is caused by one of the following conditions.

Short Child of Short Parents (Familial Short Stature)

The first and most common reason for short stature is called familial or normal variant short stature. Typically, such children are born small, but weigh more than 5 pounds 8 ounces. They're soon below the 3rd percentile (see p. 141) of all children in height, and they spend the rest of their lives there. They grow only about 4 centimeters per year, but their growth rate is constant and their growth curve is below, but perfectly parallel to, the 3rd percentile line. These youngsters look their age. Their pubertal growth spurt doesn't spurt very far, but it starts at the usual time, and their growth stops at the usual time. The final height of someone with familial short stature is below 5 feet 4 inches for a male, and below 4 feet 11 inches for a female. If the doctor knows that these are the heights normally reached in the child's family, he'll find the diagnosis easy. If the child is adopted and family height patterns aren't readily available, he'll have to perform a few tests to be sure the child's size can be called familial short stature.

There are several generalizations that we can make about predicting a child's height knowing the parents' height. When both parents are at the same end of the normal height spectrum, their offspring gravitate toward the middle. Therefore, when both parents are short, the chances are the child will also be short, but not as short as his parents. On the other hand, the height of a child with one tall and one short parent will approach one of the two parental extremes rather than settle into the middle.

If you have a child with familial or normal variant shortness, it's possible to engage in extensive testing. It will only cost money, waste time, frustrate you, and embarrass your child. There's also little to be gained by engaging the services of a seer in hopes of getting a prediction of ultimate height. Instead, why not find yourself a nice, short pediatrician who has nice, short children, and leave the rest to Mother Nature?

Small Since Birth and Not Catching Up to Peers *(Intrauterine Growth Retardation)*

Just because a baby's birth weight was under 5 pounds 8 ounces, you can't assume he was born prematurely. Some babies arrive not a minute too early, but, for a variety of reasons, they're small (see p. 140). Several years ago, the term used for these babies was *intrauterine growth retardation;* the current term is *small for gestational age* (SGA). If you want to predict a child's size, it's important to distinguish a normal infant who was born small because he was born too soon (a true premie) from an SGA baby, because the small premie will catch up with his full-term peers by early childhood, while the SGA infant may not. Many small babies who were assumed to be premature because of their size are reclassified as SGA when they don't show the expected catch-up growth.

Whatever factors operated to make the SGA baby small, such as the mother's smoking, use of alcohol or other drugs, high blood pressure, or placental insufficiency, can also limit the baby's future growth potential. Such children are perfectly proportioned, short youngsters who look their age, enter puberty at the right time, and become normal short adults. Their small stature had nothing to do with their genes, and therefore will have no effect on the size of their children.

Short Child Who Looks Much Younger Than His Age *(Constitutional Delay in Growth)*

This big group of little children tends to overlap with the group of children with familial short stature (see p. 324). In fact, some medical centers believe that the two entities are really one. The distinction is based entirely on the presence or absence of a significantly delayed "bone age." If there's no bone age delay, the child's shortness is called familial short stature. If there *is* a significant delay, it's called normal variant or constitutional maturation delay, or familial slow maturation, or constitutional delay of adolescence, or constitutional delay of growth. The key words are *familial* and *delay*. Since slow maturation inevitably means delayed pubertal development, this group will be discussed again (see p. 329).

Many children with constitutional delay are genetically coded for normal size, but a different set of genes that codes for rate of growth has dictated a slower than normal rate of maturation. It's as if their clocks were wound up to run a bit slower than the rest. At birth, their size is usually normal, but by the age of two or three years, their slower rate of growth puts them at the bottom of the growth chart. By the time these children start school, their faces, body proportions, and sizes are those of children two years younger. Teachers, parents, even their peers usually consider these children "darling," and if they do something appropriate for their age, it seems precocious. This is a good time for such children. They spend a lot of time sitting on laps and being cuddled.

If you have a family history of small children who eventually became normal-sized adults, your doctor can make the diagnosis without a lot of tests. If there's any doubt, he can confirm it by taking X rays of your child's wrist. The many bones around the wrist joint mature at different times during childhood, and do so in a consistent pattern. This makes it possible to look at a wrist X ray and estimate, within a few months, the "age" of the wrist. That age is called the bone age. In constitutional maturation delay, the bone age is typically as many years behind the chronological age as is the "height age" (the age for which the child's height would be considered average). In other words, a child of ten with maturational delay might have the height of an average eight-year-old (height age eight), and his wrist X ray would show a bone that's also eight (bone age eight).

During the years 11 to 14, when both fast and average maturers are doing their thing, maturationally delayed children fall way behind. This is *not* a very good time for such children. Although maturational delay occurs equally in boys and girls, boys are particularly vulnerable to being bullied, ridiculed, and teased at this time by their larger and more sexually mature friends, which is probably why 90 percent of all children referred to endocrinologists for maturational delay are boys.

Some children with maturational delay have double trouble if they're also genetically destined to be short. They're very short and though they make up some of their height disparity when their belated growth spurt comes, it's not enough. Ultimately, these children have to settle for "short." Many children with maturational delay, however, are destined for normal size; they just have to be patient. When their taller peers are through growing, they continue with their growth. If your child has this problem, it will help if he can relate to some tall member of the family who remembers spending the better part of his youth marching off to the front of the line in school. You can also try to cheer him up with the suggestion that his slow rate of aging will keep him youthful even when he's old.

For some children, particularly those who are still far from puberty at a time when their peers are already fabricating sexual conquests, the psychological impact of their physical immaturity is so great that something should be done. Usually, this means giving the boys testosterone (the male sex hormone) and the girls estrogen (the female hormone) to nudge them into puberty. The boys must understand that this won't increase their eventual height. It will do no more than speed up development so that they'll be taller sooner. This is tricky business and best left in the hands of an expert (see p. 328). (See p. 340, **Ref. 100**; see p. 349, **Ref. 281**; see p. 350, **Ref. 282**; see p. 350, **Ref. 283**; see p. 350, **Ref. 284**.)

MUCH TALLER THAN OTHER CHILDREN OF SAME AGE
Tall Child of Tall Parents (*Familial Tall Stature*)

The infant with familial tall stature quickly establishes her position atop the growth chart and remains there throughout her childhood. She's often taken for being older than she is, but her facial appearance and bones are normal for her age. Her puberty will start and stop at the normal times. When she's finished growing, she'll be a tall adult.

As in the case of the short child of short parents (see p. 324), your doctor will have no problem making this diagnosis. What's in doubt is the eventual height that the tall child will reach. If the child is a girl, you may be concerned about her psychological adjustment and, for this reason, seek help from an endocrinologist. (It's very rare that a tall *boy* of tall parents is disturbed enough by his condition to consult an endocrinologist.)

There's a treatment for the tall girl, and, like the treatment for maturational delay (see p. 327), it's undertaken only for psychological reasons. Not every tall girl wants to be treated. Many tall girls are thrilled with their statuesque beauty and athletic advantage, and the thought of treatment never enters their lofty heads. On the other hand, some tall girls are absolutely devastated by their height. If your youngster's predicted adult height is unacceptable to her, and if she's young enough, treatment can be found. It is perhaps a sign of our times that in recent years, very few girls have gone ahead with estrogen treatment after they've had an appointment to discuss their tallness with a pediatrician who is experienced with this problem.

As in the case of maturational delay, the treatment for tallness is designed to push the tall prepubertal child into an early puberty. If she's already in puberty, it's probably too late for her to be helped significantly. If she's too young, an early puberty would be too great a psychological burden to add to her problems of stature. The ideal time to start treatment is between 9 and 13 years of age. It consists of giving the female hormone estrogen to girls and the male hormone testosterone to boys. Since both hormones accelerate bone age, they shorten the period that remains for growth. Once the youngster's growth has stopped, the hormones are discontinued.

To date, this treatment, when handled by a specialist, has produced no reproductive problems. (See p. 340, **Ref. 100.**)

Tall, Mature-Appearing Child of Average Parents *(Familial Rapid Maturation)*

This problem is the exact opposite of maturational delay (see p. 325). The child's final-height genes are coded for average height, but his rate-of-growth genes are set on "fast." The pattern is familial and, like other members of his family, this youngster has a biological clock that runs too fast. Even as a small child, he's bigger and stronger than his friends. He also looks older, and his bone age is appropriate for his height age and the way he looks. Aside from having to pay adult prices at the movies, this boy has a great time. Leadership roles in school and sports achievements come easily to such rapidly maturing boys.

Rapidly maturing girls, on the other hand, find life a lot more difficult. They tend to be embarrassed by their large size and earlier sexual maturation.

Both boys and girls with familial rapid maturation should start sex education classes earlier than most of their peers. Puberty hits them like a ton of bricks, and before they know it, their growth is over. Their average and slow-maturing friends keep plodding along, and before too long, the rapid maturer finds himself a somewhat stocky but average-sized adult. Since there are no effective medicines to delay or slow puberty, counseling and psychological support should be provided if the child seems to need it. (See p. 340, **Ref. 100.**)

SEXUALLY LESS DEVELOPED THAN EXPECTED FOR AGE *(Delayed Pubertal Development)*

If you've ever attended an elementary school graduation, you've probably noticed that 12- and 13-year-olds can look amazingly different from each other. Some look more like their teachers than their classmates, while others still look like small children. There's so much normal variation at this age that some children have already completed their puberty before others of the same age have begun.

To understand and simplify the changes brought by normal puberty, doctors use a uniform rating system called the Tanner stages. According to this system, sexual maturation proceeds from the infantile or prepubertal (Tanner I) to adult (Tanner V). In these terms, puberty is the transitional period from Tanner I to V.

Girls begin sexual maturation before boys. A girl's growth spurt, beginning with her hands and feet, is her earliest indication of puberty. The first sexual area to mature is her breasts. In terms of Tanner stages, breast maturation proceeds as follows:

Tanner II: A widening and darkening of the areola with firm breast tissue appearing beneath the nipple. This normally occurs at 9.0 to 13.3 years of age (a mean of 11.2). As the girl's breasts begin to bud, her hips widen, and her form begins to look distinctly female.

Tanner III: The breast develops further to form a distinct mound. This happens between the ages of 10.0 and 14.3 years (a mean of 12.2).

Tanner IV: The breast forms a larger mound, which in 75 percent of girls has a second mound, the areola, atop the first breast mound. This occurs between ages 10.8 and 15.2 years (a mean of 13.1).

Tanner V: The adult breast is defined not by its size but by its shape. Its areolar area recedes to the same level as the rest of the breast, so the breast no longer has a mound-on-a-mound appearance. This stage is reached between 11.9 and 18.8 years of age (a mean of 15.3).

While most girls complete their breast development in 4 years, some take up to 9 years and are still growing after they reach the age of 20.

Though breast budding is usually the first sign of sexual maturation, 16 percent of all girls begin their maturation with pubic hair development. Regardless of which of the two comes first—breast development or pubic hair—the other follows within a year. If this doesn't occur, the girl is not experiencing true puberty. A girl's pubic hair stages proceed as follows:

Tanner II: Her pubic hair is long and sparse and curly, and is usually confined to the labia majora. This stage is reached by 9.3 to 14.1 years of age (a mean of 11.7).

Tanner III: Her hair covers the middle of the pubic area and is considerably darker, coarser, and curlier than before. The age is 10.2 to 14.6 years (a mean of 12.4).

Tanner IV: Her pubic hair grows outward toward the thighs, covering two thirds of the pubic area by age 10.8 to 15.1 years (a mean of 13.0). Girls usually begin to grow hair under their arms at this point. If the girl has acquired enough body fat (minimum weight is usually 94 pounds; the average weight is 103 pounds), the first menstrual period, the menarche (*men* means month; *arche* is beginning), usually arrives at this Tanner stage. Menarche coincides with Tanner II in only 5 percent of girls. It coincides with Tanner III in 25 percent of all girls, Tanner IV in 60 percent, and Tanner V in the remaining 10 percent. The mean age of menarche for white American girls is 12.8 years; for black American girls, 12.5 years. By menarche, a girl's growth spurt is largely over, although another 3 to 4 more inches over the next two years is still possible.

Tanner V: Adult-type hair covers the entire pubic area and there's a bit on the upper thighs. This stage is normally reached by ages 12.2 to 16.7 years (a mean of 14.4). The process of developing pubic hair normally takes 2.5 years to complete. Many girls grow hair from the middle of the pubic area toward the navel (see p. 242). This type of growth is called Tanner VI.

Overall, most girls take about four years to complete their sexual maturation.

Puberty begins for a boy with growth of his testicles, and for the rest of puberty, testicular length is used as the basis for determining a boy's genital development.

Tanner II: The length of the boy's testicles is greater than 2 centimeters, and the scrotum's skin begins to lose its fat (see p. 192). This process takes place between ages 9.5 and 13.8 years (a mean of 11.6). When a boy reaches this stage, his growth spurt begins, and his physique begins to appear masculine.

Tanner III: His testicles are longer than 3.3 centimeters, and his penis begins to get longer. The age for this stage is 10.8 to 14.9 years (a mean of 12.9).

Tanner IV: The boy's testicles measure more than 4.1 centimeters and his penis grows wider as well as longer. Boys normally reach this stage by 11.7 to 15.8 years (a mean of 13.8). A lot is going on during this stage. The good news is that the boy's growth rate is at its fastest. His voice is deepening and he's starting to have nocturnal emissions (wet dreams), indicating maturation of his prostate gland. The bad news (from the boy's point of view) is that his breasts may be enlarging (see p. 254)!

Tanner V: The boy's genitalia consist of an adult-sized, adult-shaped penis, a darkly pigmented scrotum, and a testicular length greater than 5 centimeters. Young men normally reach this stage at 12.7 to 17.1 years (an average of 14.9).

A boy takes about three years to complete his genital development. In general, his pubic hair development (pubarche) lags behind his genital growth, but since pubic hair development proceeds faster, both reach adult status at about the same time. Hair under the boy's arms appears about two years after pubic hair, and hair begins to grow on his face when his genitals are at Tanner stage III or IV.

There's reason to take note if a boy develops pubic hair before his genitals enlarge. If so, his pubarche is out of the normal order, and your doctor, seeing this, will consider what if anything might be going wrong.

Fifteen percent of older boys have their pubarche before their testicular enlargement (gonadarche). Their pubarche is age-appropriate, but since there's no testicular enlargement, they haven't truly entered puberty.

Such false starts are called pseudopuberty, and are similar to the pseudopuberty of premature thelarche (see p. 178).

If pubic hair development occurs in a boy under ten years old, it's considered premature pubarche. Like the age-appropriate variety, it's a type of pseudopuberty, since the main event of male puberty, enlargement of the testicles, hasn't taken place.

Like the unexpected presence of breasts, the unexpected presence of hair raises the question of the source of the activating hormone—in this case, the male hormone androgen (see p. 243). The growth of pubic hair is no exception and the source of the androgen can be the testicles and/or the adrenal glands. If the boy experiences pubarche without true puberty, the extra androgen responsible is of adrenal origin, and the level of the testicular androgen, testosterone, is normal (prepubertal). His adrenal glands are just jumping the gun on his testicles. When the boy's testicles are ready, normal puberty will still occur at the expected time. (For some reason, many children with premature pubarche—girls as well as boys—are either obese or show some signs of neurologic malfunction.)

Puberty can be considered delayed if it hasn't started by the usual time, or if, when it does start, it stops instead of progressing at the expected rate. The signs of delayed puberty in a girl are (1) no breast development by 13 years of age, (2) no menarche by 16, or (3) no menarche after 5 years of breast development. For a boy, the signs are (1) no enlargement of the testicles by 13.5 years of age or (2) genitals that have been developing for 5 years but still aren't adult.

According to these criteria, 2 to 3 percent of all adolescents have delayed puberty. Of these, a few have a problem with their endocrine glands, and a few others have a "silent" illness serious enough to interfere with their development. Another small minority have a pubertal delay that's a direct result of their particular life-style. For example, young female ballet dancers who are both very thin and very active can expect their menarche one to three years late. The more underweight, the later the menarche. Underweight is only part of the reason for their delay; too much muscle may be the rest. For normal menstrual function, girls seem to need a certain amount of body fat in relation to their body mass, and young ballet dancers, like top female athletes, have a lot of muscle and/or little fat. Nothing needs to be done in these cases. Pubertal delay has no long-term harmful effects in and of itself, and young, intensely competitive, dedicated girls need not give up their activity just to have a menstrual period.

The great majority (90 percent) of adolescents with pubertal delay have constitutional delay of puberty. These adolescents come in two sizes: short and regular. The short ones are older versions of the small, young-appearing children with constitutional delay of growth who are now old enough to be pubertal. Their height ages are several years behind their chronological ages, and are closer to their bone ages. Adolescents of average height with delayed puberty also have delayed bone ages, but their height ages are obviously closer to their chronological, or real, ages.

Over 60 percent of families of children with constitutional delay of puberty have other members with the same pattern, but those individuals may not be the parents. The other family members may be aunts, uncles, or grandparents. Boys and girls are affected equally, but the problem is especially apt to produce misery for boys, and thus boys are 15 times more likely to seek medical attention than girls with constitutional delay of puberty.

A boy with this problem, like the younger boys with constitutional maturational delay (see p. 325), needs information, counseling, and emotional support. For example, a male high school freshman with the size, muscle mass, and maturation level of an 11-year-old should be steered away from trying out for the football team and toward soccer, tennis, swimming, and gymnastics. Or he should be urged to take up such activities as debating and drama.

If the child sees himself as freakish, you should emphasize his normalcy and point out that, while he may be out of sync with his friends, he's perfectly synchronized with the developmental patterns of his family. If his self-esteem has become a disaster area, if he seems beyond the reach of parental reassurances, he can be judiciously nudged into puberty with hormone therapy administered by an expert (see p. 327). In any case, what he needs most is your sensitive and thoughtful support. (See p. 350, **Ref. 285**; see p. 350, **Ref. 286**; see p. 350, **Ref. 287**; see p. 350, **Ref. 288**; see p. 350, **Ref. 289**.)

References

1. M. J. Maisels. "Neonatal Jaundice." In *Neonatology*, ed. by G. B. Avery, pp. 335–377. Philadelphia: J. B. Lippincott, 1975.

2. A. Cordova. "The Mongolian Spot." *Clinical Pediatrics*, 20:714–719, November 1981.

3. K. L. Tan. "Nevus Flammeus of the Nape, Glabella and Eyelids." *Clinical Pediatrics*, 11:112–118, February 1972.

4. A. H. Jacobs and R. G. Walton. "The Incidence of Birthmarks in the Neonate." *Pediatrics*, 58:218–222, August 1976.

5. S. Hurwitz. *Clinical Pediatric Dermatology*, pp. 190–194. Philadelphia: W. B. Saunders Co., 1981.

6. N. B. Esterly and L. M. Solomon. "Blistering and Scaling Dermatoses." Neonatal Dermatology, II. *Journal of Pediatrics*, 77:1075–1088, December 1970.

7. N. B. Esterly and L. M. Solomon. "The Newborn Skin." Neonatal Dermatology, I. *Journal of Pediatrics*, 77:888–894, November 1970.

8. H. E. Evans and L. Glass. *Perinatal Medicine*, p. 81. Hagerstown, Md.: Harper and Row, 1976.

9. J. A. Davis and D. Schiff. "Bruising as a Cause of Neonatal Jaundice." *Lancet*, March 19, 1966, pp. 636–638.

10. B. M. Mogelner et al. "Subcutaneous Fat Necrosis of the Newborn." *Clinical Pediatrics*, 20:748–750, November 1981.

11. *Variations and Minor Departures in Infants*. Evansville, Ind.: Mead Johnson and Co., 1978.

12. P. J. Honig et al. "Congenital Ingrown Toenails." *Clinical Pediatrics*, 21:424–426, July 1982.

13. D. W. Smith. *Recognizable Patterns of Human Deformation*. Major Problems in Clinical Pediatrics, vol. 21. Philadelphia: W. B. Saunders Co., 1981.

14. S. Yasunaga and R. Rivera. "Cephalohematoma in the Newborn." *Clinical Pediatrics*, 13:256–260, March 1974.

15. C. Zelson, S. J. Lee, and M. Pearl. "The Incidence of Skull Fractures Underlying Cephalohematomas in Newborn Infants." *Journal of Pediatrics* 85:371–373, September 1974.

16. J. M. Graham and D. W. Smith. "Parietal Craniotabes in the Neonate: Its Origin and Significance." *Journal of Pediatrics,* 95:114, 1979.

17. H. Nishida and H. M. Risemberg. "Silver Nitrate Ophthalmic Solution and Chemical Conjunctivitis." *Pediatrics* 56:368–373, September 1975.

18. R. E. Behrman. *Neonatal-Perinatal Medicine,* 2nd ed. St. Louis: C. V. Mosby Co., 1977.

19. D. W. Smith. *Recognizable Patterns in Human Malformation.* Major Problems in Clinical Pediatrics, vol. 7. Philadelphia: W. B. Saunders Co., 1976.

20. W. W. Tunnessen. *Sign and Symptoms in Pediatrics.* Philadelphia: J. B. Lippincott Co., 1983.

21. V. McKusick. *Mendelian Inheritance in Man,* 5th ed. Baltimore: Johns Hopkins University Press, 1978.

22. G. J. Romanes. *Cunningham's Textbook of Anatomy,* 12th ed. New York: Oxford University Press, 1981.

23. G. A. Popich and D. W. Smith. "Fontanels: Range of Normal Size." *Journal of Pediatrics,* 80:749–752, May 1972.

24. H. H. Hussey. "Tongue-tie," editorial. *Journal of the American Medical Association,* 228:735, May 6, 1974.

25. K. B. Nelson and G. D. Eng. "Congenital Hypoplasia of the Depressor Anguli Oris Muscle: Differentiation from Congenital Facial Palsy." *Journal of Pediatrics,* 81:16–20, July 1972.

26. G. B. Avery. *Neonatology.* Philadelphia: J. B. Lippincott Co., 1975.

27. F. Rahbar. "Clinical Significance of Supernumerary Nipples in Black Neonates." *Clinical Pediatrics,* 21:46, 1982.

28. J. F. McKiernan and D. Hull. "Breast Development in the Newborn." *Archives of Disease in Childhood,* 56:525, 1981.

29. R. D. Harley. *Pediatric Ophthalmology,* p. 463. Philadelphia: W. B. Saunders Co., 1975.

30. M. Perlman and S. H. Reisner. "Asymmetric Crying Facies and Congenital Anomalies." *Archives of Disease in Childhood,* 48:627, 1973.

31. S. W. Gray and J. E. Skandalakis. *Embryology for Surgeons.* Philadelphia: W. B. Saunders Co., 1972.

32. P. M. Marden, D. W. Smith, and M. J. McDonald. "Congenital Anomalies in the Newborn Infant, Including Minor Variations." *Journal of Pediatrics,* 64:357, 1964.

33. J. I. E. Hoffman. "Auscultation." In *Pediatrics,* 17th ed., ed. by Abraham M. Rudolph, pp. 1241–1243. New York: Appleton-Century-Crofts, 1982.

34. E. D. Burnard. "The Cardiac Murmur in Relation to Symptoms in the Newborn." *British Medical Journal,* January 17, 1959, p. 134.

35. M. Brando and R. D. Rowe. "Auscultation of the Heart—Early

Neonatal Period." *American Journal of Diseases of Children,* 101:575–586, May 1961.

36. B. J. Alpert, E. D. Mellits, and R. D. Rowe. "Spontaneous Closure of Small Ventricular Septal Defect." *American Journal of Diseases of Children,* 125:194–196, February 1973.

37. A. S. Nadas et al. "Spontaneous Functional Closing of Ventricular Septal Defects." *New England Journal of Medicine,* 264:309–316, February 1961.

38. R. J. Illingsworth. *Common Symptoms of Disease in Children,* 7th ed. Boston: Blackwell Scientific Publications, 1982.

39. I. Arad, F. Eyal, and P. Fainmesser. "Umbilical Care and Cord Separation." *Archives of Disease in Childhood,* 57:887–888, 1982.

40. C. E. Koop. *Visible and Palpable Lesions in Children.* New York: Grune and Stratton, 1976.

41. L. Lassaletta et al. "The Management of Umbilical Hernias in Infancy and Childhood." *Journal of Pediatric Surgery,* 10:405–409, June 1975.

42. N. Mor, P. Merlob, and S. H. Reisner. "Tags and Bands of the Female External Genitalia in the Newborn Female." *Clinical Pediatrics,* 22:122, February 1983.

43. R. Kahn, B. Duncan, and W. Bowes. "Spontaneous Opening of Congenital Imperforate Hymen." *Journal of Pediatrics,* 87:768–770, November 1975.

44. K. C. Henderson, "Hydrometrocolpos in a Newborn." *American Journal of Diseases of Children,* 129:1190, October 1975.

45. J. Oster. "Clinical Phenomena Noted by a School Physician Dealing with Healthy Children." *Clinical Pediatrics,* 15:748–751, August 1976.

46. D. I. Williams. *Pediatric Urology.* New York: Appleton-Century-Crofts, 1968.

47. L. G. Lutzker, S. J. Kogan, S. B. Levitt. "Is Routine Intravenous Urography Indicated in Patients with Hypospadias?" *Pediatrics,* 59:630–633, April 1977.

48. C. G. Scorer. "Descent of the Testicle in the First Year of Life." *British Journal of Urology,* 27:374, 1955.

49. B. Fallon. "Congenital Anomalies Associated with Cryptorchidism." *Journal of Urology,* 127:91, 1982.

50. I. J. Cour-Palais. "Spontaneous Descent of the Testicle." *Lancet,* June 25, 1966, p. 1403.

51. R. Baker. "Cryptorchidism." *Hospital Medicine,* December 1967, p. 30.

52. C. T. Ryder, G. W. Mellin, and J. Caffey. "The Infant's Hip—Normal or Dysplastic?" *Clinical Orthopedics,* 22:7–15, 1962.

53. R. S. Siffert. *How Your Child's Body Grows.* New York: Grosset and Dunlap, 1980.

54. I. V. Ponseti and J. R. Becker. "Congenital Metatarsus Adductus: The Results of Treatment." *Journal of Bone and Joint Surgery,* 48-A:702–711, June 1966.

55. R. Birch and J. Wenger. "Unilateral Outward Turning of the Leg in Infancy." *British Medical Journal,* 28:776–777, March 7, 1981.

56. W. T. Boyce. "Care of the Foreskin." *Pediatrics in Review,* 5:26–30, July 1983.

57. E. Stone. "Should a Young Child's Inward-Pointing Feet Be Treated?" *The New York Times,* April 19, 1983, p. C3.

58. L. T. Staeheli. "Tortional Deformity." *Pediatric Clinics of North America,* 24:4, November 1977.

59. E. J. Sell. "Calcified Nodules in the Heel: A Complication of Neonatal Intensive Care." *Journal of Pediatrics,* 88:473, 1980.

60. K. R. Powell et al. "A Prospective Search for Congenital Dermal Abnormalities." *Journal of Pediatrics,* 87:744–750, November 1975.

61. J. Galbraith. "Little Devil." *National Wildlife,* August–September 1983, p. 23.

62. S. J. Robinson. "Treatment of Cardiac Arrythmias." *Pediatric Clinics of North America,* 11:315, May 1964.

63. E. Lipton, A. Steinschneider, and J. B. Richmond. "Cardio-pulmonary Observations." Autonomic Function in the Neonate, VIII. *Pediatrics,* 33:212–215, February 1964.

64. S. Z. Walsh. "The Esophageal Electrocardiogram During the First Week of Life." *Acta Paediatrica Scandinavica,* supp. 173, 1967.

65. R. Saken, G. L. Kates, and K. Miller. "Drug-Induced Hypertension in Infancy." *Journal of Pediatrics,* 95:1077, December 1979.

66. E. H. Watson and G. H. Lowry. *Growth and Development of Children,* 5th ed. Chicago: Year Book Publishers, 1967.

67. H. L. Barnett. *Pediatrics,* 14th ed. New York: Appleton-Century-Crofts, 1968.

68. M. Stahlman. *Neonatology,* ed. by G. Avery. Philadelphia: J. B. Lippincott, 1975.

69. H. L. Halliday, G. McClure, and M. McReed. "Transient Tachypnea of the Newborn: Two Distinct Clinical Entities?" *Archives of Disease in Childhood,* 56:322, 1981.

70. S. P. Waite and E. B. Thoman. "Periodic Apnea in the Full-Term Infant: Individual Consistency, Sex Differences, and State Specificity." *Pediatrics,* 70:79, July 1982.

71. S. Rummer and J. Fawcett. "Delayed Clearance of Pulmonary Fluid in the Neonate." *Archives of Disease in Childhood,* 57:63–67, 1982.

72. F. McSweeney, N. P. C. Cavanaugh, and P. Langeith. "Outcome

in Congenital Stridor (Laryngomalacia)." *Archives of Disease in Childhood,* 52:215–218, 1977.

73. G. Polgar and G. P. Kong. "The Nasal Resistance of Newborn Infants." *Journal of Pediatrics,* 67:557–567, October 1965.

74. M. J. Maisels. "Jaundice in the Newborn." *Pediatrics in Review,* 3:305–319, April 1983.

75. M. J. Maisels and K. Gifford. "Neonatal Jaundice in Full-Term Infants." *American Journal of Diseases of Children,* 137:561–562, June 1983.

76. K. Pryor. *Nursing Your Baby.* New York: Harper and Row, 1963.

77. M. A. Wessel et al. "Paroxysmal Fussiness in Infancy." *Pediatrics,* 14:421, 1954.

78. T. B. Brazleton. "Crying in Infancy." *Pediatrics,* 29:579, 1962.

79. W. M. Leibman. "Infantile Colic." *Journal of the American Medical Association,* 245:732, February 20, 1981.

80. D. W. Hide and B. M. Ginger. "Prevalence of Infant Colic." *Archives of Disease in Childhood,* 57:559, 1982.

81. J. L. Paradise. "Maternal and Other Factors in the Etiology of Infantile Colic." *Journal of the American Medical Association,* 197:123, July 18, 1966.

82. J. H. Imber. "Living (and Coping) with Colic." *American Baby,* August 1982.

83. C. C. Roy, A. Silverman, and F. J. Cozzetto. *Pediatric Clinical Gastroenterology,* 2nd ed. St. Louis: C. V. Mosby, 1975.

84. J. J. Herbst. "Gastroesophageal Reflux." *Journal of Pediatrics,* 98:859, June 1981.

85. A. R. Euler and M. E. Ament. "Gastroesophageal Reflux in Children: Clinical Manifestations, Diagnosis, Pathophysiology, and Therapy." *Pediatric Annals,* 22:678, November 1976.

86. La Leche League. *The Womanly Art of Breast Feeding.* Franklin Park, Ill.: La Leche League, 1981.

87. D. L. Coulter and R. J. Allen. "Benign Neonatal Sleep Convulsions." *Archives of Neurology,* 39:191–192, March 1982.

88. A. Berger, B. Sharf, and S. T. Winter. "Pronounced Tremors in Newborn Infants: Their Meaning and Prognostic Significance." *Clinical Pediatrics,* 14:834, September 1975.

89. A. H. Parmelee, H. R. Schulz, and M. D. Disbrow. "Sleep Patterns in the Newborn." *Journal of Pediatrics,* 58:241, 1961.

90. T. F. Anders. "Night-waking in Infants During the First Year of Life." *Pediatrics,* 63:860–864, 1979.

91. A. Healy. "The Sleep Patterns of Preschool Children." *Clinical Pediatrics,* 11:174, 1972.

92. T. F. Anders and P. Weinstein. "Sleep and Its Disorders in Infants and Children: A Review." *Pediatrics*, 50:312, August 1972.

93. D. Hoefnagel and B. Biery. "Spasmus Nutans." *Developmental Medicine and Child Neurology*, 10:32, 1968.

94. P. Jayalakshmi et al. "Infantile Nystagmus." *Journal of Pediatrics*, 77:177–187, August 1970.

95. A. Chutorian. "Benign Paroxysmal Torticollis, Tortipelvis and Retrocollis in Infancy." *Neurology*, 24:366, April 1974.

96. T. Deonna and D. Martin. "Benign Paroxysmal Torticollis in Infancy." *Archives of Disease in Childhood*, 56:956–959, December 1981.

97. T. G. Quattlebaum. "Benign Familial Convulsions in the Neonatal Period and Early Infancy." *Journal of Pediatrics*, 95:257, August 1979.

98. N. J. Lenn and J. S. Hamill. "Congenital Radial Nerve Pressure Palsy." *Clinical Pediatrics*, 22:388, 1983.

99. H. Kravitz and J. J. Boehm. "Rhythmic Habit Pattern in Infancy: Their Sequence, Age of Onset, and Frequency." *Child Development*, 42:399, 1971.

100. D. W. Smith. "Growth and Its Disorders." Major Problems in Clinical Pediatrics, Vol. 15. Philadelphia: W. B. Saunders Co., 1977.

101. A. D. Lascari. "Carotenemia." *Clinical Pediatrics*, 20:25–29, January 1981.

102. M. M. Mathews-Roth. "Canthaxanthin-Produced 'Skin Tan': Carotenoderma by Any Name." *Journal of the American Medical Association*, 250:1100, August 26, 1983.

103. R. M. Barkin and M. E. Pichichero. "Diphtheria-Pertussis-Tetanus Vaccine: Reactogenicity of Commercial Products." *Pediatrics*, 63:356, February 1979.

104. P. J. Knight and C. B. Reiner. "Superficial Lumps in Children: What, When and Why?" *Pediatrics*, 72:147–153, August 1983.

105. F. E. R. Simons and J. G. Schaller. "Benign Rheumatoid Nodules." *Pediatrics*, 56:29, 1975.

106. J. D. Stroud. "Hair Loss in Children." *Pediatric Clinics of North America*, 30:641–657, 1983.

107. R. E. Day and W. H. Schutt. "Normal Children with Large Heads—Benign Familial Megalencephaly." *Archives of Disease in Childhood*, 54:512–517, 1979.

108. D. D. Weaver and J. C. Christian. "Familial Variation in Head Size and Adjustment for Parental Head Circumference." *Journal of Pediatrics*, 96:990–994, 1980.

109. C. J. Sells. "Microcephaly in a Normal School Population." *Pediatrics*, 59:262–265, 1977.

110. F. Hecht and J. V. Kelly. "Little Heads: Inheritance and Early Detection. *Journal of Pediatrics,* 95:731–732, 1979.

111. S. V. Rajkumar et al. "Popsicle Panniculitis of the Cheeks." *Clinical Pediatrics,* 15:619–621, 1976.

112. H. Kravitz et al. "The Cotton-tipped Swab." *Clinical Pediatrics,* 13:965, 1974.

113. D. M. Lypscomb. "How Frequent Are Ear Lesions and Hearing Defects Among U.S. Children?" *Clinical Pediatrics,* 12:125, 1973.

114. R. E. McDonald. "Examination of the Mouth." *Pediatric Clinics of North America,* 3:853–869, November 1956.

115. S. J. Moss. *Your Child's Teeth.* Boston: Houghton Mifflin Co., 1977.

116. R. L. Van Der Horst. "On Teething in Infancy." *Clinical Pediatrics,* 12:607, 1973.

117. I. L. Swann. "Teething Complications, a Persisting Misconception." *Postgraduate Medicine,* 55:24–25, 1979.

118. P. J. Honig. "Teething: Are Today's Pediatricians Using Yesterday's Notions?" *Journal of Pediatrics,* 87:415, 1979.

119. A. Tasanen. "General and Local Effects of the Eruption of Deciduous Teeth." *Annales Paediatriae Fenniae,* 14(supp. 29):1, 1968.

120. L. Pratt. "Tonsillectomy and Adenoidectomy: Mortality and Morbidity." *Transactions of the American Academy of Ophthalmology and Otolaryngology,* 74:1146, 1974.

121. J. L. Paradise. "Why T&A Remains Moot." *Pediatrics,* 49:648, 1972.

122. J. L. Paradise. "Clinical Trials of Tonsillectomy and Adenoidectomy: Limitations of Existing Studies and a Current Effort to Evaluate Efficacy." *Southern Medical Journal,* 69:1049, 1976.

123. E. M. Mandel and C. F. Reynolds. "Sleep Disorders Associated with Upper Airway Obstruction in Children." *Pediatric Clinics of North America,* 28:897, 1981.

124. L. B. Lowe. "Cold Panniculitis in Children." *American Journal of Diseases of Children,* 115:709, 1968.

125. B. K. Devgan and A. E. Brodeur. "Apical Pneumatocele." *Archives of Otolaryngology,* 102:121, 1976.

126. B. D. Schmitt. "Cervical Adenopathy in Children." *Postgraduate Medicine,* 60:251–255, 1976.

127. L. L. Barton and R. D. Feigen. "Childhood Cervical Lymphadenitis: A Reappraisal." *Journal of Pediatrics,* 84:846–852, 1974.

128. L. E. Holt. *The Diseases of Infancy and Childhood,* pp. 816–818. New York: D. Appleton and Co., 1899.

129. W. W. Zuelzer and J. Kaplan. "The Child with Lymphaden-

opathy." *Seminars in Hematology,* 12:323, 1975.

130. E. L. Coodley. "Finding the Cause of Lymph Node Enlargement." *Consultant,* December 1979, pp. 31–42.

131. P. J. Knight, A. F. Mulne, and E. L. Vassy. "When Is Lymph Node Biopsy Indicated in Children with Enlarged Peripheral Nodes?" *Pediatrics,* 69:391–396, 1982.

132. A. Altchek. "Premature Thelarche." *Pediatric Clinics of North America,* 19:543, 1972.

133. A. M. Pasquino at al. "Transient Psuedo-Precocious Puberty by Probable Oestrogen Intake in Three Girls." *Archives of Disease in Childhood,* 57:954, 1982.

134. C. A. Caceres and L. W. Perry. *The Innocent Murmur.* Boston: Little, Brown and Co., 1967.

135. S. Freedman. "Some Thoughts About Functional or Innocent Murmurs." *Clinical Pediatrics,* 12:679, 1973.

136. A. B. Bergman and J. J. Stamm. "The Morbidity of Cardiac Nondisease in School Children." *New England Journal of Medicine,* 276:108, 1967.

137. C. K. Meador. "The Art and Science of Nondisease." *New England Journal of Medicine,* 272:92–95, 1965.

138. B. Joorabchi. "The Emergence of Cardiac Nondisease Among Children in Iran." *Israel Journal of Medical Science,* 15:202, 1979.

139. C. J. Marienfeld et al. "A 20-Year Follow-up Study of 'Innocent' Murmurs." *Pediatrics,* 30:42, 1962.

140. R. D. Greenwood. "Should Parents Be Informed About Innocent Murmurs?" *Clinical Pediatrics,* 12:468–470, 1973.

141. C. D. Benson. "Hernias of Abdominal Wall Other than Inguinal." In *Pediatric Surgery,* ed. by C. D. Benson, p. 588. Chicago: Year Book Medical Publishers, 1962.

142. W. Van Essen. "The Retractile Testis." *Postgraduate Medicine,* 42:270, 1966.

143. P. Roth. *Portnoy's Complaint.* New York: Random House, 1969.

144. B. Hanstead and H. T. John. "Idiopathic Scrotal Edema of Children." *British Journal of Urology,* 36:110, 1964.

145. N. J. Nemoy, S. Rosen, and L. Kaplan. "Scrotal Panniculitis in the Prepubertal Male Patient." *Journal of Urology,* 118:492, 1977.

146. J. S. Allen and J. L. Summers. "Meatal Stenosis in Children." *Journal of Urology,* 112:526, 1974.

147. A. S. Litvak, J. A. Morris, and J. W. McRoberts. "Normal Size of the Urethral Meatus in Boys." *Journal of Urology,* 115:736, 1976.

148. W. A. Schonfeld. "Primary and Secondary Sexual Characteristics." *American Journal of Diseases of Children,* 65:535, 1943.

149. M. L. Modalsky. "Labial Fusion: A Cause of Recurrent Urinary Tract Infections." *Clinical Pediatrics,* 12:345, 1973.

150. W. E. Nelson. *Textbook of Pediatrics,* 11th ed., p. 1813. Philadelphia: W. B. Saunders Co., 1979.

151. J. C. Jacobs. *Pediatric Rheumatology for the Practitioner.* New York: Springer-Verlag, 1982.

152. R. L. Ruff and D. Secrest. "Benign Acute Childhood Myositis." *Archives of Neurology,* 39:261–263, 1982.

153. H. Silverstein. "Induced Rotational Nystagmus in Normal Infants." *Journal of Pediatrics,* 67:432, 1965.

154. J. M. Gwaltney and W. S. Jordan. "Rhinoviruses and Respiratory Disease." *Bacteriological Reviews,* 28:409, 1964.

155. C. M. Myer and R. T. Cotton. "Nasal Obstruction in the Pediatric Patient." *Pediatrics,* 72:766, 1983.

156. G. L. Mandell. "When to Suspect Immune Defects." *Consultant,* April 1979, p. 83.

157. L. Lambert-Lagace. *Feeding Your Child.* Cambridge, Ont.: Collier-Macmillan Habitex Books, 1976.

158. M. Davidson and R. Wasserman. "The Irritable Colon of Childhood (Chronic Nonspecific Diarrhea Syndrome)." *Journal of Pediatrics,* 69:1027, 1966.

159. W. A. Walker. "Chronic Nonspecific Diarrhea of Childhood." Ross Laboratories, *Pediatric Case Reports in Gastrointestinal Disease,* vol. II, no. 4, November 1982.

160. J. A. Walker-Smith. "Toddler's Diarrhea." *Archives of Disease in Childhood,* 55:329, 1980.

161. H. L. Greene and F. K. Ghishan. "Excessive Fluid Intake as a Cause of Chronic Diarrhea in Young Children." *Journal of Pediatrics,* 102:836, 1983.

162. S. A. Cohen et al. "Chronic Nonspecific Diarrhea: Dietary Relationships." *Pediatrics,* 64:402, 1979.

163. S. Livingston. "Breath-Holding Spells in Children." *Journal of the American Medical Association,* 212:2231, 1970.

164. C. T. Lombrosco and P. Lerman. "Breath-Holding Spell (Cyanotic and Pallid Infantile Syncope)." *Pediatrics,* 39:563, 1967.

165. J. B. P. Stephenson. "Reflex Anoxic Seizures ('White Breath Holding'): Nonepileptic Vagal Attacks." *Archives of Disease in Childhood,* 53:193–200, 1978.

166. D. W. Dunn and C. H. Snyder. "Benign Paroxysmal Vertigo of Childhood." *American Journal of Diseases of Children,* 130:1099, 1976.

167. M. R. Koenigsberger et al. "Benign Paroxysmal Vertigo of Childhood." *Neurology,* 20:1108, 1970.

168. F. Sallustro and C. W. Atwell. "Body Rocking, Head Banging and Head Rolling in Normal Children." *Journal of Pediatrics,* 93:704, 1970.

169. V. de Lissovoy. "Head Banging in Early Childhood." *Journal of Pediatrics*, 58:803, 1961.

170. V. Dubowitz. "The Floppy Infant." *Clinics in Developmental Medicine*, 76, 1980.

171. E. F. Rabe. "The Hypotonic Infant." *Journal of Pediatrics*, 64:422, 1964.

172. R. S. Paine. "The Future of the 'Floppy Infant': A Follow-up Study of 133 Patients." *Developmental Medicine and Child Neurology*, 5:115, 1963.

173. M. H. Goellner, E. E. Ziegler, and S. J. Fomon. "Urination During the First Three Years of Life." *Nephron*, 28:174–178, 1981.

174. C. E. Hollerman, P. Jose, and P. L. Calgano. *Neonatology: Pathophysiology and Management of the Sick Newborn*, p. 487. Philadelphia: J. B. Lippincott Co., 1975.

175. P. P. Kelales et al. "Urinary Vaginal Reflux in Children." *Pediatrics*, 51:941, 1973.

176. L. A. Davis and W. F. Chumley. "The Frequence of Vaginal Reflux During Micturition—Its Possible Importance to the Interpretation of Urine Cultures." *Pediatrics*, 38:293, 1966.

177. L. Glicklich. "An Historic Account of Enuresis." *Pediatrics*, 8:859, 1951.

178. S. Marshall, H. H. Marshall, and R. P. Lyon. "Enuresis: An Analysis of Various Therapeutic Approaches." *Pediatrics*, 52:813, 1973.

179. T. Oppel et al. "The Age of Attaining Bladder Control." *Pediatrics*, 42:614, 1967.

180. G. I. Martin. "Imipramine Pamoate in the Treatment of Childhood Enuresis." *American Journal of Diseases of Children*, 122:42, 1971.

181. W. C. Watson, R. G. Luke, and J. A. Inall. "Beeturia: Its Incidence and a Clue to Its Mechanism." *British Medical Journal*, October 19, 1963, p. 971.

182. W. W. Tunnessen, C. Smith, and F. A. Oski. "Beeturia: A Sign of Iron Deficiency." *American Journal of Diseases of Children*, 117:424, 1969.

183. S. Shuster. "The Cause of Striae Distensae." *Acta Dermato-Venereologica*, 59(supp. 85):161–169, 1979.

184. D. Whitehouse. "Diagnostic Value of the Café au Lait Spot in Children." *Archives of Disease in Childhood*, 41:316, 1966.

185. R. G. Burwell, N. J. James, and D. I. Johnson. "Café au Lait Spots in Schoolchildren." *Archives of Disease in Childhood*, 57:631, 1982.

186. M. J. B. Dales. "Dysplastic Congenital Nevi Must Be Detected,

Followed Early Because Melanoma Risk High." *Pediatric News,* 18:22, February 1984.

187. V. M. Riccardi. "Traditional Two Types of Neurofibromatosis Too Limited." *Pediatric News,* 18:13, February 1984.

188. J. Garafalo and A. P. Kaplan. "Histamine Release and Therapy of Severe Dermatographism." *Journal of Allergy and Clinical Immunology,* 68:103, 1981.

189. A. B. Shrank. "Juvenile Plantar Dermatosis." *British Journal of Dermatology,* 100:641, 1979.

190. M. S. Wien and M. R. Caro. "Traumatic Epithelial Cysts of the Skin." *Journal of the American Medical Association,* 102:197, 1934.

191. A. P. Forbes. "Hypertrichosis." *New England Journal of Medicine,* 273:602, 1965.

192. J. J. Leng and R. B. Greenblatt. "Hirsutism in Adolescent Girls." *Pediatric Clinics of North America,* 19:681, 1972.

193. G. H. Kalish and S. S. Gellis. "Hypertrophy of the Masseter or Temporalis Muscles or Both." *American Journal of Diseases of Children,* 121:346, 1971.

194. C. F. Fergusen and E. L. Kendig. *Pediatric Otolaryngology.* Philadelphia: W. B. Saunders Co., 1972.

195. J. A. Kirchner. "Current Concepts in Otolaryngology: Epistaxis." *New England Journal of Medicine,* 307:1126, 1982.

196. A. Kullaa-Mikkonen, M. Mikkonen, and R. Kotilainen. "Prevalence of Different Morphologic Forms of the Human Tongue in Young Finns." *Oral Surgery,* 53:152, 1982.

197. R. Marks and M. J. Simons. "Geographic Tongue—a Manifestation of Atopy." *British Journal of Dermatology,* 101:159, 1979.

198. R. Marks and B. G. Radden. "Geographic Tongue: a Clinicopathologic Review." *Australian Journal of Dermatology,* 22:75, 1981.

199. W. B. Klaustermeyer. *Practical Allergy and Immunology.* New York: John Wiley and Sons, 1983.

200. C. J. Heifetz. "Let Us Leave Umbilical Hernias Alone." *Journal of Pediatrics,* 64:303, February 1964.

201. J. L. Paradise et al. "Efficacy of Tonsillectomy for Recurrent Throat Infection in Severely Affected Children." *New England Journal of Medicine,* 310:674, 1984.

202. R. D. Mercer. "Pseudogoiter: Modigliani Syndrome." *Cleveland Clinic Quarterly,* 42:319, 1975.

203. O. Steeno et al. "Changes in Areolar Size in Boys During the Growth Phase and Pubertal Development." *Andrologia,* 7(1):49, 1975.

204. H. E. Carlson. "Gynecomastia." *New England Journal of Medicine,* 303:795–799, 1980.

205. V. C. Strasburger. "Why Adolescent Medicine?" *Clinical Pediatrics,* 23:12, 1984.

206. J. H. Wulsin. "Breast Lesions in Children." *Hospital Medicine,* May 1968, pp. 54–58.

207. D. P. Goldstein and V. Miler. "Breast Masses in Adolescent Females." *Clinical Pediatrics,* 21:17–19, 1982.

208. S. M. Love, R. S. Gelman, and W. Silen. "Fibrocystic 'Disease' of the Breast—a Nondisease?" *New England Journal of Medicine,* 309:1010–1014, 1982.

209. B. J. Anson and C. B. McVay. *Surgical Anatomy,* p. 467. Philadelphia: W. B. Saunders Co., 1971.

210. R. P. Lyons, S. Marshall, and M. P. Scott. "Varicocele in Childhood and Adolescence: Implications in Adulthood Infertility?" *Urology,* 19:641, 1982.

211. O. G. Berger. "Varicocele in Adolescence." *Clinical Pediatrics,* 19:810–811, 1980.

212. R. P. Lyons, S. Marshall, and M. P. Scott. "Varicocele in Youth." *Western Journal of Medicine,* 138:832–834, 1983.

213. C. J. Dewhurst, C. A. Cowell, and L. C. Barrie. "The Regularity of Early Menstrual Cycles." *The Journal of Obstetrics and Gynecology of the British Commonwealth,* 78:1093–1095, 1971.

214. J. Orley et al. "Vaginal Discharge in Puberty." *Gynaecologia,* 168:191–202, 1969.

215. A. F. Singleton. "Vaginal Discharge in Children and Adolescents." *Clinical Pediatrics,* 19:799–804, 1980.

216. J. C. Morrison and S. A. Fish. "Adolescent Genital Dermatoses." *Southern Medical Journal,* 69:1136–1140, 1976.

217. G. A. Bachmann and E. Kemmann. "Prevalence of Oligomenorrhea and Amenorrhea in a College Population." *American Journal of Obstetrics and Gynecology,* 144:98–102, 1982.

218. P. E. Alvin and I. F. Litt. "Current Status of the Etiology and Management of Dysmenorrhea in Adolescence." *Pediatrics,* 70:516–525, 1982.

219. J. M. Dinham. "Popliteal Cysts in Children: The Case Against Surgery." *Journal of Bone and Joint Surgery,* 57-B:69–71, 1975.

220. W. Raushching and P. G. Lindgren. "Popliteal Cysts in Adults." *Acta Orthopedica Scandinavica,* 50:583–591, 1979.

221. P. P. Symeonides and C. Paschaloglou. "Localized Hypertrophy of the Semimembranous Muscle Simulating Popliteal Cyst." *Journal of Bone and Joint Surgery,* 52-B:337–339, 1970.

222. J. R. Gallagher. *Medical Care of the Adolescent,* 3rd ed. New York: Appleton-Century-Crofts, 1976.

223. E. J. Rogala, D. S. Drummond, and J. Gurr. "Scoliosis: Incidence and Natural History." *Journal of Bone and Joint Surgery,* 60-A:173–176, 1978.

224. H. A. Keim. *The Adolescent Spine.* New York: Springer-Verlag, 1982.

225. H. A. Peterson. "Leg Aches." *Pediatric Clinics of North America,* 24:731–736, 1977.

226. J. Oster and A. Nielsen. "Growing Pains." *Acta Paediatrica Scandinavica,* 61:329–334, 1972.

227. J. J. Calabro et al. "Growing Pains: Fact or Fiction?" *Postgraduate Medicine,* 59:66–72, 1974.

228. R. Gorlin. "The Hyperkinetic Heart Syndrome." *Journal of the American Medical Association,* 182:823–829, 1962.

229. L. C. Harris. "Spurious Heart Disease in Athletic Children." *Journal of Pediatrics,* 72:755–756, 1968.

230. R. A. Johnson, E. Haber, and W. G. Austen. *The Practice of Cardiology.* Boston: Little, Brown and Co., 1980.

231. W. Evans. "The Heart in Sternal Depression." *British Heart Journal,* 8:162, 1946.

232. A. C. deLeon et al. "The Straight Back Syndrome." *Circulation,* 42:193, 1965.

233. B. Hwang et al. "The Electrocardiogram in Patients with Scoliosis." *Journal of Electrocardiology,* 15:131–136, 1982.

234. S. H. Rahimtoola. "Abnormal ECG in Clinically Normal Individuals." *Journal of the American Medical Association,* 250:1321–1323, 1983.

235. R. G. Castile, B. A. Staats, and P. R. Westbrook. "Symptomatic Pectus Deformities of the Chest." *America Review of Respiratory Disease,* 126:564–568, 1982.

236. B. M. Parker. "Mitral Valve Prolapse: What 'Popping Click' and 'Crescendo Murmur' Mean." *Consultant,* February 1979, p. 78.

237. C. F. Wooley. "The Mitral Valve Prolapse Syndrome." *Hospital Practice,* June 1983, pp. 163–174.

238. S. Londe and D. Goldring. "High Blood Pressure in Children: Problems and Guidelines for Evaluation and Treatment." *American Journal of Cardiology,* 37:650–657, 1976.

239. M. J. Jesse. "Essential Hypertension in Children." *Hospital Practice,* November 1982, pp. 81–88.

240. D. Goldring and A. Hernandez. "Hypertension in Children." *Pediatrics in Review,* 3:235–246, 1982.

241. S. Londe et al. "Hypertension in Apparently Normal Children." *Journal of Pediatrics,* 78:569–577, 1971.

242. E. Lieberman. "Essential Hypertension in Children and Youth: A Pediatric Perspective." *Journal of Pediatrics,* 85:1–11, 1974.

243. L. K. Rames et al. "Normal Blood Pressures and the Evaluation of Sustained Blood Pressure Elevation in Childhood: The Muscatine Study." *Pediatrics,* 61:245–251, 1978.

244. M. C. Turner et al. "Blood Pressure Elevation in Children with

Orthopedic Immobilization." *Journal of Pediatrics,* 95:989–992, 1979.

245. M. K. Mardini, M. A. Mikati, and R. Lifeso. "Hypertensive Encephalopathy: A Rare Complication after Orthopedic Manipulation." *American Journal of Diseases of Children,* 136:1092–1094, 1982.

246. D. Pickering. "Precordial Catch Syndrome." *Archives of Disease in Childhood,* 56:401, 1981.

247. M. J. Sparrow and E. L. Bird. " 'Precordial Catch': A Benign Syndrome of Chest Pain in Young Persons." *New Zealand Medical Journal,* 88:325, 1978.

248. R. H. Pantell and B. W. Goodman. "Adolescent Chest Pain: A Prospective Study." *Pediatrics,* 71:881–886, 1983.

249. D. J. Driscoll, L. B. Glickrich, and W. J. Gallen. "Chest Pain in Children: A Prospective Study." *Pediatrics,* 57:648–651, 1976.

250. J. A. Koufman and P. D. Blalock. "Classification and Approach to Patients with Functional Voice Disorders." *Annals of Otology, Rhinology and Laryngology,* 91:372–377, 1982.

251. D. Zakim and T. D. Boyer. *Hepatology: A Textbook of Liver Disease.* Philadelphia: W. B. Saunders Co., 1982.

252. J. Apley. *The Child with Abdominal Pains,* 2nd ed. Oxford, England: Blackwell Scientific Publications, 1975.

253. F. Lifshitz. *Carbohydrate Intolerance in Infancy.* Clinical Disorders in Pediatric Nutrition. New York: Marcel Dekker, 1982.

254. F. J. Simoons, J. D. Johnson, and N. Kretchmer. "Perspective on Milk Drinking and Malabsorption of Lactose." *Pediatrics,* 59:98–109, 1977.

255. S. L. Halpern. *Quick Reference to Clinical Nutrition.* Philadelphia: J. B. Lippincott, 1979.

256. E. V. Boisaubin. "Approach to Obese Patients." *Western Journal of Medicine,* 140:794–797, 1984.

257. P. Lindner. *Childhood Obesity,* 2nd ed. Littleton, Mass.: PSG Publishing Co., 1980.

258. H. Steiner. "Anorexia Nervosa." *Pediatrics in Review,* 4:123–129, 1982.

259. G. S. Golden. "Tics in Childhood." *Pediatric Annals,* 12:821–824, 1983.

260. J. E. Schowater. "Tics." *Pediatrics in Review,* 2:55–57, 1980.

261. I. J. Schatz. "Orthostatic Hypotension: Diagnosis and Treatment." *Hospital Practice,* April 1984, pp. 59–69.

262. R. M. Katz. "Cough Syncope in Children with Asthma." *Journal of Pediatrics,* 77:48–51, 1970.

263. C. B. Lyle et al. "Micturition Syncope." *New England Journal of Medicine,* 265:982–986, 1961.

264. P. Howard et al. "The 'Mess Trick' and the 'Fainting Lark.' " *British Medical Journal,* August 18, 1951, pp. 382–384.

265. J. R. Gallagher. *Medical Care of the Adolescent.* 3rd ed. New York: Appleton-Century-Crofts, 1975.

266. H. S. Singer. "Head Trauma for the Pediatrician." *Pediatrics,* 62:819–825, 1978.

267. S. H. Greenblatt. "Posttraumatic Transient Cerebral Blindness." *Journal of the American Medical Association,* 225:1073–1076, 1973.

268. G. W. Paulson. "Benign Essential Tremor in Childhood." *Clinical Pediatrics,* 15:67–70, 1976.

269. J. H. Pincus and A. M. Chutorian. "Familial Benign Chorea with Essential Tremor: A Clinical Entity." *Journal of Pediatrics,* 70:724–729, 1967.

270. R. S. Asnes and R. L. Mones. "Pollakiuria." *Pediatrics,* 52:615–617, 1973.

271. "The Haematuria of the Long Distance Runner," editorial. *British Medical Journal,* July 21, 1979, p. 159.

272. V. M. Vehaskari et al. "Microscopic Hematuria in Schoolchildren: Epidemiology and Clinicopathologic Evaluation." *Journal of Pediatrics,* 95:676–684, 1979.

273. J. M. McConville, C. D. West, and A. J. McAdams. "Familial and Nonfamilial Benign Hematuria." *Journal of Pediatrics,* 69:207, 1966.

274. M. I. Marks, P. N. McLaine, and K. N. Drummond. "Proteinuria in Children with Febrile Illness." *Archives of Disease in Childhood,* 45:250, 1970.

275. P. N. McLaine and K. N. Drummond. "Benign Persistent Asymptomatic Proteinuria in Childhood." *Pediatrics,* 46:548–552, 1970.

276. V. M. Vehaskari and J. Rapola. "Isolated Proteinuria: An Analysis of a School-Age Population." *Journal of Pediatrics,* 101:661–668, 1982.

277. "Postural (Orthostatic) Proteinuria: No Cause for Concern," editorial. *New England Journal of Medicine,* 305:639, 1981.

278. V. M. Vehaskari. "Orthostatic Proteinuria." *Archives of Disease in Childhood,* 57:729–730, 1982.

279. M. S. Ward. "The Office Determination of Proteinuria in Adolescents." *Pediatric Annals,* 7:97–115, 1978.

280. B. E. Glahn. "Giggle Incontinence (Enuresis Risoria): A Study and an Aetiologic Hypothesis." *British Medical Journal,* 51:363–366, 1979.

281. S. Raiti. "Short Stature: Evaluation and Treatment." *Pediatric Annals,* 9:14–23, 1980.

282. S. A. Hendricks and B. M. Lippe. "Short Stature in Children: Finding the Cause." *Consultant,* September 1979, pp. 23–31.

283. R. G. Rosenfeld and R. Hintz. "Diagnosis and Management of Growth Disorders." *Drug Therapy,* May 1983, pp. 33–47.

284. R. Lanes. et al. "Are Constitutional Delay of Growth and Familial Short Stature Different Conditions?" *Clinical Pediatrics,* 19:31–33, 1980.

285. R. L. Rosenfield, B. H. Rich, and A. W. Lucky. "Adrenarche as

a Cause of Benign Pseudopuberty in Boys." *Journal of Pediatrics,* 101:1005–1009, 1982.

286. A. W. Root and E. D. Reiter. "Evaluation and Management of the Child with Delayed Pubertal Development." *Fertility and Sterility,* 27:745–755, 1976.

287. A. Prader. "Delayed Adolescence." *Clinical Endocrinology,* 4:143–155, 1975.

288. H. V. Barnes. "The Teenager with Pubertal Delay." *Primary Care,* 3:215–229, 1976.

289. R. E. Frisch, G. Wyshak, and L. Vincent. "Delayed Menarche and Amenorrhea in Ballet Dancers." *New England Journal of Medicine,* 303:17–19, 1980.

Index

for chewing, 246
flabby, 221–222
lactic acid, 276
swelling behind knee, 268
swelling in face, 246
Muscularity, increased, 243

Nails
of newborn
ingrown toenails, 56
size and shape, 104
of preschooler
biting, and lymph node enlargement, 175
Naps, 221
Nasolacrimal duct, blocked, 66–67
Natural puberty discharge, 264
Navel
healing, 86–87
oozing, 87
pain directly beneath, 295–297
umbilical hernia, 88–89
Nearsightedness, nodding and, 135
Neck
of newborn
short, 77
turned or twisted, 77–78
wry, 77–78
of preschooler
ballooning, 171
lumps, 171–178
swelling after contact with cold, 170
of older child
apparent swelling of thyroid, 253
Neonatal sleep myoclonus, 132
Nerve compression weakness, 137–138
Nervous system
of newborn

convulsions ("benign"), 126
head nodding, 135–136
jerking movements, 131–132
jittery movements, 132–133
repetitive, rhythmic movements, 138
sleep-wake periods, 133
twisting and turning, 136
weakness from nerve compression, 137–138
of preschooler
body rocking, 218–219
breath holding, 213–216
dizziness, 216–217
giving up nap, 221
head banging, 218–219
nightmares, 220
rag doll infant, 221–222
screaming, 219
sleep disturbances, 219–221
of older child
rhythmic trembling of head and hands, 315–317
temporary blindness after head injury, 314
twitching, 307–308
sleeptalking, 315
sleepwalking, 315
Neurocirculatory asthenia, 281–282
neurofibromatosis, 236–237
Neurologist, for tremors, 316
Neurotic behavior, mitral valve prolapse syndrome and, 283
Nevi, 39–42
flat salmon patch, 40–41
Mongolian spot, 39–40
port wine stain, 40–41
spider spot, 244
strawberry mark, 41–42
see also Moles
Nevus araneus, 244
Nevus flammeus, 40–41
Nevus simplex, 40–41

· ABOUT THE AUTHORS ·

Gil Simon, M.D., was born in Brooklyn, New York, and completed his premedical studies at Colgate University and his medical studies at the University of Rochester. His postgraduate and specialty training consisted of an internship in pediatrics at the Upstate Medical Center in Syracuse, New York, a fellowship in preventive medicine at the University of Virginia, and a residency in pediatrics at Babies Hospital, Columbia-Presbyterian Medical Center, New York. From 1967 until 1983, Dr. Simon was a member of the faculty of Columbia University College of Physicians and Surgeons, teaching students, interns, and residents. In 1983, he moved to Sacramento, California, where he established a general pediatric practice. He is married and has five children, ranging from 2 to 25 years of age.

Marcia Cohen's articles have appeared in such periodicals as *The New York Times Magazine, Ladies' Home Journal,* and *Reader's Digest.* She has written extensively on consumer medicine. A graduate of Harvard and Radcliffe colleges, and the mother of two children, she is the former executive editor of Hearst's *Sunday Woman* and the former editor of the "You" section of the New York *Daily News.*